CEN EXAMINATION REVIEW

ANN J. BRORSEN, MSN, RN, CCRN, CEN
COO AND DIRECTOR OF CLINICAL APPLICATIONS
PRO ED
MENIFEE, CALIFORNIA

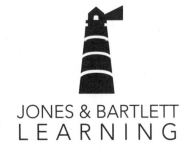

JONES & BARTLETT
LEARNING

World Headquarters
Jones & Bartlett Learning
5 Wall Street
Burlington, MA 01803
978-443-5000
info@jblearning.com
www.jblearning.com

Jones & Bartlett Learning books and products are available through most bookstores and online booksellers. To contact Jones & Bartlett Learning directly, call 800-832-0034, fax 978-443-8000, or visit our website, www.jblearning.com.

Substantial discounts on bulk quantities of Jones & Bartlett Learning publications are available to corporations, professional associations, and other qualified organizations. For details and specific discount information, contact the special sales department at Jones & Bartlett Learning via the above contact information or send an email to specialsales@jblearning.com.

Copyright © 2012 by Jones & Bartlett Learning, LLC, an Ascend Learning Company

All rights reserved. No part of the material protected by this copyright may be reproduced or utilized in any form, electronic or mechanical, including photocopying, recording, or by any information storage and retrieval system, without written permission from the copyright owner.

Some images in this book feature models. These models do not necessarily endorse, represent, or participate in the activities represented in the images.

The author, editor, and publisher have made every effort to provide accurate information. However, they are not responsible for errors, omissions, or for any outcomes related to the use of the contents of this book and take no responsibility for the use of the products and procedures described. Treatments and side effects described in this book may not be applicable to all people; likewise, some people may require a dose or experience a side effect that is not described herein. Drugs and medical devices are discussed that may have limited availability controlled by the Food and Drug Administration (FDA) for use only in a research study or clinical trial. Research, clinical practice, and government regulations often change the accepted standard in this field. When consideration is being given to use of any drug in the clinical setting, the healthcare provider or reader is responsible for determining FDA status of the drug, reading the package insert, and reviewing prescribing information for the most up-to-date recommendations on dose, precautions, and contraindications, and determining the appropriate usage for the product. This is especially important in the case of drugs that are new or seldom used.

Production Credits
Publisher: Kevin Sullivan
Acquisitions Editor: Amanda Harvey
Editorial Assistant: Sara Bempkins
Associate Production Editor: Sara Fowles
Associate Marketing Manager: Katie Hennessy
V.P., Manufacturing and Inventory Control: Therese Connell
Composition: Cenveo Publisher Services
Cover Design: Kate Ternullo
Cover Image: (left to right) © Tyler Olson/ShutterStock, Inc.; © Andrew Gentry/ShutterStock, Inc.; © YAKOBCHUK VASYL/ShutterStock, Inc.
Printing and Binding: Courier Kendallville
Cover Printing: Courier Kendallville

To order this product, use ISBN: 978-1-4496-3177-2

Library of Congress Cataloging-in-Publication Data
Brorsen, Ann J.
  CEN examination review / Ann J. Brorsen.
    p. ; cm.
  Includes bibliographical references.
  ISBN 978-1-4496-1576-5 (pbk.)
  1. Emergency nursing—Examinations, questions, etc. I. Title.
  [DNLM: 1. Emergency Nursing—Examination Questions. WY 18.2]
  RT120.E4B76 2012
  610.73'6076—dc22   2011007235

6048

Printed in the United States of America
15 14 13 12 10 9 8 7 6 5 4 3 2

Contents

	About the Author	v
	Contributors	vii
	Reviewers	ix
	Acknowledgments	xi
	Preface	xiii
Section 1:	Introduction to the CEN Credential	1
Section 2:	Test-Taking Strategies	3
Section 3:	Cardiovascular	7
Section 4:	Pulmonary	57
Section 5:	Orthopedic and Musculoskeletal	103
Section 6:	Maxillofacial and Ocular	135
Section 7:	Neurology	147
Section 8:	Obstetrics and Gynecology	173
Section 9:	Shock States	215
Section 10:	Genitourinary and Renal	233
Section 11:	Gastrointestinal	265
Section 12:	Substance Abuse, Toxicologic, and Environmental	295
Section 13:	Medical Emergencies	329
Section 14:	Psychosocial	379

About the Author

Ann J. Brorsen, RN, MSN, CCRN, CEN

Ann is a nationally known speaker and has presented certification review courses for the CEN, Adult and Pediatric CCRN, and PCCN. Ann has presented programs as diverse as advanced hemodynamics to best practice models for hospital corporations. Ann is a member of Sigma Theta Tau, the American Association of Critical-Care Nurses, the Society of Critical Care Medicine, and the Emergency Nurses' Association. Ann also works as a consultant for educational program development and management training for healthcare facilities. Ann continues clinical practice in the ED, ICU, and critical care transport. Ann is currently the COO and Director of Clinical Applications for Pro Ed in Menifee, California.

Contributors

Melissa R. Christiansen, RN, MSN, NP-C, CCRN, CNRN

Melissa has over 23 years of experience as a critical care nurse in neurological, cardiac, and trauma ICUs. She is currently working as a family nurse practitioner in Southern California. Melissa has presented programs on neurological and neuroscience topics, adult critical care, and emergency nursing certification reviews and courses in post-anesthesia nursing. Melissa is a member of Sigma Theta Tau, the American Association of Critical-Care Nurses, the American Association of Neuroscience Nurses, and the American Academy of Nurse Practitioners.

Keri R. Rogelet, RN, MSN, MBA/HCM, CCRN

Keri has presented national programs for the Neonatal CCRN, Pediatric CCRN, developmental care, and adult health issues. Keri is a regional NRP trainer for the American Academy of Pediatrics and a lead instructor for the S.T.A.B.L.E. program. Keri's professional associations include Sigma Theta Tau, the American Association of Critical-Care Nurses, and the Academy of Neonatal Nurses. In addition, she works as a consultant for pediatric and neonatal product applications. Keri is maintaining clinical practice as a neonatal intensive care nurse. She is currently the CFO and Director of Clinical Development for Pro Ed in Menifee, California.

Reviewers

Francine Boaz, RN
Emergency Department
Vanderbilt University Medical Center
Nashville, Tennessee

Mary A. Cowett, RN, RNC-BC
Riverside Community Hospital
Riverside, California

Connie Thomas, RN
Riverside Community Hospital
Riverside, California

Acknowledgments

Mary Margaret Forsythe, RN, and Nancy O. Roberts, RN

Mary Margaret and Nancy were two instructors who were ultimate professionals and who believed in their students and the profession of nursing. These women were incredible individuals and will live in the hearts of hundreds of nurses. They passed before their time and are desperately missed.

Karen S. Ehrat, RN, PhD

Karen saw potential in a new grad and made education a joy and a privilege. Her untimely death stole a piece from every soul she touched.

I am so grateful to all the nurses who provided suggestions for content of this book. The contributors worked unselfishly and through many a long night. Thank you to the reviewers who gave their time, effort, and suggestions to enhance the content of this manuscript. I would also like to express my gratitude to the editorial and production staff at Jones & Bartlett Learning.

A.J.B.

Preface

Congratulations! You are one step closer to achieving certification as an emergency nurse. Even if you plan to use this book as a study guide for emergency nursing, this will be an invaluable resource. A brief introduction to the CEN credential and test-taking strategies are presented to help you study effectively.

This book contains over 1200 test questions with rationales that cover a broad range of topics and are representative of the type of questions you will find on the actual examination. The current trend for item writers is to present a question in such a way as to not state any identifiable characteristics, such as a name, age, or gender (if possible). However, some of the questions found in this book contain first names randomly chosen from friends or lists of popular baby names. Any name or patient condition presented here is for educational purposes only. Any resemblance to any person, living or dead, is purely coincidental.

With this book purchase you will have access to an online application that allows you to create your own practice tests. The questions online are randomly selected and enable you to time yourself and practice as if you were taking the actual examination.

All of us who contributed to the content of this book are dedicated to helping you successfully pass this exam and achieve recognition as a certified emergency nurse. Please feel free to contact us if you have any questions or you would like to schedule a CEN review course for your facility or group.

Contact Information

Website: www.forproed.com
Email: proedcertify@yahoo.com

SECTION 1:

Introduction to the CEN Credential

Traditionally, nurses have worked in a variety of roles and environments. For most of the 20th century nurses had spent many hours in clinical situations and were prepared to practice in any area when they graduated from their programs. Nursing eventually had to adjust from the general practitioner to a nurse who would concentrate practice in one area. Nurses worked in emergency rooms, operating rooms, recovery rooms, obstetrics, and medical-surgical units. Only those nurses who worked in operating rooms or who administered anesthesia were considered specialized. With the advent of emerging technology, the post–World War II population boom, and a trend toward increasingly more acute patients, nursing and hospitals adjusted by placing patients in more subspecialized areas.

One critical issue that arose in the 20th century related to patients with poliomyelitis, who were increasing both in number and special needs. The "iron lung" had been around for years. In the 1930s the machine cost $1,500, which was also the median cost for a home at that time. Patients who could afford such treatment began to recover, only to develop sequelae that required specialized care. Tilt beds and hot-pack treatments were initiated. At one time even curare was used to combat the severe muscle spasms suffered by polio victims. All these treatments required time and resources, including larger numbers of nurses.

In 1931, the American Association of Nurse Anesthetist (no "s" on the end) formed. On June 4, 1945, the organization held the first-ever certification examination for a nursing specialty. In 1952, the first accredited program for nurse anesthetists was started.

In 1955 Jonas Salk announced the discovery of a vaccine for polio. The vaccine would help prevent spread of the disease, but thousands of victims still required care. Technology in general was improving and becoming more broadly available. Although the first EKG machines were available in the United States as early as 1909, they were not widely used until the late 1950s.

In the 1960s, many patients required around-the-clock specialized care that required resources and practitioners who were experts or who had a great deal of experience with the particular condition or disease process. Veterans of previous wars and the escalating Vietnam War required increasingly more medical resources. Hospitals began placing cardiac, trauma, burn, and acute medical patients in areas of the hospital designated as providing more specialized care. Patient survival rates improved so the numbers of specialized areas increased. The one constant in patient care at this time was that receiving areas of hospitals were designated "emergency rooms."

Six members of the Emergency Nurses Association met in New York in August 1979. These six nurses formed the Certification Committee and worked to establish the first certification examination designed specifically to assess the existing level of emergency nursing knowledge. This committee evolved into the Board of Certification for Emergency Nursing and today has become the BCEN. For a complete history and current information about the BCEN and all the certifications available, please visit www.ena.org.

All the requirements for the CEN examination may be found on the ENA website. In addition, the site contains a handbook that includes a content outline. This outline covers specific subject matter you will need to know for successful completion of the examination. The content outline is updated on a regular basis, so you must be familiar with the current requirements and content of the exam. Remember, thousands of nurses have passed this examination, and you can too!

REFERENCES

Retrieved January 23, 2011, from http://www.ena.org
Retrieved July 20, 2010, from http://americanhistory.si.edu/polio/howpolio/index.htm
Retrieved July 20, 2010, from http://www.anesthesia-nursing.com/wina.html

SECTION 2:

Test-Taking Strategies

When preparing for the CEN exam, the first thing to do is be absolutely honest with yourself about how you study. If you have good study habits and plenty of time, you are very fortunate. If you are a procrastinator, studying a little bit at a time might help. Nurses have to juggle so many roles that take up their time: parent, child, employee, student, teacher, and on and on. One of the biggest struggles is simply finding time and a place to study. Discovering your learning style will help you find a better way to absorb information.

Three types of learners are commonly identified: visual, auditory, and kinesthetic. There is no perfect strategy for learning because every person is unique. Not everyone has a single style of learning; you may use a mix of styles depending on your situation. *Visual learners* learn better from reading and writing than from hearing and talking about information. Background noise, such as music or television, is distracting to these types of learners. Finding a quiet space is a problem for some people. You may have to stay awake after family members have gone to bed. Flashcards often work, and some people use colored markers to highlight important information.

Auditory learners learn information effectively by listening and talking. Playing music, listening to audiotapes, or being part of a study group often works. *Kinesthetic learners* prefer to learn via a "hands-on" approach. Nurses often learn this way because we have to listen to lectures and then demonstrate skills. This approach focuses on the use of models, manikins, or patients and works well for many healthcare providers. Kinesthetic people are often "antsy" and cannot sit still for long periods of time, so lectures may be difficult for them without frequent breaks. If you are a kinesthetic learner, some of the things that might help while studying include taking frequent breaks, walking around, or riding a stationary cycle.

No matter what your personal learning style, your test-taking skills can be improved. How? Practice! That is why this book is written in a question-and-answer format. Keep practicing the questions until you can answer at least 80% correctly. Research has shown that two-thirds of study time should be spent taking sample tests and only one-third of study time should be spent reviewing content.

Studying, like regular exercise, is good for the brain. As nurses, we must always keep abreast of the professional literature and spend time studying to keep our knowledge and skills up to date. In addition, many states require continuing education to renew a professional license. Anything worthwhile takes time, effort, and sacrifice.

There is no way around studying for this certification. There are no shortcuts! If you have been out of school for a while, don't despair! It may be slow going at first, so take things a little at a time. Just like going to the gym, you should make a plan to study in one particular place and at the same time if possible. This is your space and your time—claim it. Have all your books, tapes, and other study materials handy. If you need snack food, make sure it is not all sugar and include some salty food. Caffeine tends to make people jittery, but if you need it, it may be right for you.

The CEN content outline is a blueprint of the exam's content. The major sections are broken down into subheadings and topics. If you study only a little at a time, you will be fine. One day you may feel like studying right-sided EKGs; the next day you may focus on chest tubes. You may download the current content outline at www.ena.org. The current content outline is not included in this book because the exam changes frequently and you should have a copy of the current information.

If you study with a group, you can save a lot of time and effort by breaking up the topics for that study period and having each person present his or her topic(s) and provide handouts and practice questions for the rest of the group. When you can make up a test question about a subject, you really will be prepared. Study for short periods of time, say 30 to 45 minutes, and then take a break. Set small goals, and after you have accomplished each one, reward yourself!

EXAM CONTENT

The CEN certification exam consists of 175 multiple-choice test questions. Twenty-five of those questions do not count; they are there to be validated. In other words, every question is tried first to see if it is written well and if a certain percentage of people answer it correctly. At this point in the process, a question can still be "tweaked" for use on future exams.

Your results are determined by how many answers you get correct and the version of the examination used. Some questions are a bit more difficult than others. If you do not know an answer, take your best guess, because you have at least a chance of guessing correctly. You get points only for questions answered correctly.

STUDY TIPS

A multiple-choice test question consists of three parts: an introductory statement, a stem (question), and options from which you must select the correct answer. The introductory statement provides information about a clinical issue, pathophysiology, or a nursing action or duty.

Stems are worded in different ways. Some stems are in the form of a question; others are in the form of an incomplete statement. Additionally, a stem usually requests one of two types of responses: a positive response or a negative response. The questions you will practice from in this book may have an occasional negative stem to facilitate learning. There are no longer any multiple-multiple-choice questions on the exam!

Key words are important words or phrases that help focus your attention on what the question is asking. Examples of key words include *always, most, first response, earliest, priority, first, on admission, common, best, least, not, immediately,* and *initial*.

You should always be looking for a *therapeutic response*. The nurse is *always* therapeutic. In other words, your *initial response* as a nurse is *always* the therapeutic response—you must acknowledge and validate the patient's feelings. Communication skills learned in Nursing 101 are important components of successful test-taking strategies. More than one option may contain a therapeutic response. When in doubt, validate, validate, validate. Always validate the feelings before you present information. A medical emergency would, of course, take precedence.

Who is actually the focus of the question? You need to be able to identify this person. Sometimes questions are asked about a friend, a relative, or a significant other instead of a patient. A lot of information in the question may be deliberately distracting. Also, you must, when applicable, validate that person's feelings first.

WHEN IN DOUBT

When answering questions on the examination, remember Maslow's hierarchy of needs and the ABCs (airway, breathing, circulation). When these goals are met, then safety is the priority. After safety, the psychological needs are a priority. Assessment always comes before diagnosis and treatment (intervention). Learning takes place only if the learner is motivated.

Eliminate incorrect options. This gives you a 50% chance of guessing the correct answer. Here are some hints:

- Select the most general, all-encompassing option.
- Eliminate similar options or those that contain words such as "always" or "never."
- If two options say essentially the same thing, then neither is correct. If three of the four options sound similar, choose the one that sounds different.
- Look for the longest option. It is usually the correct answer.
- Watch for grammatical inconsistencies between the stem and options.

IT'S TIME TO TAKE YOUR CERTIFICATION EXAM!

Well, you are finally ready! The night before the exam, get a good night's sleep. Do not cram the night before, although that is easier said than done. Do something relaxing and enjoyable, like going to a movie or out to dinner. Try to avoid caffeine or any other stimulant. Please email or call when you pass the exam so you can be congratulated.

REFERENCES

Kobel Lamonte, M. (2007). Test-taking strategies for CNOR certification. *Association of Operating Room Nurses. AORN Journal, 85*(2), 315–332.

Ludwig, C. (2004). Preparing for certification: Test-taking strategies. *Medical-Surgical Nursing, 13*(2), 127–128.

PRACTICE QUESTIONS AND ANSWERS

The next sections contain over 1,200 practice questions. The questions are written with four responses, like those you will find on the CEN examination.

Even though questions are divided into systems and issues, many topics will cross over to another section. For example, you will find questions about shock states in several sections.

The questions will have a variety of complexity. Some questions will be quite easy to answer and some will be quite difficult to answer and require critical thinking and integration of practices. On occasion, information previously covered within the context of one patient situation will be asked again in a slightly different way. Material on drug dosages and medications commonly in use at time of publication are included to help you prepare for the CEN examination.

Keep practicing until you can routinely answer 80% of these questions correctly. At that point you should be ready to take the certification examination.

The first section, cardiovascular, contains several questions about basic hemodynamics. You may be provided patient information on the actual CEN exam that utilizes terminology related to hemodynamics. The questions are designed to familiarize you with this information, reduce stress, and increase your probability of success.

SECTION 3:

Cardiovascular

1. Unstable angina usually associated with left anterior descending (LAD) coronary artery lesions is known as
   A. Prinzmetal's angina
   B. Wellen's syndrome
   C. Crescendo angina
   D. Ludwig's angina

2. Your patient exhibits ST segment depression on his EKG along with moderate, substernal chest pain. These findings indicate a possible
   A. Anteroseptal MI
   B. Myocardial ischemia
   C. Lateral wall MI
   D. Pericardial tamponade

3. Right ventricular preload in the heart is measured by the
   A. Left atrial pressure
   B. Pulmonary artery systolic pressure
   C. Central venous pressure
   D. Pulmonary artery occlusive pressure

4. Determine the pulse pressure for a patient who has a pulse of 75, a BP of 125/85, and a respiratory rate of 16.
   A. 20
   B. 38
   C. 40
   D. 52

5. Left ventricular preload in the heart is measured by the
   A. Left ventricular systolic pressure
   B. Pulmonary artery systolic pressure
   C. Pulmonary artery diastolic pressure
   D. Pulmonary artery wedge pressure

6. What is the MAP (mean arterial pressure) for a patient with a blood pressure of 120/60 and a heart rate of 70?
   A. 60
   B. 70
   C. 80
   D. 50

7. Which of the following percentages would be considered a normal value for an ejection fraction (EF)?
   A. 25%
   B. 30%
   C. 35%
   D. 60%

8. Calculate the cardiac output for a patient with a heart rate of 78 and a stroke volume of 60 ml.
   A. 18%
   B. 4.68 L/min
   C. 468 ml/min
   D. 0.769 L/min

9. Which of the following statements is true about events that occur during a normal cardiac cycle?
   A. Metabolism in the heart is unchanged during diastole
   B. Metabolism of the heart is decreased during diastole
   C. An increase in cardiac output increases diastole
   D. Diastole comprises about 40% of the cardiac cycle

10. Which of the following pulmonary artery pressures and CVP pressures would be considered in the normal range?
    A. PAP = 40/24   PAOP = 15   CVP 20
    B. PAP = 14/8   PAOP = 4   CVP 2
    C. PAP = 24/12   PAOP = 9   CVP 7
    D. PAP = 36/30   PAOP = 22   CVP 24

11. In patients with normal cardiac anatomy, right atrial pressure equals
    A. Right ventricular end diastolic pressure
    B. Left atrial pressure
    C. Right ventricular systolic pressure
    D. Right ventricular diastolic pressure

12. Paul was admitted to the ED for chest pain that occurred while he was sleeping and the pain has not resolved. He was diagnosed with Prinzmetal's angina. This form of angina
    A. Is caused by a blockage of the circumflex artery
    B. Is a benign form of angina
    C. Is usually caused by a coronary vasospasm
    D. Will always resolve with administration of nitroglycerin

13. Calcium channel blockers act primarily on
    A. Serotonin uptake
    B. Arteriolar tissue
    C. Lung receptors only
    D. Reduction of cardiac output

14. What are the most valuable pieces of information evaluated with a 12-lead EKG?
    A. Rate, rhythm, arrhythmias
    B. Rate, rhythm, axis, hypertrophy, infarction
    C. Rate, arrhythmias, infarction
    D. Rate, bundle branch block, hypertrophy

15. Increased preload may be caused by
    A. Hemorrhage
    B. Hyperthermia
    C. Renal problems
    D. Vomiting

16. Decreased preload may result from
    A. Hyperthermia
    B. Hypothermia
    C. Sympathetic stimulation
    D. Vasoconstriction

17. Which of the following conditions would decrease afterload?
    A. Use of nitrates
    B. Hypothermia
    C. Aortic stenosis
    D. Hypertension

18. Pulsus alternans is most often noted with
    A. Mitral stenosis
    B. Constrictive pericarditis
    C. Left ventricular failure
    D. Aortic stenosis

19. The S_2 heart sound is created by
    A. Opening of the aortic and mitral valves
    B. Closure of the pulmonic and aortic valves
    C. Opening of the pulmonic and mitral valves
    D. Closure of the pulmonic and tricuspid valves

20. Stimulation of the right vagus nerve in turn stimulates the
    A. Sinoatrial (SA) node
    B. Mandibular branch of the trigeminal nerve
    C. Acetylcholine reabsorption
    D. Chemoreceptors in the carotid arch

21. Cyanosis of the skin, mucous membranes, and nail beds can occur when deoxygenated hemoglobin is present within the circulation. This cyanosis may be observed when which of the following levels of deoxygenated hemoglobin is reached?
    A. 5 g/100 ml
    B. 50 g/500 ml
    C. 50 g/250 ml
    D. 15 g/200 ml

22. On an EKG, upright QRS complexes in leads V_1 and V_2 indicate which of the following types of bundle branch block?
    A. Right
    B. Left
    C. Dual bundle
    D. V_1, V_2 does not show bundle branch blocks

23. Marlene had an MI with second-degree heart block. She just had a VVI pacemaker inserted. What does the first V indicate?
    A. Paced, ventricular
    B. Paced, inhibited
    C. Ventricular inhibited
    D. Ventricular

24. Your patient was diagnosed with left-sided heart failure. On an EKG, left-sided heart failure results in
    A. Tall, peaked P waves
    B. Wide, notched P waves
    C. Changes in ST segments
    D. A prolonged Q wave

25. Mariah has been diagnosed with acquired valvular heart disease. The primary cause of acquired valvular heart disease is
    A. Heredity
    B. Drug abuse
    C. Rheumatic fever
    D. Fetal alcohol syndrome

26. What does the second V in a VVI pacemaker indicate?
    A. Ventricular paced
    B. Ventricular inhibited
    C. Ventricular sensed
    D. Ventricular programmed

27. If a $beta_2$ receptor in the heart is stimulated, the effect of this stimulation may be
    A. A reflex bradycardia
    B. Arterial vasoconstriction
    C. Bronchodilation
    D. Increased SVR

28. Which of the following statements is true about lidocaine?
    A. Lidocaine may cause hypotension
    B. Lidocaine administration may cause a moderate gastrointestinal intolerance
    C. Lidocaine does not impair normal contractility
    D. Lidocaine can cause nystagmus

29. Quinidine and hypomagnesemia can both lead to which of the following conditions?
    A. Monomorphic ventricular tachycardia
    B. Torsade de Pointes
    C. Ventricular fibrillation
    D. Atrial tachycardia

30. Peter is a 20 year old football player who was brought to the ED with chest pain. The EKG monitor now reveals PVCs and runs of tachycardia. Lidocaine is ordered. Which of the following symptoms of lidocaine toxicity requires immediate intervention?
    A. A respiratory rate of 7
    B. A narrowing QRS
    C. A heart rate of 70
    D. Hypertonicity

31. Matthew was started on esmolol for severe hypertension refractive to other drug regimens. Esmolol is incompatible with which of the following medications?
    A. Cimetidine
    B. Furosemide
    C. Penicillin G potassium
    D. Midazolam

32. Dilated cardiomyopathy is characterized by dilation of the ventricles and impaired systolic function. Common causes are valvular heart disease and ischemic heart disease. Other causes are idiopathic. The most common cause of idiopathic dilated cardiomyopathy is
    A. Autoimmune
    B. Alcohol
    C. Genetic
    D. Familial

33. Today you are precepting a student nurse. You are preparing to administer Lasix, 40 mg IV. The student asks you how fast the IV dose may be administered. You explain that Lasix must be given slowly because
    A. Lasix may cause nausea
    B. A rash may develop
    C. Hyperkalemia may occur
    D. A rapid infusion can lead to hearing loss

34. Diuretics are used in the treatment of CHF. A diuretic that reduces urinary calcium losses is
    A. Diamox
    B. Chlorothiazide
    C. Furosemide
    D. Spironolactone

35. Myoshi was admitted to the ED with a diagnosis of hypertrophic cardiomyopathy. Which of the following hemodynamic effects would usually be seen in a patient with hypertrophic cardiomyopathy?
    A. Increased CO, increased ejection fraction
    B. Normal CO, increased ejection fraction
    C. Increased CO, decreased ejection fraction
    D. Decreased CO, increased ejection fraction

36. Which of the following is considered an end effect of CHF?
    A. Atrial fibrillation
    B. Increased renal perfusion
    C. Pulmonary venous shrinkage
    D. Systemic venous engorgement

37. The type of cardiomyopathy that is characterized by replacement of normal cells by fatty tissue is known as
    A. Restrictive cardiomyopathy
    B. Hypertrophic cardiomyopathy
    C. Arrhythmogenic cardiomyopathy
    D. Dilated cardiomyopathy

38. Symptoms of right-sided heart failure include
    A. Orthopnea
    B. Elevated PAD, PAOP
    C. Hepatomegaly
    D. Pulmonary edema

39. If an early intra-aortic balloon pump (IABP) balloon inflation occurs, the balloon inflates
    A. Prior to closure of the aortic valve
    B. Prior to opening of the pulmonic valve
    C. Prior to closure of the mitral valve
    D. Prior to opening of the tricuspid valve

40. Your patient is being treated with an IABP. While performing an assessment, you note that the patient no longer has a palpable left radial pulse. What is the probable cause of the loss of this pulse?
    A. A malfunctioning arterial line
    B. The patient's position
    C. Hypovolemia
    D. The IABP balloon catheter has migrated upward

41. A relative contraindication for the use of an IABP is
    A. An aortic dissection
    B. An abdominal aortic aneurism
    C. Thrombocytopenia
    D. Aortic insufficiency

42. An absolute contraindication to the use of IABP therapy is
    A. An aortic dissection
    B. Thrombocytopenia
    C. Peripheral vascular disease
    D. Femur fracture

43. Marvin has required placement of an intra-aortic balloon pump in the ED prior to emergency surgery for a failed aortic valve. The IABP will have which of the following benefits for Marvin's condition?
    A. Increased diastolic fill
    B. Increased afterload
    C. Increased pulmonary pressures
    D. Increased PVR

44. The most common complication of IABP therapy is
    A. Stroke
    B. Infection
    C. Lower limb ischemia
    D. Anemia

45. Which of the following conditions predispose the patient to an increased risk for an allergic reaction to protamine sulfate?
    A. Influenza vaccine
    B. Type 2 diabetes
    C. A history of PKU
    D. Allergy to fish

46. Bertha was initially admitted to your ED for severe dyspnea and has been diagnosed with congestive heart failure. After further study it was determined that she has restrictive cardiomyopathy. A common cause of restrictive cardiomyopathy is
    A. An unknown viral infection
    B. Glycogen storage disease
    C. A history of diabetes
    D. Unknown

47. Darlene has been experimenting with multiple drugs. She was admitted to your ED after a cocaine overdose. Darlene has had an anterolateral myocardial infarction. Where do you expect to see changes on the 12-lead EKG?
    A. Leads V_1, V_2, I, and AVL
    B. Leads V_2, V_3, V_4, I, and AVL
    C. Leads V_2, V_3, V_4, II, III, and AVF
    D. Leads V_1, V_2, II, III, and AVF

48. Brendon is receiving propranolol IV for SVT and hypertension. Which of the following are life-threatening side effects of propranolol administration?
    A. Laryngospasm and bronchospasm
    B. Complete heart block and dizziness
    C. Respiratory depression and cardiovascular collapse
    D. Polymorphic VT and dyspnea

49. You are mentoring a new nurse in the ED. The patient you will be caring for is receiving lidocaine via a continuous infusion. The new ED nurse must learn that lidocaine may cause adverse effects such as
    A. Hyperexcitability
    B. CNS toxicity
    C. Ventricular tachycardia
    D. Premature atrial complexes

50. Regurgitation systolic murmurs are associated with
    A. Aortic stenosis
    B. Pulmonic valve disease
    C. Ventral septal defect
    D. Atrial septal defects

51. If the inferior wall of the heart is infarcted, the leads that will most directly reflect the injury are
    A. I and aVL
    B. II, III, and aVF
    C. V_1–V_2
    D. V_5–V_6

52. Luke is a 65 year old admitted to the ED for treatment of chest pain and severe hypertension. A nitroglycerin drip was ordered. Which of the following is true regarding nitroglycerin administration?
    A. Use only plastic IV tubing
    B. Nitroglycerine may be piggybacked to Isolyte P
    C. Nitroglycerine should be filtered prior to delivery
    D. Have normal saline or other volume expander available at bedside

53. You are teaching your patient about her Coumadin (warfarin) therapy. Part of your teaching must include foods to avoid. Which of the following foods should be avoided?
    A. Broccoli, soybean oil, spinach
    B. Olive oil, peanut butter, kale
    C. Avocado, broccoli, peas
    D. Broccoli, green beans, spinach

54. What do abnormal Q waves signify on a 12-lead EKG?
    A. Partial thickness death of myocardium
    B. Complete thickness infarction of myocardium
    C. They are of no significance
    D. Repolarization of the myocardium

55. The most common new onset dysrhythmia seen in a patient with a diagnosis of pulmonary edema is
    A. Paroxysmal atrial tachycardia
    B. Supraventricular tachycardia
    C. Sinus rhythm with a RBBB
    D. Atrial fibrillation

56. What are some common reasons for pacemaker insertion?
    A. Tachycardia, Wenckebach, and bradycardia
    B. Symptomatic bradycardia, overdrive pacing, and acute MI with sinus dysfunction
    C. Complete heart block, Wenckebach, and tachycardia
    D. Bundle branch block, Wenckebach, and tachycardia

57. Right-sided congestive heart failure signs and symptoms include
    A. Respiratory distress and hepatomegaly
    B. Rapid capillary refill and absent jugular venous distension
    C. Weak femoral pulses and abdominal tenderness
    D. Increased SVR and strong femoral pulses

58. Increased afterload would be present in a patient with which of the following conditions?
    A. Polycythemia
    B. Aortic insufficiency
    C. Hypovolemia
    D. Sepsis

59. Right ventricular afterload may be reduced by
    A. A hypoxic state
    B. Hypoventilation
    C. Inhaled nitric oxide
    D. Administration of epinephrine

60. Your patient was diagnosed with left ventricular failure. Early signs of left ventricular failure are
    A. Hypoxemia and peripheral cyanosis
    B. Tachypnea and tachycardia
    C. Dyspnea and profuse sweating
    D. Central cyanosis and paradoxical respirations

61. While auscultating heart sounds on your new patient, you hear an S_3 heart sound. The third heart sound occurs as a result of
    A. Active atrial contraction
    B. Aortic stenosis
    C. Closure of the aortic and pulmonic valves
    D. Increased blood flow across the AV valves

62. An anterior wall infarction may be seen in leads
    A. V_4, R
    B. V_5–V_6
    C. V_7–V_9
    D. V_2–V_4

63. Which of the heart valves is most rarely affected by infective endocarditis?
    A. Tricuspid
    B. Pulmonic
    C. Mitral
    D. Aortic

64. Mr. C. was admitted to the ED with cough, fever, chills, anorexia, malaise, and headache. He currently has a pericardial friction rub and has a history of rheumatic fever. While examining Mr. C., you note fine, dark lines in his nail beds and some flat lesions on his palms. These flat lesions are known as
    A. Janeway lesions
    B. Osler's nodes
    C. Roth spots
    D. Pella's sign

65. Which of the following medications should be monitored for cyanide toxicity and avoided in patients with renal problems?
    A. Propranolol
    B. Sodium nitroprusside
    C. Dopamine
    D. Verapamil

66. A definitive diagnosis of myocarditis can be made via
    A. Transmural catheterization
    B. Transesophageal ultrasound
    C. Transcutaneous ultrasound
    D. Endomyocardial biopsy

67. Your patient had a syncopal episode at work. When he arrived at the ED, he became apneic and bradycardic. After a dose of atropine and one minute of assisted ventilations, he resumed a normal sinus rhythm and normal respirations. At first, it was thought the patient had the flu. When an IV was started for fluid replacement, excessive bleeding was noted at the IV site. Further examination and tests revealed slight hepatomegaly and hepatitis. Labs showed high numbers of bands and an elevated platelet count. A diagnosis of myocarditis was made. A likely causative agent for this condition is
    A. Group B *Streptococcus*
    B. *Escherichia coli*
    C. Coxsackie B_1 virus
    D. Halothane toxicity

68. Adverse effects of procainamide include
    A. Depressing the excitability of cardiac muscle
    B. Junctional tachycardia
    C. Slowing conduction in the atria
    D. Severe hypotension

69. You are treating an elderly woman in the ED with suspected sepsis. Her blood pressure is 94/54, heart rate is 120, respiratory rate is 20, O_2 saturation is 86% on room air. Before initiating an infusion of dopamine, which of the following actions is a priority for the nurse?
    A. Obtain consent for a central line
    B. Prepare to infuse dobutamine and dopamine together
    C. Verify the number of isotonic crystalloid boluses already given in the ED
    D. Ensure phentolamine mesylate is at bedside

70. High-dose epinephrine was started for your patient after resuscitation from a cardiac arrest due to beta-blocker overdose. Which of the following lab results should you monitor closely?
    A. Glucose levels
    B. Calcium levels
    C. Chloride levels
    D. Sodium levels

71. Mort received 4 mg of morphine IV and now is unresponsive and his respiratory rate and depth are diminished. The antagonist for morphine is
    A. Naloxone
    B. Atropine
    C. Regitine
    D. Bicarbonate

72. Heather is an asthmatic in decompensated shock. You are preparing to begin vasoactive support. Which of the following is the most appropriate vasoactive drug of choice?
    A. Isuprel
    B. Dopamine
    C. Vasopressin
    D. Neosynephrine

73. You are mentoring a new nurse in the ED who is caring for a patient receiving a dopamine drip. The order is to titrate the dopamine to keep the systolic blood pressure over 80 mmHg. You note that the nurse is titrating the drip every 2 to 3 minutes. You should
    A. Praise the nurse for her diligence
    B. Verify the order for systolic blood pressure, because it should be > 70 mmHg
    C. Suggest that titrations be done only in 15-minute increments
    D. Advise the nurse to wait at least 5 minutes between titrations

74. Vittore was diagnosed with SVT. He will be discharged with amiodarone to control his SVT. Which of the following discharge instructions is true?
    A. Continue normal outside activities without restrictions
    B. Continue original theophylline regimen
    C. Avoid grapefruit
    D. Dark urine is normal during the first 3 months of treatment

75. Vasopressin was started on your patient who is suffering from diabetes insipidus. Which of the following side effects warrants immediate intervention?
    A. Unexplained weight loss
    B. Hyperactivity
    C. Abdominal cramping
    D. Confusion

76. Victor was transported to the ED because of changes in mentation, development of ascites, orthopnea, paroxysmal nocturnal dyspnea, and excessive fatigue. On physical examination, you note S_3 and S_4 gallops, basilar crackles, and the EKG shows sinus tachycardia. These symptoms are usually indicative of which of the following types of cardiomyopathy?
    A. Restrictive cardiomyopathy
    B. Dilated cardiomyopathy
    C. Alcohol-induced cardiomyopathy
    D. Hypertrophic cardiomyopathy

77. Your patient requires an infusion of dobutamine. Dobutamine improves cardiac output primarily by
    A. Increasing afterload
    B. Increasing heart rate
    C. Decreasing preload
    D. Improving contractility

78. Atropine was given to your patient during an episode of bradycardia that resulted in a heart rate in the 20s. The patient had just been deeply suctioned. The low heart rate was unresponsive to oxygen support, so assisted ventilation via a bag-valve mask was provided. The heart rate improved to prebradycardic levels. Which of the following potential complications of atropine administration may now occur?
    A. Diuresis
    B. Hypertension
    C. Rebound bradycardia
    D. Headache

79. Your patient with recurrent VT was started on intravenous amiodarone today. Which of the following signs should the ED nurse monitor closely during administration of the initial loading dose?
    A. Urine output and parathyroid levels
    B. Urine output and liver function tests
    C. Thyroid levels and hypertonicity
    D. Observe for greenish discoloration of the skin and monitor thyroid levels

80. The type of echocardiography used to evaluate the motion of the cardiac valves and detect pericardial fluid is known as _____ echocardiography
    A. M-mode
    B. Two-dimensional
    C. Contrast
    D. Continuous-wave Doppler

81. In addition to heart rate and urine output, which of the following laboratory values should be monitored closely for a patient taking diazoxide and furosemide for hypertension?
    A. Glucose levels
    B. Bilirubin levels
    C. Calcium levels
    D. Copper levels

82. A complication of high-contrast mediums used for cardiac catheterizations is
    A. Hypoglycemia
    B. High sodium content
    C. Polycythemia
    D. Seizures

83. Which of the following statements is true about pericardial effusions?
    A. Diastolic filling is increased
    B. On CXR, a "water bottle" silhouette is noted
    C. The voltage of the QRS complex is increased
    D. This is a painless, hard-to-diagnose condition

84. The type of echocardiography that shows the quantity of flow across an obstruction is called
    A. Two-dimensional echocardiography
    B. Continuous-wave Doppler echocardiography
    C. M-mode echocardiography
    D. Contrast echocardiography

85. Your patient is 48 years old and is being discharged to the care of his primary healthcare provider following treatment for a small pulmonary embolus. He will be continuing anticoagulant therapy. You are reinforcing previous teaching about his medication. Your patient takes numerous herbal remedies daily. Which ones should he avoid while he is taking an anticoagulant?
    A. Dong quai, gingko biloba, ginseng
    B. Aloe extract, bilberry, broccoli
    C. Calendula, clove, allspice
    D. Fenugreek, licorice, leeks

86. Betty has severe hypotension. Norepinephrine bitartrate (Levophed) is infusing via her central line. Which of the following orders should you question?
    A. Monitor blood pressure every 30 minutes
    B. Administer with dopamine
    C. Dilute in D_5W
    D. Administer via a central line

87. Cardiac glycosides are often used in the treatment of heart failure. A major effect of this classification of medications is
    A. Increased conductivity
    B. Positive chronotropism
    C. Its usefulness as a ventricular antiarrhythmic
    D. Inotropism

88. Which drug listed below contains a high concentration of iodine?
    A. Lidocaine
    B. Amiodarone
    C. Aminophylline
    D. Digoxin

89. Dobutamine is used to improve cardiac output primarily by
    A. Causing profound peripheral vasodilation
    B. Acting on alpha-adrenergic receptors in the heart
    C. Acting on beta$_1$ adrenergic receptors in the heart
    D. Acting on both alpha- and beta-adrenergic receptors in the cardiovascular tissue

90. Alpha-adrenergic effects of norepinephrine include
    A. Increased force of myocardial contraction
    B. Peripheral arteriolar vasoconstriction
    C. Increased AV conduction time
    D. Central venous vasodilation

91. An example of a pansystolic murmur is
    A. Pulmonic insufficiency
    B. Tricuspid insufficiency
    C. Atrial stenosis
    D. Mitral stenosis

92. A reflex tachycardia caused by stretch of right atrial receptors is known as the
    A. Herring-Sines law
    B. Bainbridge reflex
    C. Starling's law
    D. Renin angiotensin system

93. Your patient is being treated for severe dyspnea, dysphagia, palpitations, and an intractable cough. On auscultation you hear a loud S_1 and a right-sided S_3 and S_4. A pulmonary artery catheter is placed and large A waves are seen in the PA tracing. The patient probably has
    A. Mitral stenosis
    B. Myocarditis
    C. Atrial stenosis
    D. Mitral insufficiency

94. Nifedipine is classified as a
    A. Calcium channel blocker
    B. Beta-blocker
    C. MAO inhibitor
    D. Catecholamine

95. Gloria has been consuming large quantities of power drinks and has been having intermittent episodes of SVT. Today she was transported to the ED because she had a syncopal episode at dance class and requires therapy for the SVT. Which of the following medications is specific to the treatment of sustained supraventricular tachycardia?
    A. Atropine
    B. Theophylline
    C. Amiodarone
    D. Adenosine

96. The most commonly used type of ventricular assist device is the
    A. RVAD
    B. VAD
    C. BIVAD
    D. LVAD

97. Indications for use of a ventricular assist device are
    A. Extensive organ damage
    B. As destination therapy
    C. Prolonged cardiac arrest
    D. Dysrhythmias

98. You are preparing to give adenosine to a patient in SVT. Why is it important that adenosine be given rapidly?
    A. If given slowly, the adenosine will probably fail to convert the SVT
    B. Adenosine is incompatible with adrenalin
    C. If given slowly, adenosine may cause systemic vasodilation and reflex tachycardia
    D. If given slowly, adenosine may cause blurred vision

99. Which of the following statements is true regarding the fourth heart sound (S_4)?
    A. S_4 occurs just after the first heart sound
    B. The fourth heart sound occurs with ventricular contraction
    C. The fourth heart sound is benign
    D. The fourth heart sound is always pathologic after 24 hours of life

100. A heart murmur associated with acute valvular regurgitation is called
    A. S_3
    B. S_2
    C. S_1
    D. S_4

101. Eileen was diagnosed with refractive SVT that did not respond to either adenosine or cardioversion. She is being monitored before being transported for ablation therapy. Tachyarrhythmias that are refractive to conventional therapies may have to be treated with radiofrequency ablation. This treatment is usually successful on reentry tachyarrhythmias. The radiofrequency destroys myocardial tissue via
    A. Radiation
    B. Heat
    C. Cold
    D. An overriding signal to ablate the pacemaker

102. Parker has Wolf-Parkinson-White syndrome. She has experienced increasing bouts of tachycardia over the past few weeks. Parker's cardiologist has decided to use a pacemaker. How do you explain this type of pacemaker to a new orientee you are precepting in the ED?
    A. The pacemaker or AICD is set on demand mode and is asynchronous
    B. The pacemaker is at a set constant rate of 80 bpm and is synchronized
    C. The pacemaker or AICD is set on demand mode and is synchronous
    D. The pacemaker or AICD is set on inhibit mode and is synchronous

103. Randall has had an AICD for 8 months. He has come to the ED after a syncopal episode during work today. You note his pulse is very irregular and he is complaining of getting "zapped" often. Randall says he is exhausted from the repeated shocks and asks for pain medication. Randall's EKG shows sinus bradycardia with numerous pacemaker spikes. As an ED nurse, you suspect
    A. Randall's AICD has a faulty lead
    B. Randall has been in the proximity of a large magnetic field
    C. The battery in Randall's AICD is losing power
    D. Randall has a generator failure of his AICD

104. What type of pacemaker/AICD program code would you expect for a patient with complete heart block?
    A. VVT
    B. DDI
    C. VVI
    D. DDD

105. Bart had a DDD pacemaker inserted 3 years ago. His college schoolwork has been declining, and he has not been participating in activities with his friends. He now has Pacemaker syndrome. What symptoms do you expect to see with this condition?
    A. Fatigue, agitation, forgetfulness
    B. Fatigue, dizziness, confusion
    C. Fatigue, agitation, dyspnea
    D. Fatigue, dizziness, syncope

106. The most common infection in patients with a ventricular assist device is
    A. Septicemia
    B. Pericarditis
    C. Pneumonia
    D. Pericardial effusion

107. Quincke's sign is usually observed in patients who have a diagnosis of
    A. Mitral stenosis
    B. Endocarditis
    C. Aortic insufficiency
    D. Pericarditis

108. Which of the following hemodynamic changes will occur in a patient with a cardiac tamponade?
    A. Contractility increases
    B. Decreased heart rate
    C. Stroke volume decreases
    D. Increased cardiac output

109. Beck's triad is a combination of symptoms useful in diagnosing a cardiac tamponade. These symptoms include
    A. Increased pulse pressure, increased JVD, and tachycardia
    B. A pericardial friction rub, hypertension, and RV failure
    C. LV failure, tachycardia, and hypertension
    D. Distended neck veins, muffled heart sounds, and hypotension

110. Stroke volume is comprised of which of the following factors?
    A. Viscosity, blood volume, and impedance
    B. Cardiac output, heart rate, and compliance
    C. Contractility, preload, and afterload
    D. Systemic impedance, heart rate, and compliance

111. During evaluation of CVP pressure monitoring tracings, the c wave represents
    A. Mechanical atrial diastole
    B. The decrease in RA volume during relaxation
    C. Emptying of the right atrium into the RV
    D. The increase in RA pressure from closure of the tricuspid valve

112. A low CVP reading may represent
    A. Pulmonary hypertension
    B. Increased contractility
    C. Biventricular failure
    D. Cardiac tamponade

113. New-onset atrial fibrillation frequently develops as a sequela to
    A. Pulmonary edema
    B. Left heart failure
    C. Use of PPIs
    D. Tricuspid regurgitation

114. If a dopamine infusion infiltrates, the suggested treatment is to inject which of the following medications into the affected area?
    A. Epinephrine
    B. Phentolamine
    C. Lidocaine
    D. Atropine

115. Your patient has developed diffuse chest pain and tachycardia. Upon auscultation you hear muffled heart sounds and note an increased JVD. You suspect the patient has developed a cardiac tamponade. If your patient does have a cardiac tamponade, which of the following findings would you expect on a chest X-ray?
    A. A dilated superior vena cava
    B. A pneumothorax
    C. Narrowed mediastinum
    D. Delineation of the pericardium and epicardium

116. Your patient has an arterial line and is being mechanically ventilated after a respiratory arrest. You note very pronounced phasic variations in the arterial line and suspect that
    A. The ETT tube is becoming dislodged
    B. The patient has tricuspid regurgitation
    C. The patient is suffering from heart failure
    D. The arterial line is kinked

117. Bryce is in cardiogenic shock. At this time he is awaiting placement on an intra-aortic balloon pump. In any patient with cardiogenic shock, an undesirable outcome would produce
    A. Increased cardiac output
    B. Increased systemic vascular resistance
    C. Decreased ventricular preload
    D. Decreased pulmonary artery pressures

118. Jayden was diagnosed with left ventricular failure. Early signs of left ventricular failure are
    A. Hypoxemia and peripheral cyanosis
    B. Tachypnea and tachycardia
    C. Dyspnea and profuse sweating
    D. Central cyanosis and paradoxical respirations

119. John was admitted to the ED with aortic insufficiency. During his initial assessment, you note the popliteal BP is higher than the brachial BP by at least 30 mmHg. This phenomenon is known as
    A. DeRoge's sign
    B. Hill's sign
    C. Holmes' sign
    D. Rochelle's sign

120. Intravenous hydralazine is incompatible with
    A. Furosemide
    B. Hydrocortisone
    C. Potassium chloride
    D. Heparin

121. Ginger and her family just returned from a vacation in Europe. She has been complaining to her husband about leg cramping for the past 3 days. Ginger's nurse practitioner sent her to the ED for further evaluation. During your initial assessment you found Ginger sitting on the side of the gurney, leaning forward. She states the position relieved her newly developed chest pain. She also states that the pain is worse on inspiration. You notify the ED physician, and he orders a CXR and lab work. The sed. rate and WBCs are elevated. Ginger most likely is suffering from
    A. A thoracic aneurysm
    B. Pericarditis
    C. Pulmonary hypertension
    D. A pulmonary embolus

122. Mike is a 22 year old football player. When he returned home from school this afternoon, he was short of breath and overly fatigued. His roommate mentioned that Mike's ankles were quite swollen at that time. Mike uncharacteristically went to bed, and when his roommate could not arouse him, he called paramedics. Mike arrived in your ED about 30 minutes ago. He is being mechanically ventilated at TV 750, FiO2 .80, AC 14. He remains unresponsive. A pulmonary artery catheter was placed. His assessment findings are as follows:
EKG: ST at 124
Art line BP 68/42 cuff BP 64/46 Doppler only to Dorsalis Pedis, no pressure obtained
Skin pale, cool, clammy
RR 15, breath sounds = crackles LLL, RLL   Marked pretibial and pedal edema
Mentation: Unresponsive to painful stimuli
Pulmonary artery catheter readings:
    PAP 46/28
    PAOP 26
    RAP 18
Cardiac Output 3.2   Cardiac Index 1.2
Mike is probably developing
    A. Pulmonary hypertension
    B. A cardiac tamponade
    C. Cardiogenic shock
    D. Right heart failure

123. Chris took his brother's motorcycle out for a ride. Chris lost control of the motorcycle in the rain. He was wearing a helmet and protective gear and suffered a fractured left femur, left flail chest, a cervical sprain, and road rash on his face and neck. He is admitted with a blood pressure of 82/42, HR 102, RR 26 and shallow, T 98.2°F. His 12-lead EKG shows ST elevation in the anterior leads. His CXR shows a normal cardiac silhouette and no infiltrates. His HgB is 9.0, Hct is 31. MB is 18%. He is restless and complains of pain in the chest and left leg. Chris is probably suffering from
    A. Pulmonary edema
    B. Hypovolemic shock
    C. Systolic dysfunction
    D. Pulmonary hypertension

124. Your patient is in decompensated shock. You have dobutamine infusing via a peripheral IV line. You have just received an order to give sodium bicarbonate intravenously and to give ampicillin intravenously as well. As an ED nurse, you know the most appropriate actions to take are to
    A. Stop the dobutamine and infuse the sodium bicarbonate while waiting for pharmacy to send the ampicillin
    B. Start a peripheral heparin lock to infuse the sodium bicarbonate and follow with the ampicillin infusion
    C. Ask the physician to place a central line or PICC line for additional venous access ports
    D. Piggyback the ampicillin on the main IV line and start another peripheral line on the other arm

125. Mario was seen in the ED after falling from his roof. He sustained a left fractured tibia and fibula and a fractured left clavicle. Mario will require a splenectomy and was just admitted to your care at shift change. The surgeon is 15 minutes from the hospital. Your initial assessment results are as follows:
    EKG: ST at 110 with isolated PVCs
    Art line BP 70/50 cuff BP 76/50 skin pale, cool, clammy
    RR 26, breath sounds clear, slightly diminished RLL O_2 2 L/min via NC
    Mentation: Responds to questions slowly, oriented to self and time
    Pulmonary artery catheter readings:
      PAP 24/8
      PAOP 5
      RAP 4
    Cardiac Output 3.3   Cardiac Index 1.7
    Which of the following conditions do you believe Mario is developing?
    A. Cardiogenic shock
    B. Hypovolemic shock
    C. Septic shock
    D. Left ventricular failure

126. Snyder has been huffing freon and experimenting with crack cocaine. Yesterday, he was snorting cocaine when he became short of breath and felt diffuse chest discomfort. He went inside for lunch and the pain disappeared. Snyder tried watching TV because he felt more fatigued than ever. Today, he was admitted to your ED with orthopnea and profound dyspnea. Snyder agreed to placement of a pulmonary artery catheter and the following information was obtained:
    EKG: Borderline ST at 100 with rare PACs
    Cuff BP 142/74 skin warm, pale capillary refill 4 seconds
    2+ pitting edema (pretibial)
    RR 20, breath sounds: crackles in posterior lobes O_2 2 L/min via NC
    ABGs were drawn, but results are unavailable
    Mentation: Alert, oriented × 4
    Pulmonary artery catheter readings:
      PAP 40/20
      PAOP 20
      RAP 5
    Cardiac Output 3.6   Cardiac Index 2.0

Snyder probably has developed

A. A chylothorax
B. A mild pericarditis
C. Pulmonary edema (noncardiac)
D. Left ventricular failure

127. Magda is 71 years old and was alert and active last evening, playing cards with her friends. This morning, her daughter found Magda just sitting on the side of her bed, hardly able to move. At first, the paramedics and the personnel in the ED thought Magda had suffered a stroke, but because her EKG showed large R waves in leads V_1 and V_2, a pulmonary artery catheter was placed without incident. Physical parameters include

EKG: SR at 92, no ectopy
Cuff BP 94/62 skin pale, cool, clammy
RR 18, breath sounds clear, slightly diminished LLL O_2 2 L/min via NC
Moderate jugular venous distension, no bruits
Mentation: Lethargic
Pulmonary artery catheter readings:
   PAP 24/10
   PAOP 9
   RAP 20
Cardiac Output 4.9   Cardiac Index 2.4
Expected diagnosis for Magda is

A. Pericarditis
B. LV hypertrophy
C. RV infarction
D. Aortic insufficiency

128. Lars is a 25 year old hockey player. He is being evaluated for cardiomyopathy. His initial ejection fraction was 24%, and he has been confused most of the time since admission to the ED 2 hours ago. On admission his EKG showed ST depression in leads V_1–V_4. He has become more dyspneic and is getting restless. Current vital signs and parameters are

EKG: ST at 116
Art line BP 110/64 cuff BP 102/70 skin pale, cool   +4 bilateral pretibial and pedal
edema   +3 Sacral edema   Temp 99°F
RR 30, breath sounds clear, slightly diminished RLL O_2 4 L/min via mask
Mentation: Oriented to self, confused at times
Pulmonary artery catheter readings:
   PAP 48/22
   PAOP 20
   RAP 16
Cardiac Output 3.4   Cardiac Index 2.0

What condition does Lars appear to be suffering from at this time?
A. Anterior MI
B. Inferior wall MI
C. Biventricular failure
D. Right ventricular failure

129. Your patient is in fulminant CHF. What is the purpose of administering vasoactive and inotropic medications to this patient?
    A. Decrease preload, decrease afterload, increase contractility
    B. Increase preload, increase afterload, decrease contractility
    C. Increase myocardial oxygen demand, decrease contractility, increase afterload
    D. Decrease myocardial oxygen demand, decrease contractility, increase preload

130. Your patient was found in the ED waiting room in full arrest. After placing the patient on a monitor, you discover the patient is in ventricular fibrillation. Your first priority is to
    A. Cardiovert the patient with 200 Joules
    B. Administer 1 mg of 1:10,000 epinephrine IV
    C. Administer 300 mg of amiodarone IV
    D. Defibrillate the patient with 200 Joules

131. Which of the following drugs is classified as both a negative chronotrope and a positive inotrope?
    A. Amiodarone
    B. Digoxin
    C. Pronestyl
    D. Epinephrine

132. Your patient just had a temporary atrial pacemaker placed. On the EKG you note pacemaker spikes that are not followed by p waves. Which of the following nursing actions should be performed at this time?
    A. Turn off the pacemaker
    B. Make certain the pacemaker is in the demand mode
    C. Increase the milliamperes
    D. Nothing—the pattern is normal

133. Which of the following statements is true regarding a type I aortic aneurysm?
    A. Type I aneurysms are the rarest form of aneurysm
    B. Tears begin in the ascending aorta
    C. Type I aneurysm tears are in the intimal lining
    D. Type I tears are in the descending aorta

134. Type III aneurysms
    A. Begin in the thoracic arch
    B. Are the rarest form of aneurysm
    C. Involve intimal tears
    D. Occur in the descending aorta

135. A risk factor for an aortic aneurysm would not include
    A. Connective tissue disorders
    B. Medial necrosis of the aorta
    C. Hypotension
    D. Coarctation of the aorta

136. A patient has had a pulmonary artery catheter placed and is receiving a vasodilator for a hypertensive crisis. Suddenly, he develops ventricular fibrillation and then becomes asystolic. The most probable cause of his cardiovascular collapse is
    A. A CVA
    B. A malfunctioning catheter
    C. A saddle embolus
    D. Left ventricular hypertrophy

137. If a patient is suffering from cardiogenic shock, which of the following therapies could be administered to improve cardiac contractility without an increase in the SVR?
    A. Epinephrine
    B. Dopamine
    C. Fluids
    D. Norepinephrine

138. Your patient was injured when a tree fell on his car following a rainstorm. The paramedics had to cut the patient out of his car. On initial assessment you note a 20 mmHg difference in the blood pressures of both arms. His feet are pale and cool and the lower extremity pulses are weak. This patient is probably suffering from a
    A. Flail chest
    B. Ruptured aorta
    C. Ruptured right ventricle
    D. Ruptured abdominal aortic aneurysm

139. Your patient was admitted to the ED complaining of diffuse abdominal pain. On initial assessment you notice a pulsatile mass in his abdomen. The next action you should take is to
    A. Palpate the mass to determine its size
    B. Immediately report this finding to the physician
    C. Auscultate the mass
    D. Prepare the patient for a biopsy of the mass

140. Your patient has pericarditis and the physician has prescribed colchicine. Your patient teaching should include dietary restrictions. Which food should the patient avoid if taking colchicine?
    A. Diet Coke
    B. Pears
    C. Grapefruit
    D. Bananas

141. If a patient becomes tachycardic, what happens to the QT and RR intervals?
    A. No change occurs
    B. The QT interval lengthens and the RR interval remains constant
    C. The QT interval shortens and the RR interval lengthens
    D. The QT and the RR intervals shorten

142. If your patient is experiencing cannon "a" waves, this phenomenon is due to
    A. A powerful atrial wave
    B. A pneumothorax impinging on the inferior vena cava
    C. Pulsations seen on an arterial pressure tracing
    D. A stenotic aortic valve

143. When should you suspect a patient has suffered a right ventricular MI?
    A. When the patient has right arm pain or paresthesias with substernal chest pain
    B. When the patient has an inferior wall MI and ST elevation in leads V_1 and V_2
    C. When anginal pain is unrelieved with sublingual NTG
    D. With EKG changes in leads V_5 and V_6

144. Under the new 2010 American Heart Association guidelines for chest compressions, the rescuer should compress the sternum of an adult to a depth of
    A. 1 inch
    B. 1½ inches
    C. 2 inches
    D. 3 inches

145. The 2010 BLS sequence for adults receiving CPR is
    A. ABC
    B. CAB
    C. AOB
    D. BAC

146. Which of the following statements is true regarding routine application of cricoid pressure during cardiac arrest?
    A. Cricoid pressure is not recommended as a routine action
    B. Cricoid pressure should be applied whenever possible during cardiac arrest
    C. Cricoid pressure must be used when there are two or more rescuers
    D. Cricoid pressure must be applied only by a paramedic, MICN, or a physician

147. The most reliable method of confirming and monitoring correct placement of an ETT is by use of
    A. Auscultation
    B. Visualization of the cords
    C. Use of an end tidal CO_2 monitor
    D. Continuous wave capnography

148. The single, most important component of a successful outcome for a patient requiring advanced cardiac life support is
    A. Early defibrillation
    B. Use of epinephrine in place of vasopressin
    C. Therapeutic hypothermia
    D. High-quality CPR

149. According to the 2010 American Heart Association Guidelines for CPR and Emergency Cardiovascular Care, which of the following medications is no longer recommended for routine use in the management of PEA or asystole?
    A. Epinephrine
    B. Adenosine
    C. Atropine
    D. Vasopressin

150. Withdrawal of life support is a difficult decision. If an adult post–cardiac arrest patient is treated with therapeutic hypothermia, the patient should be evaluated via neurologic signs, biomarkers, electrophysiologic studies, and imaging where available at _____ after cardiac arrest.
    A. 24 hours
    B. 48 hours
    C. 72 hours
    D. 96 hours

151. Which of the following statements about drowning victims is true?
    A. There is no evidence that water acts as an obstructive foreign body
    B. CPR should be performed while the patient is in the water
    C. Immediate maneuvers to relieve foreign body airway obstruction should precede BLS
    D. Spinal cord injuries are common among drowning victims

152. How does STEMI differ from NSTEMI?
    A. STEMI involves myocardial cell death
    B. They are the same except for the EKG tracing
    C. The cardiac enzymes are elevated in the STEMI only
    D. The cardiac enzymes are elevated only in NSTEMI

153. A 66 year old man who drove himself to the ED has been having substernal chest pain radiating to his jaw and left arm for the last 45 minutes. He is diaphoretic and short of breath. His EKG tracing shows ST elevation in leads V_2–V_4. Which of the following actions or treatments should you anticipate being ordered for this patient?
    A. STAT cardiac enzymes
    B. Fibrinolytic therapy as soon as possible
    C. Percutaneous coronary intervention
    D. Admission to the intensive care unit

154. Which of the following parameters is considered diagnostic of a STEMI on the 12-lead EKG?
    A. A STEMI must be diagnosed by the cardiac enzymes results, not an EKG
    B. A 1-mm ST elevation of the affected coronary vessel
    C. A 5-mm ST elevation of the affected coronary artery
    D. A large R wave with ST elevation in an anterior lead

155. What is the purpose of a right-side 12-lead EKG?
    A. It allows a view of the pulmonary blood flow
    B. It looks at the inferior wall of the heart
    C. It looks at the right ventricle and the posterior heart
    D. It assesses for left ventricle aneurysm

SECTION 3: CARDIOVASCULAR ANSWERS

1. **Correct answer: B**
   Unstable angina usually associated with left anterior descending (LAD) coronary artery lesions is known as Wellen's syndrome. Characteristic changes include inverted symmetric T waves and/or biphasic waves with little or no ST elevation and the absence of Q waves. However, the most dangerous aspect of this syndrome is that the EKG changes appear only when the patient is pain free. Sometimes, staff may believe the resolution of pain means the patient can be scheduled for a stress test. The stress test may initiate an impending MI, so it must not be performed. When a patient has Wellen's syndrome, an MI may occur in as little as a few minutes to a few days.

2. **Correct answer: B**
   ST segment depression usually indicates myocardial ischemia. This patient also exhibited substernal chest pain, another finding seen with ischemia.

3. **Correct answer: C**
   Right ventricular preload in the heart is measured by the central venous pressure (CVP). The normal range for a CVP is 2–10 mmHg. The CVP is also known as the right atrial pressure.

4. **Correct answer: C**
   A pulse pressure is the difference between the systolic blood pressure and the diastolic blood pressure—in this case, 40. This measurement is significant because if the patient has a narrow pulse pressure, it would indicate systemic compensatory vasoconstriction due to a decrease in arterial pressure (the stroke volume falls and the systolic pressure decreases). Another way to look at this phenomenon is to think of the high systemic vascular resistance causing an increase in diastolic pressure.

5. **Correct answer: D**
   Left ventricular preload in the heart is measured by the pulmonary artery wedge pressure (PAWP). When a pulmonary artery catheter is inserted, a balloon is inflated and carries the tip of the catheter into the pulmonary artery where it "wedges." The tip senses pressure ahead of it, which is the pressure from the left side of the heart. This pressure can also be called the pulmonary artery occlusive pressure (PAOP) or the left ventricular end diastolic pressure (LVEDP). The normal range is 4–12 mmHg.

6. **Correct answer: C**
   The MAP is a mean pressure that takes into account that the diastolic phase of the cardiac cycle comprises two-thirds of the cycle. The calculation for the MAP is MAP = 2(DBP) + (SBP) / 3; in this case, 80. If you took the average of the two pressures, it would not account for the importance of the diastolic phase. The heart rate is not entered into this calculation. Patients should maintain a MAP of at least 60 to ensure perfusion to the brain and kidneys.

7. **Correct answer: D**
   The ejection fraction should be over 50%. This is the amount of blood ejected from the left ventricle compared to the total amount available. This amount is expressed as a percentage. For example, if the ventricle contains 90 ml of blood and 50 ml are

ejected, the amount would be represented as a percentage, in this case 55%. An ejection fraction of 35% or less indicates a problem with contractility, outflow, or filling.

8. **Correct answer: B**
Normal cardiac output should be 4 to 8 L/min. The formula for calculating this value is CO = HR × SV. In this case, 78 (HR) × 60 (SV) = 4680 ml/min. Converted to liters, this value would equal 4.68 L/min.

9. **Correct answer: B**
Metabolism of the heart is decreased during diastole, which comprises about one-half of the cardiac cycle at birth. Shortly after birth the diastolic phase lengthens to comprise two-thirds of the cardiac cycle. An increase in cardiac output decreases diastole.

10. **Correct answer: C**
Normal pulmonary artery pressures and CVP pressures are as follows:
CVP (RAP) = 2–8 mmHg
PAS = 20–30 / 6–10 mmHg
PAD = 5–12 mmHg
PAM = 10–20 mmHg
PAOP (PCWP) = 4–12 mmHg

11. **Correct answer: A**
In patients with normal cardiac anatomy, right atrial pressure equals right ventricular end diastolic pressure (RVEDP), which equals central venous pressure. This question refers back to CVP = RAP and now the value of RVEDP is added, and all these terms refer to right ventricular preload.

12. **Correct answer: C**
Prinzmetal's angina is also known as variant angina and is usually caused by a coronary vasospasm. It may occur at rest, long after exercise, or during sleep.

13. **Correct answer: B**
Calcium channel blockers act primarily on arteriolar tissue. Large lumen vessels in the arterial system are affected. The advantage of this action is that both systolic and diastolic pressures are reduced and the patient will not have a drop in blood pressure. The blood pressure may be lowered slightly and cause a reflex baroreceptor response to speed up the heart rate to maintain cardiac output.

14. **Correct answer: B**
Rate, rhythm, axis, hypertrophy, and infarction are the most valuable areas examined in a 12-lead EKG.

15. **Correct answer: C**
Increased preload may be caused by renal problems. An overload of fluid is present in the intravascular space. Preload may also be increased in cases where resistance is increased, such as in valve dysfunctions or vasoconstriction. Anything that blocks fluid from progressing forward or prevents elimination of fluids is a potential cause of increased preload. If the heart fails and the myocardium cannot pump out, such as in damage from surgery, cardiomyopathies, or decreased stretch following heart surgery, preload increases.

16. **Correct answer: A**
    Decreased preload may result from hyperthermia (vasodilation), diuresis, hemorrhage, surgery, vomiting, and diarrhea. Any condition(s) that may result in a loss of fluid within the intravascular space will decrease preload.

17. **Correct answer: A**
    Afterload is the resistance the heart must pump against. Nitrates are vasodilators, so their use decreases resistance. Aortic stenosis increases afterload because the ventricle has to work harder to overcome a dysfunctional valve. Hypothermia vasoconstricts vessels and increases resistance, and hypertension is usually the result of narrowing of vessels, producing increased resistance.

18. **Correct answer: C**
    Pulsus alternans occurs in left ventricular failure when a weakened myocardium cannot maintain an even pressure with each contraction. The pulses alternate between strong and weak. This condition is also seen in CHF.

19. **Correct answer: B**
    The S_2 heart sound is created by closure of the pulmonic and aortic valves. S_2 is best heard in the upper left sternal border or pulmonic area.

20. **Correct answer: A**
    When the parasympathetic and sympathetic nervous systems stimulate the right vagus nerve, the SA node is affected and slows the heart rate. Acetylcholine is a neurotransmitter.

21. **Correct answer: A**
    Cyanosis may be observed when at least 5 g/100 ml of deoxygenated hemoglobin is present in circulation.

22. **Correct answer: A**
    Upright QRS complexes in leads V_1, V_2 show right bundle branch blocks. A simple way to remember which type of bundle branch block with a QRS wider than 0.12 seconds is to think of the turn signals on your car. For a right turn you must push the lever up, for a left turn the lever must go down. So looking at V_1 and V_2 if the QRS is upright, then there is a right bundle branch block. If V_1 and V_2 are downward in force, then it is a left bundle branch block.

23. **Correct answer: A**
    Using ICHD nomenclature, the first V is the chamber paced.

24. **Correct answer: B**
    On an EKG, left-sided heart failure results in wide, notched P waves. A tall, peaked P wave is indicative of right-sided heart failure. Changes in ST segments (or T waves) usually indicate myocardial ischemia.

25. **Correct answer: C**
    Rheumatic fever remains the most common cause of acquired valvular disease. The valves are a perfect place for bacteria to colonize. Blood is a perfect medium for bacterial growth. The causative organism is beta-hemolytic streptococcus.

26. **Correct answer: C**
    Using ICHD nomenclature, the second V is the chamber sensed.

27. **Correct answer: C**
If a beta$_2$ receptor in the heart is stimulated, it may cause bronchodilation, vasodilation (lowered SVR), and smooth muscle relaxation.

28. **Correct answer: C**
Lidocaine does not impair normal contractility. Lidocaine may shorten the QT interval, and the side effects usually involve the CNS: slurred speech, drowsiness, confusion, paresthesias, seizures, and convulsions. Hypotension, nystagmus, and gastrointestinal intolerance are effects of phenytoin, another class 1B drug.

29. **Correct answer: B**
Quinidine and hypomagnesemia can lead to Torsade de Pointes (also known as polymorphic ventricular tachycardia), a recurrent ventricular tachycardia that turns on its axis every 6-8 beats, giving the EKG a twisting or "turning on point" look. Hypomagnesemia may occur when the patient receives total parenteral nutrition.

30. **Correct answer: A**
Lidocaine infusion may cause respiratory arrest. A respiratory rate of 7 indicates impending failure and immediate action is required to provide respiratory support via a resuscitation bag, and staff should prepare for intubation. The infusion should be stopped if respiratory failure occurs, if a widening QRS is noted, or the heart rate drops below 60. The infusion must also be stopped if the patient becomes hypotensive, has difficulty speaking, or experiences numbness and tingling. These are symptoms of lidocaine toxicity.

31. **Correct answer: B**
Esmolol is incompatible with furosemide. Furosemide administration requires alternative venous access or oral administration. Esmolol is compatible with cimetidine, penicillin, and midazolam.

32. **Correct answer: B**
Even though the exact causes are unknown, a large number of alcoholics develop dilated cardiomyopathy. Three possible reasons have been identified:
   1. The alcohol itself, or the metabolites, have a toxic effect
   2. Alcohol sometimes contains additives, such as cobalt
   3. The cause may be nutritional in origin, such as a thiamine deficiency

   New research shows a possible viral link to the chronic alcoholism. It is interesting that this type of cardiomyopathy might reverse itself if the drinking is stopped. Other types of cardiomyopathy are not reversible.

33. **Correct answer: D**
Rapid infusion of Lasix can cause tinnitus and hearing loss.

34. **Correct answer: B**
Chlorothiazide reduces urinary calcium losses and does not result in profound potassium losses.

35. **Correct answer: B**
Hypertrophic cardiomyopathy results in a normal cardiac output and an increased ejection fraction. In hypertrophic cardiomyopathy the myocardium thickens, but it is not symmetrical. There is more thickening of the ventricular septum than the ventricle. If you were to look at a heart with this condition, it could appear normal externally.

When the septum is thicker, it creates a hyperdynamic state by increasing contractility, so the ejection fraction is increased. In rare conditions where the septum is asymmetrically thickened, the left ventricular outflow is impaired, so the cardiac output would be decreased.

36. **Correct answer: D**
Congestive heart failure results in a systemic venous engorgement because blood does not flow forward and is allowed to pool in organs and peripheral circulation. Tissues become hypoxic and further diminish function until complete failure and death.

37. **Correct answer: C**
The type of cardiomyopathy characterized by replacement of normal cells by fatty tissue is known as arrhythmogenic cardiomyopathy. This is a relatively new classification of cardiomyopathy. The normal myocardial cells are replaced by fatty tissue and fibrous tissue. The right ventricle is primarily affected. Conduction cannot occur normally, and the patient will have multiple ventricular arrhythmias and right ventricular failure. Young people are at risk for sudden death. The cause of this condition is unknown, but some research has shown a possible link to an autosomal dominant gene.

38. **Correct answer: C**
Symptoms of right-sided heart failure include hepatomegaly. When the right side of the heart fails it is often due to left-sided failure. The right ventricle cannot adequately pump blood out, so filling pressures rise and the blood backs up, resulting in the hepatomegaly. Thus, the CVP and RV pressures are elevated. Additional symptoms can include splenomegaly, ascites, abdominal pain, S_3, S_4, and weight gain. Pulmonary edema, an elevated PAD and PAOP, and orthopnea are symptoms of left-sided heart failure.

39. **Correct answer: A**
If an early IABP balloon inflation occurs, the balloon inflates prior to closure of the aortic valve. The result is aortic regurgitation and reduced stroke volume. Additionally, myocardial oxygen demand and end-diastolic volumes increase.

The IABP may be inserted in the ED. The important thing to remember is that the balloon is threaded up through the femoral artery and sits in the thoracic aorta. The balloon inflates during diastole, augmenting diastolic fill. The balloon deflates during systole and reduces the workload of the heart by actually providing a suction that helps blood flow from the heart.

40. **Correct answer: D**
The loss of the left radial pulse during treatment with an IABP is due to upward migration of the balloon catheter. The catheter is probably occluding the left subclavian artery and requires immediate repositioning.

41. **Correct answer: C**
A relative contraindication for the use of an IABP is thrombocytopenia. A relative contraindication is one where the potential risk is weighed against the potential benefit. Additional relative contraindicates to IABP therapy are coagulopathies, peripheral vascular disease, end-stage cardiomyopathies, and terminal diseases.

42. Correct answer: A
An absolute contraindication to the use of IABP therapy is an aortic dissection. In addition, irreversible brain damage, abdominal aortic aneurism, and aortic insufficiency are reasons the patient should not undergo IABP therapy.

43. Correct answer: A
The IABP will decrease the workload of the heart, resulting in increased diastolic fill, decreased afterload, and reduced myocardial oxygen consumption.

44. Correct answer: C
The most common complication of IABP therapy is lower limb ischemia. Other less common complications of IABP therapy include bleeding, thrombocytopenia, anemia, catheter migration, infection, aortic dissection, and compartment syndrome.

45. Correct answer: D
An allergy to fish places the patient at an increased risk for an allergic reaction to protamine sulfate. Patients who have undergone prior cardiac procedures or diabetics who have used protamine insulin are also at risk for an allergy reaction to protamine sulfate. Protamine may also cause rebound bleeding up to 18 hours postoperatively. FYI: men who have had a vasectomy or who are infertile may have developed antibodies to protamine.

46. Correct answer: B
A common cause of restrictive cardiomyopathy is glycogen storage disease. Amyloidosis is an additional cause of restrictive cardiomyopathy. The myocardium (especially the left ventricle) becomes rigid from fibrosis. This results in inadequate left ventricular filling and increased atrial dilatation. Left ventricular diastolic dysfunction occurs, and the LVEDP is markedly increased. Systolic function remains normal in this type of cardiomyopathy. Fluid backs up into the lungs and the patient appears to have congestive heart failure. There is no cure, and symptoms are treated as they occur.

47. Correct answer: B
Leads V_2, V_3, V_4, I, and AVL are indicative of an anterolateral MI. The MI could also include V_5 and V_6, which are also lateral leads.

48. Correct answer: A
Life-threatening side effects of propranolol include laryngospasms and bronchospasms in addition to bradycardia, bone marrow suppression, and hypotension. Complete heart block and dizziness are side effects of propaferone (Rythmol). Lidocaine may cause respiratory depression and cardiovascular collapse. Polymorphic VT and dyspnea are life-threatening side effects of sotalol (Betapace).

49. Correct answer: B
Signs of CNS toxicity from lidocaine may include agitation, vomiting, drowsiness, and muscle twitching. Later signs may include loss of consciousness, seizures, respiratory depression, and apnea. Cardiac toxicity may develop and cause hypotension, bradycardia, and heart block, and may lead to cardiovascular collapse.

50. Correct answer: C
Regurgitation systolic murmurs are associated with VSD, tricuspid regurgitation, and mitral valve regurgitation. Regurgitation systolic murmurs are caused by blood flow from an area of higher pressure throughout systole to an area of lower pressure.

51. **Correct answer: B**
Leads II, III, and aVF show damage to the inferior wall of the heart. Leads I and aVL show damage to the higher areas of the lateral wall. V_1 and V_2 show septal wall damage. V_5 and V_6 show damage to the apical area.

52. **Correct answer: D**
When administering nitroglycerin it is important to have normal saline or other volume expander at bedside in case of vascular collapse. The potential collapse is related to peripheral venous and arterial dilation (relative hypovolemia). Only nonpolyvinyl chloride tubing may be used for infusion because PVC may be absorbed by the nitroglycerin. Filtration is not required before infusion. Nitroglycerin is only compatible with D_5W, normal saline, lactated Ringers, D_5NS, and half normal saline for infusion.

53. **Correct answer: A**
Many foods should be avoided when taking warfarin. Those highest in vitamin K (the antagonist to warfarin) are broccoli, brussels sprouts, cabbage, spinach, turnip greens, endive, scallions, and parsley. Additional foods to be avoided are red leaf lettuce, watercress, oils such as soybean and canola, and salads in general. All these foods decrease the effectiveness of warfarin.

54. **Correct answer: B**
Abnormal Q waves on an EKG signify a complete thickness infarction of myocardium. When the tissue dies due to myocardial infarction, it becomes electrically dead, causing the opposing energy to become the dominant feature. Partial thickness myocardial death would be a non–Q wave MI.

55. **Correct answer: D**
The most common new-onset dysrhythmia seen in a patient with a diagnosis of pulmonary edema is atrial fibrillation. Atrial fibrillation is the result of the constant stretching and disruption of normal pathways in the atrium due to increased preload from the pulmonary congestion.

56. **Correct answer: B**
There are multiple reasons for pacemaker insertion, including symptomatic bradycardia, bradycardia with escape beats, overdrive pacing, bradycardia/arrest, and acute MI with sinus dysfunction. In addition, Mobitz type II, complete heart block, and development of a new bundle branch block are reasons for pacemaker insertion.

57. **Correct answer: A**
Right-sided congestive heart failure signs and symptoms include respiratory distress and hepatomegaly. The respiratory distress is the result of blood's failure to flow to the lungs, causing hypoxemia. As blood backs up into the hepatic system, hepatomegaly and splenomegaly may result.

58. **Correct answer: A**
Polycythemia increases afterload due to the excess circulation of red blood cells. Hypovolemia and sepsis decrease afterload, as does aortic insufficiency. Aortic stenosis increases afterload, as do peripheral vasoconstriction and hypertension.

59. **Correct answer: C**
Right ventricular afterload may be reduced by inhaled nitric oxide. Use of inhaled nitric oxide, nitroglycerin, nitroprusside, PGE_1, or hyperventilation reduce right

ventricular afterload. Epinephrine increases systemic afterload due to vasoconstriction and promotes increased PVR because of the increased left heart pressures. Hypoventilation and subsequent hypoxia also increase right heart afterload.

60. **Correct answer: B**
Early signs of left ventricular failure are tachypnea and tachycardia. Severe left ventricular failure also causes dyspnea.

61. **Correct answer: D**
The third heart sound, S_3, occurs when increased blood flow travels across the AV valves secondary to rapid passive ventricular filling from the atria. This is easy to remember if you associate the S_3 sound with fluid. It is prominent in CHF, mitral valve insufficiency, anemia, and left-to-right shunts like ASD and VSD.

62. **Correct answer: D**
Leads V_2–V_4 indicate damage to the anterior wall of the heart. Leads V_4 and R indicate right ventricular damage. V_5 and V_6 indicate apical injury. Leads V_7–V_9 are specific to the posterior wall.

63. **Correct answer: B**
The pulmonic valve is rarely affected by infective endocarditis. The mitral valve is the most common site affected by infective endocarditis. The aortic valve is the next most common valve affected. The tricuspid valve is often involved secondarily as a result of IV drug abuse.

64. **Correct answer: A**
Mr. C. has endocarditis. Janeway lesions are flat and painless erythematous areas found on palms and soles of the feet predominantly. Osler's nodes are small painful nodules also associated with endocarditis and found on fingers and toes. Roth spots are seen when examining the retina. They are rounded and white and associated with endocarditis. It is thought that microvascular clots form in the heart and pass through the microcirculation and impede peripheral circulation, sometimes causing necrosis. Pella's sign is not a medical term.

65. **Correct answer: B**
Patients receiving sodium nitroprusside should be monitored for cyanide toxicity, and use of sodium nitroprusside should be avoided in patients with renal problems. Cyanide toxicity may result in tachycardia and severe hypotension. Monitor venous O_2 concentration and acid-base balance. If nitroprusside extravasates from an IV, it will cause tissue sloughing and necrosis. The RBC cyanide level should be less than 50 mcg/ml.

66. **Correct answer: D**
The only definitive way to diagnose myocarditis is via an endomyocardial biopsy.

67. **Correct answer: C**
Myocarditis is clinically defined as inflammation of the myocardium. Coxsackie B_1 virus has been more prevalent as a frequent cause of myocarditis. Numerous infections, systemic diseases, drugs, and toxins are associated with the development of myocarditis. Viruses, bacteria, protozoa, and even worms have been implicated as infectious agents. The absolute band count is not sensitive enough to predict sepsis, but a ratio of immature-to-total polymorphonuclear leukocytes < 0.2 has a very high

negative predictive value. A rapid fall in a known absolute eosinophil count and morphologic changes in neutrophils may indicate sepsis.

68. **Correct answer: D**
Procainamide's adverse effects include severe hypotension (usually because of a rapid infusion) and AV block. Procainamide may also widen the QRS complex due to slow impulse conduction through the Purkinje fibers and ventricular myocardium. If the QRS widens more that 35–50%, the drug should be discontinued. Adverse effects usually disappear when the drug is discontinued. Two of the actions of procainamide are depression of the excitability of cardiac muscle and slowing the conduction in the atria.

69. **Correct answer: C**
When starting dopamine, it is important to ensure that hypovolemia has been treated appropriately. In septic shock, the patient may receive as many as 3 to 10 fluid boluses until pulmonary edema is noted or the boluses fail to impact blood pressure. Central venous access is the preferred route. If central access is unavailable, peripheral access is acceptable. However, the site must be monitored closely for infiltration and additional IV access points must be available. Phentolamine mesylate should be available in case infiltration does occur, but it is not the first action to be performed.

70. **Correct answer: A**
In patients receiving high-dose epinephrine, glucose levels should be monitored closely for potential hyperglycemia. There is an even greater risk for hyperglycemia if the patient is diabetic. Potassium, not calcium, chloride, or sodium, should also be monitored for potential hyperkalemia or hypokalemia.

71. **Correct answer: A**
The antagonist for morphine or other opioids is Narcan (naloxone). Generally, the naloxone dose is 0.4 mg IV. This dose can be repeated about every 3 to 4 minutes three times. When giving Narcan you must always be alert for the patient to relapse once the dose wears off. Administering multiple follow-up doses is not uncommon.

72. **Correct answer: A**
Isuprel (isoproterenol) is the better choice for vasoactive support for the asthmatic patient in decompensated shock. Isuprel is a catecholamine that causes smooth muscle relaxation, bronchodilation, and pulmonary vasodilation to decrease PVR and increase heart rate and contractility. Dopamine causes increased peripheral vasoconstriction to increase blood pressure but does not affect pulmonary blood flow. Vasopressin results in systemic vasoconstriction and acts on the renal tubules to increase water reabsorption. Neosynephrine causes arteriolar vasoconstriction resulting in greater PVR and more VQ shunting. There is also the possibility of the patient becoming hypoxemic.

73. **Correct answer: D**
Dopamine should not be titrated any faster than every 5 minutes because onset of action is 5 minutes and duration is 10 minutes. Titrating more frequently than every 5 minutes may result in greater hemodynamic instability and more difficulty in determining the effective dosage.

74. **Correct answer: C**

Discharge instructions for a patient prescribed amiodarone include avoiding grapefruit and grapefruit juice because they increase blood amiodarone levels. Outside activities should restrict contact sports and require use of sunscreen and clothing to protect the skin from exposure to sunlight. Amiodarone may impair liver function and lead to thrombocytopenia. Sunlight exposure may lead to a bluish gray cast to the skin. If the patient normally uses theophylline to treat asthma, the dosage may need to be decreased as amiodarone increases serum theophylline levels. However, in this case, nothing was mentioned about this patient having asthma. Dark urine, respiratory distress, and/or edema should be reported immediately to the physician as these are signs of renal and pulmonary impairment.

75. **Correct answer: D**

Patient confusion, listlessness, and headache should be reported to the ED physician immediately due to the potential for water intoxication. You would also expect to see a sudden weight gain, anuria, and hyponatremia. Monitor urine output closely as well as serum electrolytes. Abdominal cramps and nausea are expected side effects. This patient requires admission and further tests to determine the origin of the DI.

76. **Correct answer: B**

Victor has dilated cardiomyopathy that is causing systolic dysfunction. Patients with this type of cardiomyopathy will have S_3 and S_4 gallops, and the EKG may show atrial fibrillation, ventricular dysrhythmias, or a sinus tachycardia most of the time. The patient may have a systolic murmur of the AV valves. The patient will probably also have peripheral edema or ascites, hepatomegaly, and pale, cool extremities. It is possible to have changes in mentation. Hypertrophic and restrictive cardiomyopathies are diastolic dysfunctions.

77. **Correct answer: D**

Dobutamine improves cardiac output primarily by increasing cardiac contractility. Unlike dopamine, dobutamine does not increase heart rate and can be used in tachycardic patients.

78. **Correct answer: D**

Atropine administration may result in headaches, dizziness, and coma. You should also observe for urinary retention and hypotension and tachycardia due to blocking of parasympathetic receptor sites.

79. **Correct answer: B**

The ED nurse should monitor closely the urine output and liver function tests of a patient receiving a loading dose of amiodarone. The high concentration of amiodarone may cause renal necrosis and impaired output leading to vascular congestion and respiratory distress. Amiodarone has been linked to hepatocellular damage and impaired liver function. Other side effects include anemia, neutropenia, pancytopenia, and thrombocytopenia. Thyroid levels should also be monitored because amiodarone may cause hypo- or hyperthyroidism. Amiodarone has been linked to bluish gray pigmentation in long-term patients exposed to sunlight.

80. **Correct answer: A**

    Motion of cardiac valves and detection of pericardial fluid is done with M-mode echocardiography. M-mode echocardiography enables evaluation of anatomic relationships and the relative sizes of each.

81. **Correct answer: A**

    Patients taking both diazoxide and furosemide should have their glucose levels monitored closely for possible hyperglycemia. Diazoxide inhibits pancreatic release of insulin and stimulates the liver to release glucose.

82. **Correct answer: B**

    The high-contrast mediums used in cardiac catheterizations also have high sodium content.

83. **Correct answer: B**

    The classic description of an X-ray showing a pericardial effusion is the "water bottle" silhouette. In patients with a pericardial effusion, QRS amplitude is decreased. Diastolic filling is decreased as well.

84. **Correct answer: B**

    The type of echocardiography that shows the quantity of flow across an obstruction is known as continuous-wave Doppler echocardiography. This type of echocardiography is used to detect direction of shunting, estimating cardiac output, and assessing ventricular diastolic function. This type of echocardiography provides a good estimate of pressure gradients.

85. **Correct answer: A**

    Dong quai, gingko biloba, and ginseng can increase bleeding times. Saw palmetto decreases the effectiveness of Plavix.

86. **Correct answer: A**

    Norepinephrine bitartrate (Levophed) infusions require blood pressure monitoring at least every 5 minutes. Direct arterial monitoring is preferred for more accurate evaluation. The solution should be clear without particulates and mixed in D_5W, D_5W with normal saline, or normal saline and covered from direct light. Levophed may be infused with dopamine, but monitor peripheral circulation closely due to severe vasoconstriction and possible extravasation.

87. **Correct answer: D**

    Cardiac glycosides possess positive inotropic activity, which is mediated by inhibition of sodium-potassium adenosine triphosphatase. Also, cardiac glycosides reduce conductivity in the heart, particularly through the atrioventricular node, and therefore have a negative chronotropic effect. The cardiac glycosides have very similar pharmacologic effects but differ considerably in their speed of onset and duration of action. They are used to slow the heart rate in supraventricular arrhythmias, especially atrial fibrillation, and also are used in patients with chronic heart failure.

88. **Correct answer: B**

    The high iodine content of amiodarone can actually exert an effect on the thyroid and thus produce an antiarrhythmic action. It is always a good idea to ask if the patient has an allergy or sensitivity to iodine prior to administering this medication.

89. **Correct answer: C**

    Dobutamine is used to improve cardiac output by acting on beta$_1$ adrenergic receptors in the heart. It may cause minimal peripheral vasodilation but primarily acts to increase contractility, coronary blood flow, and heart rate to improve cardiac output. Dopamine acts on alpha-adrenergic receptors in the heart. Norepinephrine is a catecholamine that acts on both alpha- and beta-adrenergic receptors in the cardiovascular tissue.

90. **Correct answer: B**

    Alpha-adrenergic effects of norepinephrine include peripheral arteriolar vasoconstriction. Increased force of myocardial contraction and increased AV conduction time are the effects of beta-adrenergic sympathetic stimulation.

91. **Correct answer: B**

    By definition, pansystolic means the murmur is heard throughout systole. The only systolic murmur listed is tricuspid insufficiency. All the others are diastolic murmurs.

92. **Correct answer: B**

    A reflex tachycardia caused by stretch of right atrial receptors is known as the Bainbridge reflex. It is believed that the Bainbridge reflex exists to speed up the heart rate if the right side becomes overloaded and helps equalize pressures in both sides.

93. **Correct answer: A**

    On a pulmonary catheter tracing, large A waves may be seen with increased pressure during atrial contraction. This could be caused by mitral stenosis, an ischemic left ventricle, or failure of a left ventricle.

94. **Correct answer: A**

    Nifedipine is a calcium channel blocker.

95. **Correct answer: D**

    Adenosine is used for the suppression/elimination of sustained supraventricular tachycardia. It can also be used in diagnostic studies to establish the cause of the SVT. Adverse effects may include transient arrhythmias, flushing, dyspnea, and, rarely, apnea. It is important to note that in approximately 30% of patients, SVT recurs. Caffeine and theophylline act by competitive antagonism to diminish the effect of adenosine.

96. **Correct answer: D**

    The left ventricular assist device (LVAD) is the most commonly used because left heart failure is more common and usually precedes right ventricular failure.

97. **Correct answer: B**

    Ventricular assist devices (VAD) are used as destination therapy as well as a bridge to transplant. Prolonged cardiac arrest, especially with neurologic damage, is a contraindication to use of a VAD. Extensive organ damage is another contraindication. VADs are not indicated for dysrhythmias. Other indications for a VAD include cardiogenic shock and inability to wean from cardiopulmonary bypass. Always be aware of the possibility of device failure.

98. **Correct answer: C**

    It is important that adenosine be given rapidly because if adenosine is given slowly, it may cause systemic vasodilation and reflex tachycardia, further compromising cardiac output. Blurred vision is an expected adverse reaction. The patient should be monitored for development of atrial fibrillation, bradycardia, and heart blocks. Withhold adenosine if the patient is in atrial fibrillation, atrial flutter, and second-degree type II or complete heart block. Adenosine slows conduction via the AV node, and these rhythms may degrade to ventricular fibrillation.

99. **Correct answer: D**
The fourth heart sound, S_4, is always pathologic after the first 24 hours of life and indicates a decreased ventricular compliance. The S_4 is produced when an atrial contraction fills up the ventricle. S_4 is rarely heard in the newborn and occurs just before the S_1 heart sound. During the first 24 hours of life the S_4 may be heard just after the first heart sound and sounds like a clicking noise.

100. **Correct answer: D**
A heart murmur associated with acute valvular regurgitation is called S_4. S_1 and S_2 are normal sounds. S_3 is associated with fluid status. S_4 is associated with ventricular compliance.

101. **Correct answer: B**
Radiofrequency waves destroy myocardial tissue with heat. These waves actually heat the tissue around the active sites and prevent reentry looping. Once the temperature reaches 50°C, cell damage and death occur. The continuing heat creates a lesion about 2–5 mm in diameter. This "burned" area causes necrosis and will not conduct electricity.

102. **Correct answer: A**
It is important to explain that Parker needs a pacemaker or AICD that can deliver a more powerful impulse when needed (demand). The asynchronous mode will override Parker's internal pacemaker.

103. **Correct answer: A**
Randall has probably dislodged a lead or the lead was damaged on insertion. Either way, Randall needs a new AICD or new leads.

104. **Correct answer: D**
A dual-lead pacemaker/AICD is necessary to maintain the atrial kick. Single chamber pacing can lead to pacemaker syndrome. The letters on pacemaker modes are as follows:

Chamber Paced	Chamber Sensed	Mode of Response	Programmability, Rate modulation	Anti-Tachyarrhythmia Function
V = Ventricle	V = Ventricle	I = Inhibit	P = Simple programmable	P = Pacing
A = Atrium	A = Atrium	T = Triggered	M = Multiprogrammable	S = Shock
D = Dual chamber	D = Dual chamber	D = Dual (T & I)	R = Rate modulation	Dual = Dual (P & S)

105. **Correct answer: A**
Pacemaker syndrome is due to a loss of atrial kick or regurgitation against a closed AV valve. Fatigue, agitation, and forgetfulness are primary symptoms of this condition. It would be possible Bart's atrial lead was damaged or has failed.

106. **Correct answer: C**

    Pneumonia secondary to immobility is the primary reason for infection with VADs. Some type of ventilatory support may also be needed. Just the fact that tubes are placed into the body is a potential source of infection, but this is usually minimized by good handwashing and aseptic technique.

107. **Correct answer: C**

    Patients who have aortic insufficiency often exhibit Quincke's sign. This sign is elicited by pressing upward from underneath the nail bed on the fingertip. A visible pulsation is seen in the nail bed. This results from a pulse with a rapid initial hard pulsation followed by a sudden collapse as blood flows back through an incompetent valve.

108. **Correct answer: C**

    In a patient with a cardiac tamponade, stroke volume decreases. Because the heart cannot adequately fill or eject its contents adequately, stroke volume decreases and causes a decreased cardiac output. Contractility decreases because the muscle cannot adequately stretch and therefore contract effectively.

109. **Correct answer: D**

    Beck's triad consists of distended neck veins, muffled heart sounds, and hypotension. In tamponade, tachycardia is an early sign. A narrowed pulse pressure occurs; fluid cannot be ejected from the heart. The muffled heart sounds occur because the fluid in the sac minimizes the transmission of sound waves.

110. **Correct answer: C**

    Stroke volume is comprised of contractility, preload, and afterload. Viscosity, blood volume, and impedance represent the components of afterload. Myocardium is sensitive to changes, especially increased afterload. With only minute changes in afterload, the stroke volume can fall significantly.

111. **Correct answer: D**

    During CVP pressure monitoring, the c wave represents the increase in RA pressure from closure of the tricuspid valve.

112. **Correct answer: B**

    A low CVP reading may represent increased contractility or hypovolemia. A high reading may indicate LV, RV or biventricular failure, tricuspid regurgitation or stenosis, hypertension, hypervolemia, or cardiac tamponade.

113. **Correct answer: A**

    New-onset atrial fibrillation frequently develops as a sequela to pulmonary edema.

114. **Correct answer: B**

    Phentolamine (Regitine) 1 mg/ml solution should be injected into the affected area if dopamine infiltrates. It may take as much as 5 ml to treat the area.

115. **Correct answer: A**

    A dilated superior vena cava would appear on X-ray if a patient had a cardiac tamponade. The vena cava is dilated because blood cannot empty into the right atrium. The mediastinum would be widened. A CXR will not show delineation of the pericardium or epicardium. A pneumothorax may exist but would not be an expected finding on X-ray.

Cardiovascular | 47

116. **Correct answer: C**

Phasic variations in an arterial pressure waveform during mechanical ventilation usually indicate hypovolemia or heart failure.

117. **Correct answer: B**

In any patient with cardiogenic shock, an undesirable outcome produces increased systemic vascular resistance. A primary goal in cardiogenic shock is to improve the pumping action of the heart (improve myocardial contractility), reduce the workload (decrease SVR) and oxygen demand, and improve cardiac output. If possible, systemic vascular resistance should be decreased and the left ventricle augmented with an inotrope. Nitroprusside reduces preload and afterload. The cardiac workload is decreased as is the myocardial oxygen demand.

118. **Correct answer: B**

Early signs of left ventricular failure are tachypnea and tachycardia. Severe left ventricular failure also causes dyspnea and retractions (seen in infants predominately).

119. **Correct answer: B**

A popliteal blood pressure at least 20 mmHg higher than a brachial blood pressure is known as Hill's sign. Hill's sign reflects the rapid rise in pulsation found in patients with aortic insufficiency. DeMusset's sign is also found in aortic insufficiency (the bobbing of the head in time with the forceful pulse).

120. **Correct answer: A**

Hydralazine is incompatible with furosemide, phenobarbital, aminophylline, and ampicillin. Hydralazine is compatible with heparin, dobutamine, hydrocortisone, potassium chloride, prostaglandin E_1, and Dex/AA.

121. **Correct answer: B**

Ginger is probably suffering from pericarditis. The CXR will probably show a pericardial effusion. The elevated sed. rate and WBCs indicate infection. In pericarditis, leaning forward often relieves chest pain and lying supine makes it worse. If the pain worsens on inspiration, it is because the lungs expand and come in contact with the pericardium. The patient will probably also have a fever. One of the things to monitor is any sign of a cardiac tamponade and to make certain anticoagulants are discontinued.

122. **Correct answer: C**

Mike is developing cardiogenic shock. When the left ventricle fails, fluid backs up into the pulmonary vasculature. Because the wedge pressure is high, it means the fluid is already backed up in the left heart. The PAP and RAP are high, indicating pulmonary congestion. Cardiac output and cardiac index are low, and BP is not being maintained.

123. **Correct answer: C**

Chris is in the first stage of cardiogenic shock secondary to systolic dysfunction. The injuries to the chest may have caused a pulmonary artery laceration or a cardiac contusion, which is more likely. His blood pressure is low, and the EKG shows ST segment elevation in the anterior leads. If the myocardium is contused, it will react the same way as if an MI had occurred. The ST elevation may be the result of a physiologic insult to a coronary artery and an area of the myocardium is ischemic. The pumping function of the myocardium is compromised and may need additional support with inotropes and possibly an intra-aortic balloon pump (IABP). Chris may undergo angiography and/or surgery. Volume replacement will be necessary.

124. **Correct answer: B**
    Dobutamine is not compatible with either sodium bicarbonate or ampicillin, so the nurse cannot infuse the medications together. The appropriate choice is to start another peripheral line to administer sodium bicarbonate while waiting for the ampicillin to arrive from pharmacy. If the patient remains hemodynamically unstable and unable to obtain or maintain peripheral venous access, then it is appropriate to speak with the physician regarding more stable access such as a central line or a PICC line.

125. **Correct answer: B**
    Mario's blood pressure, PAS/PAD pressures, and RAP are low. The cardiac output and cardiac index are low, and the heart rate and respiratory rate are low. Mario's mentation is diminished. The values indicate hypovolemic shock.

126. **Correct answer: D**
    Snyder has increased exercise intolerance, edema, dyspnea, and increased PAP and wedge pressures. The RAP is normal. These are all signs of left ventricular failure.

127. **Correct answer: C**
    Magda's problem is in the right ventricle. An expected diagnosis for Magda is an RV infarction. The PAP and wedge pressures are normal. The RAP is high and there is some jugular distension. This indicates a problem with the right ventricle—it cannot pump effectively. The lungs do not seem to be the problem because the pulmonary artery pressures are normal. The lethargy may be unrelated and needs to be evaluated because it is a significant change for this patient.

128. **Correct answer: C**
    Lars is probably suffering from biventricular failure. All the pulmonary pressures are elevated. The heart cannot pump the fluid out and the lungs are congested (dyspnea). Edema is a sign of pump failure. The patient will probably develop ascites and hepatomegaly.

129. **Correct answer: A**
    The purpose of treating a patient who has CHF with vasoactive and inotropic medications is to decrease the workload of the heart by vasodilation (reduce preload and afterload) and improve contractility. These medications will decrease preload and afterload and increase contractility.

130. **Correct answer: D**
    Your first priority is to defibrillate the patient with 200 Joules with a biphasic defibrillator or 360 Joules with a monophasic defibrillator.

131. **Correct answer: B**
    Digoxin is classified as both a negative chronotrope and a positive inotrope.

132. **Correct answer: C**
    The pacemaker is not sensing. The first thing the nurse should do is increase the milliamperes. The nurse should also check the pacemaker connections and try turning the patient on the side if tolerated.

133. **Correct answer: B**

    Type I aneurysms are the most common type of aortic aneurysms. Tears begin in the ascending aorta, and the dissection extends beyond the aortic arch.

134. **Correct answer: D**

    A type III aneurysm involves a tear in the descending aorta, with distal dissection only. They are not the rarest form of aneurysm, occurring in 20–30% of cases.

135. **Correct answer: C**

    A risk factor for an aortic aneurysm would not include hypotension. Risk factors include connective tissue disorders, medial necrosis of the aorta, coarctation of the aorta, blunt chest trauma, pregnancy, family history of aortic aneurysm, and hypertension.

136. **Correct answer: C**

    The most probable cause of this patient's cardiovascular collapse is a saddle embolus. A saddle embolus is found at the bifurcation of the pulmonary artery. Prior to the patient receiving the vasodilator, the pulmonary artery was kept open by the high right-sided pressures seen with the hypertensive crisis. The decreased pressures as a result of the actions of the vasodilator allowed the embolus to migrate and obstruct the pulmonary artery.

137. **Correct answer: C**

    Administering fluids will improve contractility. Ideally, if the PAOP pressure was kept about 18–19 mmHg, contractility will improve without an increase in SVR.

138. **Correct answer: B**

    The disparity of the upper extremity blood pressures and pulses, plus the weaker lower extremity pulses, is a classic presentation for a ruptured aorta. If the patient had a ruptured abdominal aortic aneurysm, the upper extremity pulses would not differ from each other.

139. **Correct answer: B**

    This patient most likely has an abdominal aortic aneurysm that could dissect at any moment. Make the patient comfortable with a minimum of movement and inform the physician immediately.

140. **Correct answer: C**

    Patients taking colchicine should not eat grapefruit or drink grapefruit juice.

141. **Correct answer: D**

    If a patient becomes tachycardic, the QT and the RR intervals shorten.

142. **Correct answer: A**

    If your patient is experiencing cannon "a" waves, this phenomenon is due to a powerful atrial wave in the jugular venous pulse caused by the contraction of the right atrium against a closed (stenosed) tricuspid valve. The ears may actually "flap" because the wave is so powerful. A less powerful wave may occur secondary to pulmonary hypertension.

143. **Correct answer: B**

    The right ventricle infarction is often seen in the patient with an inferior wall MI and ST elevation in leads V_1 and V_2. A right-side 12-lead EKG should be done to verify the right ventricular infarction.

144. **Correct answer: C**

Under the new 2010 American Heart Association Guidelines for CPR and Emergency Cardiovascular Care guidelines for chest compressions, the rescuer should compress the sternum of an adult to a depth of 2 inches (5 cm).

145. **Correct answer: B**

The sequence for adults receiving basic life support is CAB. The 2010 American Heart Association Guidelines for CPR and Emergency Cardiovascular Care have changed the BLS sequence to compressions, airway, and breathing.

146. **Correct answer: A**

The 2010 American Heart Association Guidelines for CPR and Emergency Cardiovascular Care do not recommend routine use of cricoid pressure during cardiac arrest. There is some evidence that the use of cricoid pressure impedes the airway when performed incorrectly.

147. **Correct answer: D**

Continuous wave capnography is the most reliable method of confirming and monitoring correct placement of an ETT. Capnography can monitor the effectiveness of chest compressions and detect the return of spontaneous circulation. Use of capnography is a recommendation of the 2010 American Heart Association Guidelines for CPR and Emergency Cardiovascular Care.

148. **Correct answer: D**

According to the 2010 American Heart Association Guidelines for CPR and Emergency Cardiovascular Care, high-quality CPR is the single most important component of a successful outcome for a patient requiring advanced cardiac life support.

149. **Correct answer: C**

According to the 2010 American Heart Association Guidelines for CPR and Emergency Cardiovascular Care, atropine is no longer recommended for routine use in the management of PEA or asystole.

150. **Correct answer: C**

If an adult post–cardiac arrest patient is treated with therapeutic hypothermia, the patient should be evaluated via neurologic signs, biomarkers, electrophysiologic studies, and imaging where available at 72 hours (3 days) after cardiac arrest.

151. **Correct answer: A**

There is no evidence that water acts as an obstructive foreign body, so no maneuvers are needed to remove a foreign body. Victims should be pulled from the water prior to initiating CPR, and spinal injuries are rare among fatal drowning victims.

152. **Correct answer: B**

STEMI and NSTEMI are both myocardial infarctions. The essential fact is that the NSTEMI does not have ST elevation on the EKG tracing and is identified by the cardiac enzymes. The STEMI diagnosis is based on symptoms, clinical examination, and the EKG tracing. Treatment is not delayed for the patient presenting with STEMI.

153. **Correct answer: C**

Because the patient's symptoms have lasted more than 30 minutes, the best option for him is percutaneous coronary intervention (PCI). The PCI should not be delayed for cardiac enzyme results because the ST elevation on his EKG is sufficient evidence of an MI.

154. **Correct answer: B**
A 1-mm ST elevation, with or without a pathologic Q wave, is diagnostic for STEMI. A large R wave in lead V_1 or V_2 may indicate a posterior wall MI. An NSTEMI has no ST elevation and must have cardiac enzymes for diagnosis.

155. **Correct answer: C**
The right-side 12-lead EKG looks at the right ventricle and the posterior heart. Some facilities have the capability of performing 16-lead EKGs, which look at the entire heart without having to move the precordial leads. This complete view of the heart's vasculature status allows for pinpointing the site of the myocardial infarction.

SECTION 3: CARDIOVASCULAR REFERENCES

Abul, Y., Karakurt, S., Ozben, B., Toprak, A., & Celikel, T. (2011). C-reactive protein in acute pulmonary embolism. *Journal of Investigative Medicine, 59*(1), 8–14.

Allocca, G., Slavich, G., Nucifora, G., Slavich, M., Frassani, R., Crapis, M., & Badano, L. (2007). Successful treatment of polymicrobial multivalve infective endocarditis: Multivalve infective endocarditis. *International Journal of Cardiovascular Imaging, 23*(4), 501.

American Association of Critical Care Nurses. (2009). Pulmonary artery pressure monitoring: AACN practice alert. Retrieved November, 2, 2010, from http://www.aacn.org

American Heart Association. (2010). *Congenital cardiovascular defects: Statistics.* Retrieved September 12, 2010, from http://www.americanheart.org/presenter.jhtml?identifier=4576

Anonymous. (2002). Exercise-induced bidirectional ventricular tachycardia with alternating right and left bundle branch block-type patterns: A case report. *Angiology, 53*(5), 593–598.

Anonymous. (2005). Magnesium deficiency in critical illness. *Journal of Intensive Care Medicine, 20*(1), 3–17.

Anonymous. (2008). Medication-related complications in the trauma patient. *Journal of Intensive Care Medicine, 23*(2), 91–108.

Anonymous. (2010). Poisoning severity score, Glasgow coma scale, corrected QT interval in acute organophosphate poisoning. *Human & Experimental Toxicology, 29*(5), 419–425.

Aronow, W. S. (2010). Implantable cardioverter-defibrillators. *American Journal of Therapeutics, 17*(6), e208–e220.

Ashworth, S. W., Levsky, M. E., Marley, C. T., & Kang, C. S. (2005). Bradycardia-associated torsade de pointes and the long-QT syndromes: A case report and review of the literature. *Military Medicine, 170*(5), 381–386.

Barone, J. A., and Peppers, M. P. (1989). Therapeutic drug monitoring in emergency room toxicology settings. *Journal of Pharmacy Practice, 2*(6), 347–356.

Barrett, M. J., Lacey, C. S., Sekara, A. E., Linden, E. A., & Gracely, E. J. (2004). Mastering cardiac murmurs: The power of repetition. *Chest, 126*(2), 470–475.

Baur, L. H. B. (2008). Three dimensional echocardiography: A valuable tool to assess left atrial function in non-compaction cardiomyopathy! *International Journal of Cardiovascular Imaging, 24*(3), 243.

Berg, R. A, Hemphill, R., Abella, B. S., Aufderheide, T. P., Cave, D. M., Hazinski, M. F., . . . Swor, R. A. (2010). Part 5: Adult basic life support: 2010 American Heart Association guidelines for cardiopulmonary resuscitation and emergency cardiovascular care. *Circulation, 122*(suppl 3), S685–S705.

Bradbury-Golas, K., Campo, T. M., & Chiccarine, A. (2010). Getting to the heart of back and shoulder pain. *Advanced Emergency Nursing Journal, 32*(2), 127–136.

Bucaretchi, F., de Capitani, E. M., Hyslop, S., Mello, S. M., Madureira, P. R., Zanardi, V., . . . Fernandes, L. C. (2010). Compartment syndrome after Bothrops jararaca snakebite: Monitoring, treatment, and outcome. *Clinical Toxicology, 48*(1), 57–60.

Burgdorf, C., Nef, H. M., Haghi, D., Kurowski, V., & Radke, P. W. (2010). Tako-tsubo (stress-induced) cardiomyopathy and cancer. *Annals of Internal Medicine, 152*(12), 830–831.

Caforio, A. L. P, Daliento, L., Angelini, A., Bottaro, S., Vinci, A., Dequal, G., . . . McKenna, W. J. (2005). Autoimmune myocarditis and dilated cardiomyopathy: Focus on cardiac autoantibodies. *Lupus, 14*(9), 652–655.

Calkins, H., Reynolds, M. R., Spector, P., Sondhi, M., Xu, Y., Martin, A., . . . Sledge, I. (2009). Treatment of atrial fibrillation with antiarrhythmic drugs or radiofrequency ablation: Two systematic literature reviews and meta-analyses. *Circulation: Arrhythmia and Electrophysiology, 2*(4), 349–361.

Carabello, B., & Paulus, W. (2009). Aortic stenosis. *Lancet, 373*(9667), 956–966.

Chen, C. Y., Wang, F. L., & Lin, C. C. (2006). Chronic hydroxychloroquine use associated with QT prolongation and refractory ventricular arrhythmia. *Clinical Toxicology, 44*(2), 173.

Chernecky, C., & Berger, B. (2004). *Laboratory tests and diagnostic procedures* (4th ed.). Philadelphia: Saunders.

Choo, E. K., Weber, F. S., & Schmidt, T. A. (2009). Torsade de pointes after administration of droperidol for nausea and vomiting. *Prehospital Emergency Care, 13*(2), 261–265.

Craig, K. J. (2010). Symptomatic bradycardia. *Nursing, 40*(12), 72.

Crandall, M. A., Bradley, D. J., Packer, D. L., & Asirvatham, S. J. (2009). Contemporary management of atrial fibrillation: Update on anticoagulation and invasive management strategies. *Mayo Clinic Proceedings, 84*(7), 643–662.

D'Andrea, A., Salerno, G., Scarafile, R., Riegler, L., Gravino, R., Castaldo, F., . . . Calabro, R. (2009). Right ventricular myocardial function in patients with either idiopathic or ischemic dilated cardiomyopathy without clinical sign of right heart failure: Effects of cardiac resynchronization therapy. *Pacing and Clinical Electrophysiology, 32*(8), 1017–1029.

Darovic, G. O. (2002). *Hemodynamic monitoring: Invasive and noninvasive clinical application* (3rd ed.). Philadelphia: Saunders.

Dehnert, C., & Bartsch, P. (2010). Can patients with coronary heart disease go to high altitude? *High Altitude Medicine & Biology, 11*(3), 183.

DeMaria, S., & Weinkauf, J. L. (2011). Cocaine and the club drugs. *International Anesthesiology Clinics, 49*(1), 79–101.

den Uil, C. A., Lagrand, W. K., Valk, S. D., Spronk, P. E., & Simoons, M. L. (2009). Management of cardiogenic shock: Focus on tissue perfusion. *Current Problems in Cardiology, 34*(8), 330–349.

Douglas, R. J., & Cadogan, M. (2008). Cardiac arrhythmia during propofol sedation. *Emergency Medicine Australasia, 20*(5), 437–440.

Emergency Nurses Association, Newberry, L., & Criddle, L. M. (2005). *Sheehy's manual of emergency care* (6th ed.). St. Louis, MO: Mosby.

Farooq, M. U., Bhatt, A., & Patel, M. (2009). Neurotoxic and cardiotoxic effects of cocaine and ethanol. *Journal of Medical Toxicology, 5*(3), 134–138.

Gandhi, S. K., Powers, J. C., Nomeir, A. M., Fowle, K., Kitzman, D. W., Rankin, K. M., & Little, W. C. (2001). The pathogenesis of acute pulmonary edema associated with hypertension. *New England Journal of Medicine, 344*(1), 17–22.

Gasparis Vonfrolio, L., & Noone, J. (1997). *Emergency nursing examination review* (3rd ed.). Staten Island, NY: Power Publications.

George, A., & Figueredo, V. M. (2010). Alcohol and arrhythmias: A comprehensive review. *Journal of Cardiovascular Medicine, 11*(4), 221–228.

Goldhaber, J. I., & Hamilton, M. A. (2010). Role of inotropic agents in the treatment of heart failure. *Circulation, 121*(4), 1655–1660.

Hakuno, D., Kimura, N., Yoshioka, M., & Fukuda, K. (2009). Molecular mechanisms underlying the onset of degenerative aortic valve disease. *Journal of Molecular Medicine, 87*(1), 17–24.

Hardin, S. R., & Kaplow, R. (Eds.). (2010). *Cardiac surgery essentials for critical care nursing*. Sudbury, MA: Jones & Bartlett Learning.

Hartog, C. S., Bauer, M., & Reinhart, K. (2011). The efficacy and safety of colloid resuscitation in the critically ill. *Anesthesia & Analgesia, 112*(1), 156–164.

Hill, E. E., Vanderschueren, S., Verhaegen, J., Herjgers, P., Claus, P., Herregods, M. C., & Peetermans, W. E. (2007). Risk factors for infective endocarditis and outcome of patients with *Staphylococcus aureus* bacteremia. *Mayo Clinic Proceedings, 82*(10), 1165.

Ho, J. K., & Mahajan, A. (2010). Cardiac resynchronization therapy for treatment of heart failure. *Anesthesia & Analgesia, 111*(6), 1353–1361.

Holleran, R. S. (2005). *Emergency transport nursing* (4th ed.). St. Louis, MO: Mosby.

Jacobs, B. B., & Hoyt, K. S. (2007). *Trauma nursing core course provider manual* (6th ed.). Bedford, IL: Emergency Nurses Association.

Jeger, R. V., Radovanovic, D., Hunziker, P. R., Pfisterer, M. E., Stauffer, J. C., Erne, P., & Urban, P. (2008). Ten-year trends in the incidence and treatment of cardiogenic shock. *Annals of Internal Medicine, 149*(9), 618–626.

Joglekar, S. B., & Rehman, S. (2009). Delayed onset thigh compartment syndrome secondary to contusion. *Orthopedics, 32*(8), 624–709.

Jones & Bartlett Learning (2011). *2011 nurse's drug handbook* (10th ed.). Sudbury, MA: Jones & Bartlett Learning.

Josephson, L. (2010). Hypertrophies and intraventricular conduction defects: Causes, presentation, and significance. *Dimensions of Critical Care Nursing, 29*(6), 259–275.

Karthikesalingam, A., Holt, P. J., Hinchliffe, R. J., Thompson, M. M., & Loftus, I. M. (2010). The diagnosis and management of aortic dissection. *Vascular and Endovascular Surgery, 44*(3), 165–169.

Kaul, P., Chang, W. C., Westerhout, C. M., Graham, M. M., & Armstrong, P. W. (2007). Differences in admission rates and outcomes between men and women presenting to emergency departments with coronary syndromes. *Canadian Medical Association Journal, 177*(10), 1193–1199.

Kawasaki, T., Akakabe, Y., Yamano, M., Miki, S., Kamitani, T., Kuribayashi, T., & Sugihara, H. (2008). R-wave amplitude response to myocardial ischemia in hypertrophic cardiomyopathy. *Journal of Electrocardiology, 41*(1), 68.

Keehn, S., Weinstein, L., Levy, D., & Zimmerman, S. (2010). Back pain that takes your breath away. *Emergency Medicine News, 32*(4), 4.

Kelly, N. F. A., Walters, D. L., Hourigan, L. A., Burstow, D. J., & Scalia, G. M. (2010). The relative atrial index (RAI): A novel, simple, reliable, and robust transthoracic echocardiographic indicator of atrial defects. *Journal of the American Society of Echocardiography, 23*(3), 275–281.

Kessenich, C. R. (2011). BNP and heart failure: What is the connection? *Nurse Practitioner, 36*(1), 13–14.

Kirkpatrick, A.W., Ball, C. G., Nickerson, D., & D'Amours, S. K. (2009). Intraabdominal hypertension and the abdominal compartment syndrome in burn patients. *World Journal of Surgery, 33*(6), 1142–1149.

Kline, C. M. (2010). Focus: The deceptively complex rib cage, part I. *Journal of the American Chiropractic Association, 47*(2), 2–5.

Kumar, A., & Cannon, C. P. (2009). Acute coronary syndromes: diagnosis and management, part I: Mayo clinic proceedings. *Mayo Clinic, 84*(10), 917–938.

Kuppasani, K., & Reddi, A. S. (2010). Emergency or urgency? Effective management of hypertensive crises. *Journal of the American Academy of Physician Assistants, 23*(8), 44.

Lemon, S. J., Winstead, P. S., & Weant, K. A. (2010). Alcohol withdrawal syndrome. *Advanced Emergency Nursing Journal, 32*(1), 20–27.

Lin, C. C., Hsiang, J. T., Wu, C-Y., Oyang, Y-J., Juan, H-F., & Huang, H-C. (2010). Dynamic functional modules in co-expressed protein interaction networks of dilated cardiomyopathy. *BMC Systems Biology, 4*, 138.

Lippincott. (2010). *Professional guide to signs and symptoms* (6th ed.). Philadelphia, PA: Lippincott.

MacDonald, R. D., & Farquhar, S. (2005). Case conferences. Transfer of intra-aortic balloon pump-dependent patients by paramedics. *Prehospital Emergency Care, 9*(4), 449–453.

Madershahian, N., Liakopoulos, O. J., Wippermann, J., Salehi-Gilani, S., Wittwer, T., Choi, Y. H., . . . Wahlers, T. (2009). The impact of intraaortic balloon counterpulsation on bypass graft flow in patients with peripheral ECMO. *Journal of Cardiac Surgery, 24*(3), 265–268.

Martin, B. (2010). Family presence during resuscitation and invasive procedures: AACN practice alert. Retrieved from http://www.aacn.org

McCalmont, V., & Ohler, L. (2008). Cardiac transplantation: Candidate identification, evaluation, and management. *Critical Care Nursing Quarterly, 31*(3), 216–231.

Menon, T., Nandhakumar, B., Jaganathan, V., Shanmugasundaram, S., Malathy, B., & Nisha, B. (2008). Bacterial endocarditis due to group C streptococcus. *Journal of Postgraduate Medicine, 54*(1), 64.

Morrison, L. J., Deakin, C. D., Morley, P. T., Callaway, C. W., Kerber, R. E., Kronick, S. L., . . . Nolan, J. P. (2010). Advanced life support: 2010 international consensus on cardiopulmonary resuscitation and emergency cardiovascular care services with treatment recommendations. *Circulation, 122*(suppl 2), S345–S421.

Namasivayam, M., Adji, A., & O'Rourke, M. F. (2011). Influence of aortic pressure wave components determined noninvasively on myocardial oxygen demand in men and women. *Hypertension, 57*(2), 193–200.

Noheria, A., Anderson, P. W., Tapia-Zegarra, G. G., Baddour, L. M., & Wilson, W. R. (2010). Infective endocarditis due to Neisseria elongata. *Infectious Diseases in Clinical Practice, 18*(6), 355–358.

NoorZurani, M. H., Vicknasingam, B., & Narayanan, S. (2009). Itraconazole-induced torsade de pointes in a patient receiving methadone substitution therapy. *Drug and Alcohol Review, 28*(6), 688–690.

O'Shea, L. (2010). Differential diagnosis of chest pain. *Practice Nurse, 40*(6), 13.

Peel, D. A. (2007). Endocarditis due to a nutritionally variant *Streptococcus*: A lesson in recognition and isolation. *British Journal of Biomedical Science, 64*(4), 175.

Prescribing reference. (2009). *NPPR: Nurse practitioner's prescribing reference, 16*(2). Sanofi Aventis.

Proehl, J. A. (2008). *Emergency nursing procedures* (4th ed.). St. Louis, MO: Saunders.

Pyxaras, S. A., Lardieri, G., Milo, M., Vitrella, G., & Sinagra, G. (2010). Chest pain and ST elevation: Not always ST-segment-elevation myocardial infarction. *Journal of Cardiovascular Medicine, 11*(8), 615–618.

Qing-kun, F., Wen-wu, W., Zhen-lu, Z., Ze-jin, L., Jun, Y., Geng-sheng, Z., & Shu-zheng, C. (2010). Evaluation of D-dimer in the diagnosis of suspected aortic dissection. *Clinical Chemistry and Laboratory Medicine, 48*(12), 1733.

Radenkovic, D.V., Bajec, D., Ivancevic, N., Bumbasirevic, V., Milic, N., Jeremic, V., . . . Cijan, V. (2010). Decompressive laparotomy with temporary abdominal closure versus percutaneous puncture with placement of abdominal catheter in patients with abdominal compartment syndrome during acute pancreatitis: Background and design of multicenter, randomised, controlled study. *BMC Surgery, 10,* 22.

Reichlin, T., Hochholzer, W., Bassetti, S., Steuer, S., Stelzig, C., Hartwiger, S., . . . Mueller, C. (2009). Early diagnosis of myocardial infarction with sensitive cardiac troponin assays. *New England Journal of Medicine, 361*(9), 858–867.

Romp, R. L., & Lau, Y. R. (2010). Congenital heart disease. In R. E. Rakel & E. T. Bope (Eds.), *Conn's current therapy 2010* (pp. 337–342). Philadelphia: Saunders Elsevier.

Sen, B., McNab, A., & Burdess, C. (2009). Identifying and managing patients with acute coronary conditions. *Emergency Nurse, 17*(7), 18–23.

Shaikh, N. (2010). An obstetric emergency called peripartum cardiomyopathy! *Journal of Emergencies, Trauma and Shock, 3*(1), 39–42.

Singh, A., Khaja, A., & Alpert, M. A. (2010). Cocaine and aortic dissection. *Vascular Medicine, 15*(2), 127–133.

Stieb, D. M., Szyszkowicz, M., Rowe, B. H., & Leech, J. A. (2009). Air pollution and emergency department visits for cardiac and respiratory conditions: A multi-city time-series analysis. *Environmental Health: A Global Access Science Source, 8,* 25.

Thavendiranathan, P., Bagai, A., Khoo, C., Dorian, P., & Choudhry, N. (2009). Does this patient with palpitations have a cardiac arrhythmia? *JAMA, 302*(19), 2135–2143.

Thom, S. (2011). Hyperbaric oxygen: Its mechanisms and efficacy. *Plastic & Reconstructive Surgery, 127,* 131S–141S.

University of California Davis. (2003). Safety of droperidol in the emergency department reviewed. *Biotechnology Weekly, 16,* 327.

Urdem, L. D., Stacy, K. M., & Lough, M. E. (2005). *Thelan's critical care nursing* (5th ed.). St. Louis, MO: Mosby.

Wandling, M. W., & An, G. C. (2010). A case report of thoracic compartment syndrome in the setting of penetrating chest trauma and review of the literature. *World Journal of Emergency Surgery, 5,* 22.

Wang, E. E., Baran, E., Kharasch, M., Vozenilek, J. A., Pettineo, C., & Berg, A. (2008). The emergent transvenous pacemaker. *Academic Emergency Medicine, 15*(5), 487.

Watson, S., & Gorski, K. A. (2011). *Invasive cardiology: A manual for cath lab personnel* (3rd ed.). Sudbury, MA: Jones & Bartlett Learning.

Wessels, M. W., De Graaf, B. M., Cohen-Overbeek, T. E., Spitaels, S. C., de Groot-de Laat, L. E., Ten Cate, F. J., . . . Willems, P. J. (2008). A new syndrome with noncompaction cardiomyopathy, bradycardia, pulmonary stenosis, atrial septal defect and heterotaxy with suggestive linkage to chromosome 6p. *Human Genetics, 122*(6), 595.

SECTION 4:

Pulmonary

1. The FIO$_2$ for a nasal cannula set at a flow rate of 6 L/min is
   A. 21%
   B. 24%
   C. 30%
   D. 40%

2. Your patient has been on a nasal cannula and now requires a nonrebreather mask to maintain his oxygenation saturation at acceptable levels. A nonrebreather mask can deliver what percentage of oxygen when the O$_2$ flow rate is set at 10–15 L/min?
   A. 24–40%
   B. 30–40%
   C. 60–80%
   D. 50–60%

3. A 44 year old woman comes into the ED with a cough that has lasted 3 weeks. She reports the coughing comes in long episodes that continue until she vomits. What little sputum she produces is very thick and white. What condition do you suspect?
   A. Asthma
   B. Gastroesophageal reflex
   C. Pertussis
   D. Pneumonia

4. What is the drug of choice for treating pertussis?
   A. Penicillin VK
   B. Amoxicillin
   C. Azithromycin
   D. Doxycycline

5. A patient recently admitted to the ED requires immediate intubation. The physician orders succinylcholine. Which of the following conditions is not a side effect of succinylcholine?
   A. Hypotension
   B. Malignant hypothermia
   C. Hypokalemia
   D. Smooth muscle contraction

6. A complication/contraindication of a nasal endotracheal intubation could be
   A. It cannot be used for a patient with a cervical injury
   B. Easy access to right mainstem bronchus
   C. The patient cannot drink
   D. It may cause otitis media

7. Vecuronium (Norcuron) is eliminated primarily via the
   A. Hepatic/biliary system
   B. Spleen
   C. Renal glomerulus
   D. Large bowel

8. Gas exchange in the lungs requires movement of gas between the atmosphere, alveoli, and pulmonary vasculature. This movement of gases is via
   A. Passive diffusion
   B. Osmotic pressure
   C. Airway resistance
   D. Hydrostatic pressure

9. You are asked to draw an arterial blood gas sample. You prepare a glass syringe with heparin. What effect will too much heparin have on the sample, if any?
   A. Increase the $PaCO_2$
   B. No effect
   C. Decrease the bicarbonate
   D. Totally prevent clotting

10. You are attempting to draw an arterial blood gas sample from an arterial line. The syringe requires a lot of force to move the cylinder. What effect will this high friction on the syringe have on blood gas results, if any?
    A. It will put the artery into spasm
    B. The high friction will increase the $PaCO_2$
    C. The high friction will decrease the PaO_2
    D. There will be no effect on the results

11. Your patient was admitted to the ED and is septic. You have just drawn an ABG sample from an arterial line and handed the sample to the respiratory therapist. The respiratory therapist asks if the patient has a fever. The possibility of fever will have what effect on the sample you collected?
    A. The PO_2 will be falsely elevated
    B. The pH will rise
    C. Fever has no effect
    D. The HCO_3 will be elevated

12. The driving pressure of air divided by airflow rate determined by airway diameter is known as
    A. A V-Q mismatch
    B. A compliance curve
    C. Airway resistance
    D. Driving force curve

13. The cells responsible for forming a barrier for alveoli are
    A. Histocytes
    B. Type II alveolar epithelial cells
    C. Macrophages
    D. Type I alveolar epithelial cells

14. In the lungs, communicating channels through holes in the alveolar wall allowing gas movement between alveoli are called
    A. A preacinar artery
    B. Alveolar pores of Kohn
    C. A cylindric canae of Smolder
    D. The palmar artery

15. Accessory pathways connecting a small airway to an airspace normally supplied by another pathway is called
    A. A cartilaginous bronchus
    B. A membranous bronchiole
    C. A canal of Lambert
    D. The portal of Menifer

16. Falsely low readings on a pulse oximeter may be due to
    A. Vasodilation
    B. Vascular dyes
    C. Patient motion
    D. Fever

17. Type II alveolar cells produce
    A. Surfactant
    B. Phagocytes
    C. Macrocytes
    D. CO_2

18. A diagnosis of asthma may be made by
    A. A PEFR of 100–125
    B. An FEF of 80%
    C. A decreased FEV_1
    D. Wheezing

19. Patients with uncontrolled asthma may receive steroids and neuromuscular blocking agents in an attempt to mitigate their symptoms. These patients are at increased risk for
    A. Hypertension
    B. Prolonged muscle weakness
    C. Renal failure
    D. Hepatic failure

20. Congenital lobar emphysema predominantly affects which lung field?
    A. The right upper lobe
    B. The right middle lobe
    C. The left upper lobe
    D. The left lower lobe

21. An intrinsic factor that may contribute to the pathogenesis of congenital lobar emphysema is
    A. An adenoma
    B. Pulmonary artery dilation
    C. Lymph node compression
    D. Hyperplasia

22. Your patient required placement of chest tube after aspiration of a pleural effusion. When assessing a patient with a chest tube drainage system, which of the following statements is correct?
    A. Check for subcutaneous emphysema around the insertion site by auscultation
    B. If using a Pleur-Evac with autotransfusion connection, make certain all clamps are open
    C. The average chest tube size for an adult is 20 Fr
    D. If using a chest tube drainage system with a one-way value and suction, water is required to maintain a seal

23. The patient you are caring for will require oxygen therapy at home, so it is important the patient is taught
    A. To secure oxygen tanks in a vertical position
    B. To wear synthetic clothing to reduce the risk of static electricity
    C. To use alcohol-based swabs to reduce oral dryness
    D. To use only a nasal cannula and not a mask

24. The volume of gas remaining in the lungs at the end of one normal expiration is called
    A. Residual volume
    B. Capacitance
    C. Total lung capacity
    D. Functional residual capacity

25. The volume of gas left in the lung following a maximal respiratory effort is known as the
    A. Vital capacity
    B. Total lung capacity
    C. Residual volume
    D. Dead airspace

26. When utilizing transcutaneous PO_2 measurements, some conditions may make the results unreliable. Underestimation of oxygenation may
    A. Occur if the patient is febrile
    B. Occur when the alignment is improper
    C. Occur when skin is hypoperfused
    D. Occur when there is an air bubble between the electrode and the skin

27. Which of the following conditions is most likely to lead to inaccurate oxygen saturation values on a pulse oximeter?
    A. Probe placement on an earlobe
    B. Hyperthermia
    C. Decreased peripheral perfusion
    D. Cyanotic heart disease

28. Which of the following considerations should the ED nurse know prior to the administration of vancomycin?
    A. Vancomycin is nephrotoxic
    B. Vancomycin must be administered intramuscularly
    C. Vancomycin should always be given with an aminoglycoside
    D. Vancomycin is specific for *Staphylococcus aureus*

29. Precautions used when handling respiratory equipment or providing respiratory treatments in the ED include
    A. Using an alcohol-based antiseptic agent if your hands are visibly soiled before, during, and after patient care
    B. Using an alcohol-based antiseptic solution only if you have worn gloves during contact with the patient
    C. Using an antimicrobial soap and water before and after providing patient care
    D. Only decontaminating your hands after providing care if gloves are worn

30. Paula has contracted a wound infection secondary to an appendix removal 6 days ago. She presented to the ED complaining of incisional pain and elevated temperature. She was started on intravenous gentamicin. Gentamicin is useful in the treatment of
    A. Otitis media
    B. Gram-positive rods
    C. *Pseudomonas aeruginosa*
    D. *Bacillus*

31. Pulse oximetry readings are considered unreliable when oxygen saturation levels fall below
    A. 55%
    B. 60%
    C. 80%
    D. 70%

32. The ED nurse caring for your patient reported that your patient had been previously intubated by paramedics with an LMA. The patient is now conscious and is on a nasal cannula at 2 L/min. Which of the following statements is true regarding the use of laryngeal mask airways (LMAs)?
    A. Nurses routinely insert these airways
    B. There is a low risk of aspiration
    C. It is a temporary airway
    D. The vocal cords must be visualized

33. The oxyhemoglobin dissociation curve may be shifted to the right by
    A. Alkalosis, hyperthermia, and hypercapnia
    B. Acidosis, hypocarbia, and hypothermia
    C. Acidosis, hypercarbia, and hyperthermia
    D. Alkalosis, hypothermia, and hypercapnia

34. If the oxyhemoglobin curve shifts to the right, one factor that will affect this shift is
    A. A decrease in 2,3 DPG
    B. A decrease in temperature
    C. A decrease in pH
    D. A decrease in CO_2

35. If the oxyhemoglobin dissociation curve shifts to the left, which of the following conditions could precipitate this change?
    A. Increased temperature, increased pH
    B. Increased $PaCO_2$
    C. Increased 2,3 DPG
    D. Decreased temperature

36. Your patient required endotracheal intubation. Which of the following statements is true regarding the use of capnography to verify endotracheal tube placement?
    A. Placement of the device can be difficult to learn initially
    B. It is not necessary to auscultate lung sounds when this device is used
    C. $ETCO_2$ is a moderately reliable indicator of correct tube placement
    D. It is not a substitute for pulse oximetry

37. A measurement of total oxygen consumption is
    A. SvO_2
    B. $EtCO_2$
    C. $PtCO_2$
    D. SjO_2

38. Your patient has a confirmed flail chest. What alteration in acid-base balance would you expect with this condition?
    A. Metabolic alkalosis
    B. Metabolic acidosis
    C. Respiratory acidosis
    D. Respiratory alkalosis

39. Tyrone had 1,250 ml of pleural effusion removed via thoracentesis and immediately began coughing and was dyspneic. You believe he has developed
    A. Reexpansion pulmonary edema
    B. A pneumothorax
    C. A cardiac tamponade
    D. A hemothorax

40. Myron was referred to your ED by his physician. Myron aspirated an unknown substance at home. One of the factors to be considered when assessing a patient for possible aspiration and chemical/aspiration pneumonitis is
    A. The possibility of using syrup of Ipecac
    B. The pH of the aspirate
    C. The type of infiltrates on CXR
    D. ABG results

41. PEEP is useful in ARDS (acute respiratory distress syndrome) because
    A. PEEP decreases cardiac output
    B. PEEP decreases venous return so lungs drain more effectively
    C. PEEP prevents barotraumas
    D. PEEP can open collapsed alveoli

42. Your patient has had 2 cm H_2O PEEP added on his ventilator. The use of PEEP may cause an increase in
    A. SVR
    B. PVR
    C. PAOP
    D. CO

43. Increased PEEP may cause which of the following conditions?
    A. Barotrauma
    B. Increased cardiac output
    C. Hemothorax
    D. A decrease in left atrial pressure

44. An indication for the use of PEEP is
    A. To help reduce the need for FiO_2
    B. To help assess mean arterial pressure
    C. To increase surfactant
    D. To reduce mediastinal bleeding post-CABG

45. You suspect your patient is developing a pulmonary embolism. Signs and symptoms of a pulmonary embolus can include
    A. Sinus bradycardia or a normal EKG
    B. Pleuritic chest pain, decreased cardiac output
    C. ABGs show respiratory acidosis, increased respiratory rate
    D. Decreased PAS pressure

46. Which of the following statements is true when a patient has a pulmonary embolism?
    A. Respiratory acidosis occurs
    B. Heparin is used to dissolve clots
    C. Normal D-dimer results can rule out a pulmonary embolism
    D. Metabolic alkalosis develops

47. Pulmonary embolism is actually considered a complication of deep venous thrombosis. To assess for deep venous thrombosis, which of the following signs should be assessed?
    A. Moses'
    B. Davis'
    C. Corrigan's
    D. Hamman's

48. Georgia was admitted to the ED after a fall from a tree. She complains of stabbing substernal pain each time she changes her position. She has been diagnosed with a pneumomediastinum. A common significant finding is
    A. Cullen's sign
    B. Grey-Turner's sign
    C. Hamman's sign
    D. Handes' sign

49. You ask an orientee to carry a newly drawn ABG specimen to the lab. She does not place the sample on ice and walks away. What effect will the lack of icing have on the sample?
    A. None
    B. It invalidates the sample
    C. The pH will rise
    D. The PaO_2 will rise

50. Which of the following drugs is classified as a methylxanthine?
    A. Morphine
    B. Theophylline
    C. Prednisone
    D. Atropine

51. Jack has been hypoxic since admission to the ED for a tension pneumothorax. What potential imbalance would be expected with his hypoxic state?
    A. Hypochloremia
    B. Respiratory alkalosis
    C. Decreased bicarbonate levels
    D. Hypokalemia

52. A student nurse asks you to explain the concept of hypoxemia. Hypoxemia is best defined as
    A. A decrease in oxygen at the cellular level
    B. A decrease in oxygen at the alveolar level
    C. A decrease in oxygen levels in venous blood
    D. A decrease in oxygen levels in arterial blood

53. Martin was finally released from the hospital 2 weeks ago after a difficult course of treatment for sepsis. He is being seen in the ED for follow-up on a small laceration. He plans to visit his family in Colorado Springs. Part of the patient teaching for Martin should include information on the effects of high altitude

on his ability to oxygenate effectively. Which of the following changes would be expected on his blood gas results?
   A. The PaO$_2$ increases
   B. No effect would occur
   C. O$_2$ saturation would decrease
   D. The pH would decrease

54. Which of the following conditions is the most probable cause of the acid-base imbalance of uncompensated respiratory alkalosis?
   A. Kidney failure
   B. A side effect of theophylline
   C. Hyperventilation
   D. Hypoventilation

55. Your patient needs to be placed on mechanical ventilation. The anesthesiologist uses pancuronium bromide (Pavulon) to paralyze the respiratory muscles. Which of the following drugs counteract the effects of Pavulon?
   A. Atropine
   B. Neostigmine
   C. Narcan
   D. Regitine

56. A possible treatment to best improve airflow in status asthmaticus is the use of
   A. PEEP
   B. Heliox
   C. Norepinephrine
   D. Nebulizer treatments

57. If you hear faint breath sounds on the left side of the chest and normal sounds on the right side immediately after your patient has been intubated, most likely
   A. The ETT has an air leak
   B. The physician has intubated the esophagus
   C. The ETT is at the carina
   D. The right mainstem bronchus has been intubated

58. Which of the following pulmonary dilators is used for the treatment of pulmonary hypertension?
   A. Dobutamine
   B. Dopamine
   C. Inhaled nitric oxide
   D. Epinephrine

59. An action of nitric oxide includes which of the following effects?
   A. Vascular smooth muscle relaxation
   B. To augment prostaglandin synthesis
   C. To release macrophages
   D. To increase pulmonary vascular resistance

60. Which of the following statements is true regarding the administration of CPAP?
    A. CPAP cannot be delivered via an endotracheal tube
    B. CPAP allows for a decrease in functional residual capacity
    C. CPAP provides decreased pressure to the posterior pharynx
    D. CPAP may be administered via nasal prongs

61. An adverse effect of excessive CPAP is
    A. Continuous need to increase oxygen over time
    B. A rise in intrathoracic pressure
    C. Intraventricular hemorrhage
    D. A sudden change in cerebral blood flow

62. Charles requires mechanical ventilation. If positive inspiratory pressure (PIP) is increased on a mechanical ventilator, what effect should this have on your patient's blood gases?
    A. It raises the $PaCO_2$ and decreases the PaO_2
    B. It lowers the $PaCO_2$ and lowers the PaO_2
    C. It decreases the $PaCO_2$ and increases the PaO_2
    D. It decreases the pH and decreases the $PaCO_2$

63. One means of decreasing pCO_2 when using a pressure ventilator is to
    A. Increase FiO_2
    B. Add PEEP
    C. Increase the ventilator rate
    D. Decrease the tidal volume

64. A disadvantage of using a pressure ventilator is
    A. Laryngeal deviation
    B. Possible overdistention
    C. Changes in pressure are done on a timed cycle
    D. That PEEP cannot be adjusted

65. In a volume-limited ventilator, an increase in ventilation may be achieved by
    A. Decreasing the ventilator rate
    B. Increasing the delivered tidal volume
    C. Decreasing the PEEP
    D. Increasing the FiO_2

66. An advantage of high-frequency ventilators over conventional ventilators is
    A. Mean airway pressures do not have to be monitored
    B. HF ventilators can transport CO_2 out of the lungs utilizing smaller pressures
    C. HF ventilators should not cause barotrauma because of lower pressures
    D. HF ventilators only have an advantage over pressure ventilators

67. Which of the following statements is true about high-frequency jet ventilators?
    A. Exhalation is an active function
    B. High-frequency jet ventilators deliver high-flow, short-duration pulses
    C. Exhalation is active and forced
    D. No conventional breaths can be delivered during HFJV

68. High-frequency ventilators have a "sigh" setting. This setting is used to
    A. Allow time for proper suctioning
    B. Decrease microatelectasis and recruit alveoli
    C. Assess lung sounds apart from ventilator sounds
    D. Deliver respirations to fully exchange gases within the lungs

69. Analyze the following arterial blood gas results from a patient on 2 L O_2 via a nasal cannula
    pH   7.47
    CO_2 33
    HCO_3 21
    A. Normal
    B. Compensated respiratory acidosis
    C. Uncompensated respiratory alkalosis
    D. Uncompensated metabolic alkalosis

70. Analyze the following arterial blood gas values
    pH   7.39
    CO_2 28
    HCO_3 19
    A. Compensated metabolic acidosis
    B. Compensated respiratory acidosis
    C. Uncompensated metabolic acidosis
    D. Uncompensated respiratory acidosis

71. Analyze the following capillary blood gas results on a patient in room air
    pH   7.42
    CO_2 41
    HCO_3 23
    A. Compensated respiratory acidosis
    B. Compensated respiratory alkalosis
    C. Normal
    D. Compensated metabolic acidosis

72. Analyze the following arterial blood gas results from a patient with a ventricular septal injury from a stab wound
    pH   7.57
    CO_2 22
    HCO_3 31
    A. Uncompensated (mixed) respiratory/metabolic alkalosis
    B. Compensated respiratory acidosis
    C. Compensated metabolic alkalosis
    D. Uncompensated respiratory alkalosis

73. Analyze the following arterial blood gas values
    pH   7.38
    CO_2 65
    HCO_3 36
    A. Uncompensated metabolic alkalosis
    B. Compensated respiratory acidosis
    C. Compensated metabolic acidosis
    D. Uncompensated respiratory acidosis

74. Analyze the following arterial blood gas from an adult patient with tetralogy of Fallot
    pH   7.17
    CO_2 41
    HCO_3 14
    A. Normal
    B. Compensated respiratory acidosis
    C. Uncompensated respiratory acidosis
    D. Uncompensated metabolic acidosis

75. Interpret the following arterial blood gas result from a victim of a gunshot wound to the chest
    pH   7.23
    CO_2 61
    HCO_3 23
    A. Compensated respiratory acidosis
    B. Uncompensated metabolic acidosis
    C. Uncompensated respiratory acidosis
    D. Normal

76. Analyze the following arterial blood gas values
    pH   7.52
    CO_2 42
    HCO_3 37
    A. Uncompensated metabolic alkalosis
    B. Compensated metabolic acidosis
    C. Uncompensated respiratory alkalosis
    D. Uncompensated mixed respiratory/metabolic alkalosis

77. Analyze the following arterial blood gas values
    pH   7.43
    CO_2 36
    HCO_3 25
    A. Compensated respiratory acidosis
    B. Normal
    C. Compensated metabolic acidosis
    D. Compensated metabolic alkalosis

78. Analyze the following arterial blood gas values
    pH   7.11
    CO_2 67
    HCO_3 15
    A. Uncompensated respiratory acidosis
    B. Uncompensated metabolic alkalosis
    C. Compensated metabolic acidosis
    D. Uncompensated (mixed) respiratory/metabolic acidosis

79. Analyze the following blood gas values
    pH   7.38
    CO_2 25
    HCO_3 16
    A. Compensated respiratory alkalosis
    B. Compensated metabolic acidosis
    C. Uncompensated metabolic acidosis
    D. Uncompensated respiratory acidosis

80. Analyze the following blood gas values
    pH   7.49
    CO_2 29
    HCO_3 23
    A. Uncompensated respiratory alkalosis
    B. Compensated respiratory acidosis
    C. Compensated metabolic alkalosis
    D. Uncompensated metabolic acidosis

81. Analyze the following arterial blood gas values
    pH   7.43
    CO_2 29
    HCO_3 22
    A. Uncompensated metabolic alkalosis
    B. Uncompensated respiratory alkalosis
    C. Compensated respiratory alkalosis
    D. Compensated metabolic alkalosis

82. Analyze the following arterial blood gas values
    pH   7.32
    CO_2 67
    HCO_3 25
    A. Uncompensated metabolic alkalosis
    B. Uncompensated respiratory acidosis
    C. Compensated metabolic acidosis
    D. Compensated respiratory acidosis

83. Analyze the following arterial blood gas values
    pH   7.37
    CO_2 36
    HCO_3 24
    A. Normal
    B. Compensated respiratory acidosis
    C. Compensated metabolic acidosis
    D. Compensated respiratory alkalosis

84. Analyze the following arterial blood gas from a patient on room air
    pH   7.16
    CO_2 54
    HCO_3 21
    A. Uncompensated metabolic alkalosis
    B. Uncompensated (mixed) respiratory/metabolic acidosis
    C. Compensated metabolic acidosis
    D. Uncompensated respiratory acidosis

85. You are part of the patient safety team for your ED and are responsible for evaluating compliance with hospital-acquired infection procedures. To prevent ventilator-associated pneumonia (VAP) in the ED, the Centers for Disease Control and Prevention (CDC) recommends that respiratory equipment that comes in direct contact with patient mucosal membranes be
    A. Cleaned with an alcohol-based solution prior to autoclaving
    B. Washed with sterile normal saline at 90°F for 5 minutes prior to use
    C. Steam sterilized or autoclaved by the facility regardless if the item is multiuse or single use
    D. Wet-heat pasteurized at temperatures > 158°F for 30 minutes and packaged sterile for next use

86. Fluid therapy in ARDS is directed toward
    A. Keeping a high CO state
    B. Maintaining a low protein content
    C. Maintaining hyponatremia
    D. Maintaining a low circulating fluid volume

87. The nurse just coming on shift to care for your patient brought several ampules of normal saline to the bedside in preparation for suctioning your patient. Research has shown that use of normal saline does not thin secretions and may cause which of the following adverse effects?
    A. Decreased mean arterial pressure
    B. Decreased intrathoracic pressure
    C. Anxiety
    D. Bronchodilation

88. In the ED, patients may be mechanically ventilated by a variety of ventilator modes. Which of the following ventilator modes allows the patient to breathe spontaneously?
    A. HFV
    B. SIMV
    C. CMV
    D. Oscillator

89. A patient with acute respiratory failure will benefit from the use of which of the following ventilator strategies?
    A. Limiting plateau pressure
    B. Hyperventilation
    C. Lower CO_2 levels
    D. Maintain PEEP < 5 cm H_2O

90. One cause of decreased SvO_2 in a patient is
    A. An increased metabolic rate
    B. Sedation
    C. A decreased metabolic rate
    D. Increased cardiac output

91. Many of the ventilator circuits used in an ED utilize a closed catheter suction system. Which of the following is a disadvantage of closed catheter suctioning of a mechanically ventilated patient?
    A. The patient does not receive oxygen during the procedure
    B. The extra weight of the inline tubing
    C. Cost is higher with a single-use catheter
    D. Cost is effective if used sporadically

92. Your patient will require long-term ventilatory support via a tracheostomy. A disadvantage of using a tracheostomy tube is
    A. Subcutaneous emphysema
    B. Increases airway resistance
    C. The airway is less stable
    D. Allows for right mainstem intubation

93. Your patient requires a stoma stent. The function of a stoma stent is
    A. To prevent aspiration
    B. To avoid translaryngeal intubation
    C. To provide the ability for the patient to speak.
    D. To keep the stoma tract open

94. Which of the following statements about silicone or plastic tracheostomy tubes is true?
    A. Silicone holds up to repeated cleaning
    B. Wire reinforced tubes cannot be used in MRI imaging
    C. A one-way speaking valve is easy to use
    D. The tubes offer a lower cost to the facility

95. Ella has severe bronchitis. She has been treated at her extended care facility with a nonrebreather mask for 5 days. Today, she is exhibiting increased distress with chest discomfort, restlessness, a dry hacking cough with dyspnea, and numbness in her extremities. Pulmonary function tests (PFTs) indicate a decreased vital capacity (VC), decreased compliance, and decreased functional residual capacity (FRC). As the nurse caring for this patient, you should
    A. Administer Lasix 40 mg IV
    B. Prepare for intubation with 100% FiO_2
    C. Take the patient for a CT scan and prepare to give tPA
    D. Check the pulse oximeter correlation with an arterial blood gas and decrease the FiO_2

96. Garrett has developed ARDS. He has been on mechanical ventilation for 4 days at a rehabilitation facility for veterans. During your assessment you note that Garrett has a temperature of 100.6° F, a heart rate of 126, and a respiratory rate of 28. Garrett also has an increased cough and decreased breath sounds on the right side without tracheal deviation. You suspect his symptoms are the result of
    A. Pulmonary edema
    B. A pneumothorax
    C. Sepsis
    D. Atelectasis

97. As patients age from birth through old age, chest wall compliance decreases. One of the reasons for this change is
    A. Arterial oxygen tension increases
    B. Total lung capacity decreases
    C. Costal cartilage degeneration
    D. Decreased residual volume

98. The nursing student assigned to you for the day asks you to explain the oxyhemoglobin dissociation curve. You reply that the oxyhemoglobin dissociation curve is
    A. A relationship between dissolved oxygen and the affinity for oxygen by the hemoglobin molecule
    B. A graphic representation of carbon dioxide content versus oxygen content in arterial blood
    C. A measure of methemoglobin
    D. A way to calculate gas transport across the alveoli

99. Dewey is a 74 year old gentleman with end-stage mesothelioma. He came to the ED because of severe respiratory distress. Which of the following occupations is more likely to be associated with a diagnosis of mesothelioma?
    A. Bricklayer
    B. Gardener
    C. Office manager
    D. Shipbuilder

100. Your patient has just been intubated with an ETT. Documentation of the procedure usually would not include
    A. The time the intubator took to complete the task
    B. The size of the tube
    C. The depth of the tube
    D. If a CXR was taken

101. Mask continuous positive airway pressure (CPAP) should be used with caution if a patient has
    A. Low functional residual capacity (FRC)
    B. A basilar skull fracture
    C. Sinusitis
    D. Pneumonia

102. Which of the following medications is given orally to inhibit rapid rise in pulmonary artery pressure secondary to hypoxia?
    A. Calcium channel blockers
    B. Nitric oxide
    C. Sildenafil
    D. Prostacycun

103. Which medication listed below is both an analgesic and an amnestic?
    A. Barbiturates
    B. Propofol
    C. Atropine
    D. Ketamine

104. Which of the following statements about cyanosis is true?
    A. Cyanosis is directly related to increased $PaCO_2$
    B. Fingertip clubbing is an indication of chronic hypoxia
    C. Cyanosis may be observed when 1 to 3 grams of Hgb is desaturated
    D. Cyanosis may be easily observed in cases of anemia and polycythemia

105. Your patient had a mixed venous sample drawn from his pulmonary artery catheter with a PaO_2 result of 38 mmHg. This result indicates
    A. Acute respiratory acidosis
    B. Hypoxemia
    C. A normal value
    D. Hypoxia

106. Scott's endotracheal tube cuff has been requiring increasing pressures to maintain a good air seal. The cuff now requires 61 mmHg. What is the probable cause for the increasing pressure?
    A. Tracheal stenosis
    B. A cuff leak
    C. Tracheal atresia
    D. A wider endotracheal tube is necessary

107. The respiratory therapist tells you he is covering too many patients and cannot perform postural drainage on your patient. He says your patient needs the left upper lobes drained if possible. The correct position to help this patient is
    A. Flat on left side
    B. Flat with hips elevated
    C. Supine
    D. Semireclining

108. Your patient has a hemothorax. What is the proper location of a chest tube for evacuation of a hemothorax?
    A. In the second intercostal space, midclavicular line
    B. Second intercostal space, midaxillary line
    C. Fifth intercostal space, midaxillary line
    D. Fifth intercostal space, midclavicular line

109. An example of the hypoxemic type of respiratory failure is
    A. Increased dead air space
    B. ARDS
    C. PaO_2 < 60 mmHg while person is at rest, at sea level, on room air
    D. Right heart failure

110. A patient who is being mechanically ventilated with continuous end-tidal CO_2 ($ETCO_2$) monitored develops a pulmonary embolism. An expected change in parameters would include
    A. Increased PaO_2
    B. Decreased CVP
    C. Decreased pet CO_2
    D. Increased $PaCO_2$

111. Douglas had a pulmonary artery catheter placed to closely monitor fluid status. The physician ordered PAOP pressures now, at 1 hour, and q 8 hours thereafter while the patient is in the ICU. You obtain the initial readings during insertion of the catheter. The patient remains in the ED after another hour has passed, so you attempt to obtain another wedge pressure reading. During the next attempt for another wedge pressure, you notice decreased resistance to the syringe. Which of the following complications may have occurred?
    A. Syringe malfunction
    B. Embolization
    C. Balloon rupture
    D. This is an expected finding

112. Where does the hypoxemic drive to breathe originate?
    A. The cerebellum
    B. The aortic and carotid arteries
    C. The hypothalamus
    D. The medulla

113. The functional residual capacity is defined as
    A. The amount of air in lungs after normal expiration
    B. The amount of gas that can be forcefully exhaled after maximum inspiration
    C. The amount of gas normally exhaled after a maximum inhalation
    D. The amount of gas left in the lungs after a maximum exhalation

114. Severe carbon monoxide poisoning occurs when carboxyhemoglobin levels are higher than which of the following percentages?
    A. 10–15%
    B. 20–40%
    C. 40–50%
    D. 50–60%

115. Carbon monoxide has an affinity for hemoglobin thought to be 200–300 times greater than oxygen. Elimination of carbon monoxide from the body is via the
    A. Kidneys
    B. Liver
    C. Spleen
    D. Lungs

116. The nurse reporting to you on a new patient states that the patient has developed subcutaneous emphysema. Subcutaneous emphysema usually occurs in the area of the
    A. Head
    B. Neck
    C. Abdomen
    D. Thorax

117. Pulse oximetry should never be used
    A. To determine oxygen saturation values
    B. During a cardiac arrest
    C. As a determinant for predicting hemoglobin affinity for oxygen
    D. To help determine a patient's activity tolerance

118. A SpO_2 value of 95% correlates with which of the following PaO_2 values?
    A. 75
    B. 80
    C. 90
    D. 98

119. To prevent complications with chest tube drainage systems, the suction level should not be higher than
    A. -20 cm/H_2O
    B. -30 cm/H_2O
    C. -40 cm/H_2O
    D. -50 cm/H_2O

120. Which of the following statements is true regarding chest tube drainage systems?
    A. Drainage of frank blood in amounts > 100 ml/hour is not significant
    B. Drainage tubing should be placed horizontally on the bed and down to the collection chamber
    C. All drainage tubing should be dependent to the insertion site
    D. Chest tube drainage from a mediastinal tube should not bubble in the water seal chamber

121. Which of the following drugs is considered to be a mucolytic agent?
    A. Atropine
    B. Terbutaline
    C. Acetyl-cysteine
    D. Albuterol

122. Side effects of acetyl-cysteine include
    A. Red urine
    B. Headache
    C. Hypertension
    D. Bronchospasms

123. Patients often have decreases in lung compliance simply from the effects of aging. Which of the following conditions actually increases lung compliance?
    A. Pulmonary edema
    B. Pleural effusions
    C. Obesity
    D. Emphysema

124. Which of the following statements about laryngeal mask airways is true?
    A. It may be inserted by any nurse
    B. It may cause hoarseness after removal
    C. The patient must have an absent gag reflex
    D. The laryngeal mask airway (LMA) eliminates the risk of aspiration

125. One of the most effective ways to relieve bronchospasms is
    A. To use adrenalin
    B. Use of an antihistamine
    C. Use prednisone
    D. To use a B_2 receptor agonist

126. During a cardiac arrest your patient aspirated gastric contents. Which of the following statements is true regarding this type of aspiration?
    A. If the pH of the material is < 2.5, necrosis will be minimal
    B. The patient always develops ARDS
    C. Onset of symptoms is gradual
    D. There is little danger of atelectasis

127. When the resident attempts to place a central line, air is accidentally introduced into the line when the IV tubing becomes disconnected. The best position in which to place this patient to minimize a venous air embolism is
    A. Reverse Trendelenburg
    B. Right side
    C. Trendelenburg with left decubitus tilt
    D. Left side

128. A venous air embolism may be caused by
    A. Hemodialysis
    B. Pulmonary artery catheters
    C. Radial arterial catheters
    D. Peritoneal dialysis

129. A risk factor for thrombolic emboli includes
    A. A patient who is 1 week postpartum
    B. Carcinoma
    C. Long bone fractures
    D. Heparin administration

130. The definitive study for determination of thrombolic emboli is a
    A. Pulmonary ventilation-perfusion scan
    B. Mixed venous oxygen saturation
    C. Pulmonary angiography
    D. PAWP

131. Blood gases you would expect to see for a patient with thrombotic emboli are
    A. pH 7.42 PaO_2 88 $PaCO_2$ 28 HCO_3 22
    B. pH 7.50 PaO_2 74 $PaCO_2$ 52 HCO_3 24
    C. pH 7.32 PaO_2 86 $PaCO_2$ 29 HCO_3 26
    D. pH 7.32 PaO_2 90 $PaCO_2$ 30 HCO_3 24

132. Blood gas results you would expect to find in a pregnant woman without complications indicate
    A. Compensated respiratory alkalosis
    B. Compensated metabolic acidosis
    C. Compensated respiratory acidosis
    D. Compensated metabolic alkalosis

133. The best position for a patient with ARDS is
    A. Prone
    B. On right side
    C. On left side
    D. Supine

134. Pulmonary hypertension is generally defined as a mean pulmonary artery pressure of
    A. ≥ 10 mmHg
    B. ≥ 15 mmHg
    C. ≥ 25 mmHg
    D. ≥ 35 mmHg

135. You are receiving report on Josh, a patient with pulmonary hypertension. Which of the following symptoms is consistent with presentation of pulmonary hypertension?
    A. A prominent S_4
    B. Decreased respiratory rate
    C. Dyspnea with exertion
    D. Left-side heart failure

136. Carl is suffering from primary pulmonary hypertension. Which of the following medication groups would be used to treat this condition?
    A. Beta-blockers
    B. Calcium channel blockers
    C. MAOs
    D. Catecholamine

137. If left untreated, pulmonary hypertension may result in which of the following sequelae?
    A. Increased left atrium pressures
    B. Irreversible thinning of the medial smooth muscles in the arterioles
    C. Reversible thickening of the lateral smooth muscle in the arterioles
    D. Increased right ventricular pressures

138. What is the purpose of screening for collagen vascular disease and coagulation disorders in a patient with suspected pulmonary hypertension?
    A. Hypoxemia triggers a decrease in collagen creation
    B. Hypoxia results in decreased elastin production
    C. Decreased blood flow results in blood pooling
    D. Hypoxemia destroys collagen

139. An absolute contraindication for use of rapid sequence intubation is
    A. Total loss of facial and/or oropharyngeal landmarks, which requires a surgical airway
    B. An airway where intubation may not be successful
    C. A "crash" airway where the patient is in arrest
    D. There is no absolute contraindication for the use of rapid sequence intubation

140. Which of the following situations is not an indication for the use of rapid sequence intubation?
    A. Prolonged respiratory effort that results in fatigue or failure
    B. Uncooperative trauma patient with life-threatening injuries
    C. Stab wound to neck with expanding hematoma
    D. All cervical spine injuries

141. During rapid sequence intubation, cricoid cartilage pressure is often used to help prevent vomiting and aspiration of gastric contents. The esophagus is obstructed by the pressure to the anterior neck. This maneuver is known as the
    A. Hamman's maneuver
    B. King maneuver
    C. Sellick maneuver
    D. Pitt maneuver

142. You are caring for a patient with an acute exacerbation of reactive airway disease. The patient has a history of asthma. Which of the following signs indicate this patient is suffering from acute respiratory distress?
    A. Expiratory wheezes
    B. Grunting
    C. Sternocleodomastoid retractions
    D. Inspiratory wheezes

143. Your patient has ceased wheezing during his asthma attack. This change in his condition
    A. Indicates the patient is improving
    B. Only means the nebulizer treatment is working
    C. Indicates the patient is in complete respiratory failure
    D. Means the patient's anxiety has decreased

144. Wheezing is present in a number of medical conditions. In which of the following conditions is wheezing not present?
    A. Smoke inhalation
    B. Pneumonia
    C. Near drowning
    D. Bronchitis

145. Your patient tells you he has been taking Slo-Bid® for his asthma. Side effects of this medication include
    A. Lethargy
    B. Flaccidity
    C. Bradycardia
    D. Muscle cramps

146. Long-acting forms of B_2 agonists used in the treatment of asthma include
    A. Salmeterol (Serevent®)
    B. Albuterol (Proventil® HFA, Ventolin® HFA, Accuneb®, ProAir®)
    C. Metaproterenol (Alupent®)
    D. Levalbuterol (Xoponex® HFA, Xoponex® nebulizer solution)

147. Your patient presents to the ED with moderate dyspnea and neck swelling. He states he developed these symptoms over the past 4 hours after visiting his dentist. When auscultating his neck and chest, you hear a "crunching" sound. The sound

varied with the heartbeat and was more pronounced in the left lateral decubitus position. You suspect this patient has
   A. A partially fractured larynx
   B. A pneumomediastinum
   C. An infiltrated jugular IV
   D. A fractured sternum

148. Which of the following are symptoms of active tuberculosis?
   A. Dry cough, weight loss, night sweats
   B. Hemoptysis, fever, night sweats, weight loss
   C. Chest pain, wheezing, hemoptysis
   D. Weight loss, hemoptysis, wheezing

149. Your patient has a 14-mm induration at the site of his PPD. What does this mean?
   A. He has a positive PPD
   B. He has latent TB
   C. His results are indeterminate
   D. He has a false-positive result

150. Which of the following medications is not used to treat TB?
   A. Isoniazid
   B. Pyrazidamide
   C. Rimantadine
   D. Rifampin

SECTION 4: PULMONARY ANSWERS

1. **Correct answer: D**
   The FIO_2 for a nasal cannula set at a flow rate of 6 L/min is 40%. The nasal cannula is generally considered a low-flow oxygen device unless connected to a high-flow system. If using a flow > 4 L/m the oxygen should be humidified to prevent drying of the mucosal membranes.

2. **Correct answer: C**
   A nonrebreather mask can deliver 60–80% of oxygen when the O_2 flow rate is 10–15 L/min. If both exhalation ports have one-way valves, then near 100% oxygen may be reached. To prevent suffocation in patients where the oxygen is disconnected, nonrebreathing masks now have only one one-way valve to prevent/limit inhalation of room air. This results in decreasing the highest concentration of actual inspired oxygen to 60–80%.

3. **Correct answer: C**
   This patient's symptoms are indicative of pertussis. A PCR nasal probe should be done as soon as possible. Her family should be examined for signs of pertussis, especially if there are infants or children under the age of 2 or those who have not had a TDaP booster in the past 5 years.

4. **Correct answer: C**
   Macrolide antibiotics such as azithromycin, clarithromycin, and erythromycin are recommended treatments for pertussis. Penicillins and tetracyclines are ineffective in treating pertussis.

5. **Correct answer: D**
   Succinylcholine combines with acetylcholine to cause smooth muscle relaxation, not contraction. Prolonged use may cause a change in blocking action and result in potassium regulated alterations in electrical activity. Side effects of succinylcholine include malignant hyperthermia and hypertension or hypotension, hyperkalemia, anaphylaxis, and increased intraocular pressure.

6. **Correct answer: D**
   Because of the direct connection via the Eustachian tube, infection in the ear is possible. If a cervical injury has been stabilized, it is certainly possible for a skilled intubator to place the tube. Additional complications of the nasal endotracheal tube include nasal bleeding, sinusitis, accidental esophageal intubation, vocal cord injuries, necrosis, cuff leak or failure, and obstruction.

7. **Correct answer: A**
   Norcuron is eliminated via the hepatic/biliary system. Use with caution in patients with known or suspected hepatic or biliary compromise such as cirrhosis or hepatitis because it may take up to two times as long to clear a patient's system.

8. **Correct answer: A**
   Gas exchange in the lungs requires passive diffusion of gas between the atmosphere, alveoli, and pulmonary vasculature.

9. **Correct answer: C**
Too much heparin in a glass syringe has dilutional effects and decreases the bicarbonate and the $PaCO_2$.

10. **Correct answer: C**
Using a vacutainer or a high-friction syringe creates a vacuum. When that occurs, dissolved gases come out of solution, which decreases PaO_2 and $PaCO_2$. The increased effort to move the cylinder may cause the artery to spasm and impede obtaining the sample but will not directly affect results.

11. **Correct answer: B**
Fever causes the pH to rise. Most ABG machines are calibrated to 37° C. If the patient has a fever, the oxyhemoglobin curve will be shifted to the right. More oxygen will be given off to the tissues, so the machine has to be calibrated to account for the temperature.

12. **Correct answer: C**
The driving pressure of air divided by airflow rate determined by airway diameter is known as airway resistance.

13. **Correct answer: D**
The cells that are responsible for forming a barrier for alveoli are type I epithelial cells. Type I cells line the outside of the alveoli and are easily inflamed by inhaled toxins or heated air. In addition, type I cells maintain the blood–gas interface. Type II cells produce surfactant.

14. **Correct answer: B**
In the lungs communicating channels through holes in the alveolar wall allowing gas movement between alveoli are called alveolar pores of Kohn.

15. **Correct answer: C**
Accessory pathways connecting a small airway to an airspace normally supplied by another pathway are called canals of Lambert.

16. **Correct answer: C**
Falsely low readings on a pulse oximeter may be due to patient motion. If the patient is hypothermic or has decreased peripheral perfusion, the results will be inaccurate. Phototherapy, position of the probe, and patient motion can also cause inaccurate readings on a pulse oximeter.

17. **Correct answer: A**
Type II alveolar cells produce surfactant. Surfactant is a lipoprotein and functions by increasing surface tension of alveoli and allows alveoli to expand and contract. There should be some residual pressure in the alveoli at the end of respiration to keep the alveoli open (physiologic PEEP). If surfactant production is impaired, the alveoli's ability to exchange O_2 is compromised. Type I cells line the outside of the alveoli.

18. **Correct answer: C**
A diagnosis of asthma may be made by a decreased FEV_1. The forced expiratory volume (FEV) is how much air is exhaled during the first second of effort. This amount should be ≥75% of the predicted normal. In asthmatics this value is decreased because of obstruction. The forced vital capacity (FVC) is the total amount of gas exhaled as forcefully and rapidly as possible after taking a maximal inspiration. The result should be above 80%.

19. **Correct answer: B**
    Uncontrolled asthma symptoms during an attack may lead to prolonged and extensive muscle use to maintain independent respirations. Prolonged effort may result in respiratory failure due to respiratory muscle fatigue. Administration of a neuromuscular blocking agent further inhibits the smooth muscle retractions. Long-term steroid use has been linked to muscle wasting. Ventilatory weaning may be prolonged as respiratory muscles recover from both the disease process and pharmacologic intervention.

20. **Correct answer: C**
    In congenital lobar emphysema, the left upper lobe is affected 41% of the time, the right middle lobe 34% of the time, and the right upper lobe 21% of the time. There are rare cases of both lungs affected. Congenital lobar emphysema has two forms: hypoalveolar (affecting less than the expected number of alveoli) and polyalveolar (affecting greater than the expected number of alveoli).

21. **Correct answer: A**
    An intrinsic factor that may contribute to the pathogenesis of congenital lobar emphysema is an adenoma. Pulmonary artery dilation and lymph node compression are extrinsic factors to the development of congenital lobar emphysema. Other intrinsic factors are infection, tuberculosis, retained secretions, absence of cartilage, stenosis, and hypoplasia.

22. **Correct answer: B**
    If using a Pleur-Evac with autotransfusion connection, make certain all clamps are open. When using any autotransfusion drainage system make sure to connect the system per the manufacturer's recommendations. Most connections are color coded for easy connecting. Clamps must remain open to allow for blood collection and prevent increased intrathoracic pressures. Subcutaneous air should be checked by palpation and borders marked for further monitoring. If a one-way valve system and suction is used, water is not required to maintain a seal because the valve meets this function.

23. **Correct answer: A**
    It is important the patient be taught to store oxygen tanks in the upright position. Synthetic materials often cause static electricity. Only lemon-glycerin swabs and not alcohol-based swabs should be used if the patient has dry lips. In this case we do not know if the patient will use O_2 via a mask or cannula.

24. **Correct answer: D**
    Functional residual capacity is the volume of gas remaining in the lungs at the end of one normal expiration.

25. **Correct answer: C**
    Residual volume is the volume of gas left in the lung following a maximal respiratory effort.

26. **Correct answer: C**
    When utilizing transcutaneous PO_2 measurements, underestimation of oxygenation may occur when the skin is hypoperfused or the calibration is improper. Overestimation of oxygenation may occur if there is an air bubble or leak between the electrode and the skin.

27. **Correct answer: C**

    Adequate perfusion must exist for the probe on a pulse oximeter to register an accurate evaluation of hemoglobin saturation. If the patient is hypothermic or has decreased peripheral perfusion, the results will be inaccurate. Phototherapy, position of the probe, and patient motion can also cause inaccurate readings on a pulse oximeter.

28. **Correct answer: A**

    Prior to the administration of vancomycin, the ED nurse should know that vancomycin is nephrotoxic, especially if used in combination with aminoglycosides. Vancomycin is used in the treatment of methicillin-resistant strains (*Staphylococcus epidermidis*) and must be administered by slow intravenous drip.

29. **Correct answer: C**

    Antimicrobial soap and water may be used to decontaminate hands before, during, and after patient care regardless of glove use, visible soiling, or no apparent soiling. Hands should always be decontaminated using soap and water, waterless soap, or alcohol-based antiseptic agent before and after patient care to prevent the spread of organisms from patient to patient or from surfaces. Alcohol-based antiseptic agents should only be used if no visible soiling is observed.

30. **Correct answer: C**

    Gentamicin is effective against gram-negative rods and penicillin-resistant staphylococci, *Escherichia coli* strains, and *Pseudomonas aeruginosa*. Gentamicin may cause ototoxicity and nephrotoxicity. Gentamicin must never be given as IV push—only as a drip over at least 30–60 minutes. If the patient has oliguria or anuria, the dose must be decreased or discontinued.

31. **Correct answer: D**

    Pulse oximetry readings are considered unreliable when oxygen saturation levels fall below 70%. Pulse oximetry accuracy is impacted by patient motion, low perfusion, venous pulsation, light, poor probe positioning, edema, anemia, and carbon monoxide levels. It is important to compare pulse oximetry values against arterial blood gases to validate values below 70% on the pulse oximeter.

32. **Correct answer: C**

    The laryngeal mask airway was intended as a temporary airway. It requires minimal training to insert, but cannot be placed by RNs as a matter of course. The patient must be unconscious and/or without gag reflex. The seal around the mask is a low pressure seal, so it cannot be used on patients with high peak ventilator pressures. The LMA has a significant risk of aspiration. Advantages with use of this airway are that it is simply blindly inserted into the hypopharynx, does not require visualization of the vocal cords, and does not traumatize the trachea. Patients will not have hoarseness or lose their voice altogether. At best, patients will complain of a mild sore throat.

33. **Correct answer: C**

    Acidosis, hypercarbia, and hyperthermia all lead to a right shift in the oxyhemoglobin dissociation curve. Hemoglobin in this instance has a decreased affinity for oxygen and enhances tissue uptake of oxygen.

34. **Correct answer: C**

    If the oxyhemoglobin curve shifts to the right, one of the factors that affects this shift is a decrease in pH. A shift to the right in the oxyhemoglobin dissociation curve means hemoglobin has less affinity for oxygen. 2,3 DPG (2,3 diphosphoglyceride) is necessary to help force O_2 off the hemoglobin molecule. So if 2,3 DPG is decreased, the hemoglobin will hang onto the O_2. If the temperature is increased, the tissues need more O_2. If the PCO_2 is elevated, the tissues need more oxygen.

35. **Correct answer: D**
If the oxyhemoglobin dissociation curve shifts to the left, hemoglobin holds onto the oxygen, so the 2,3 DPG is lacking, CO_2 is decreased, and temperature is decreased. Tissues would not need as much O_2.

36. **Correct answer: D**
Capnography ($PetCO_2$) is not a substitute for pulse oximetry. A pulse oximeter measures the availability of sites on the hemoglobin molecule for oxygen transport versus how many sites are occupied. The end tidal CO_2 ($ETCO_2$) measures whether gas exchange is taking place at the cellular level. If CO_2 is being given off, the CO_2 will react with chemically treated paper in the detector. If the esophagus has been intubated, the $ETCO_2$ can give a false-positive reading if the patient has consumed a carbonated beverage within the past few hours.

37. **Correct answer: A**
SvO_2 is a measurement of total oxygen consumption.

38. **Correct answer: C**
This is a very painful condition that limits respiratory effort because of the pain or from analgesia and sedation that may be required. CO_2 will increase, PaO_2 will decrease and the pH will be below 7.35. The patient will develop respiratory acidosis.

39. **Correct answer: A**
This patient has developed reexpansion pulmonary edema. Removal of large amounts of pleural fluid increases negative intrapleural pressure. Edema occurs when the lung does not reexpand. The patient then develops a severe cough and dyspnea. If the symptoms occur during a thoracentesis, the procedure should be stopped.

40. **Correct answer: B**
The pH of the aspirate is very important. If the aspirate is acidic, there is an almost immediate creation of pulmonary edema. This is due to the collapse and breakdown of the alveoli, capillaries, and their interface. Atelectasis, possible intra-alveolar hemorrhage, and some interstitial edema lead to hypoxia. Alkalotic aspirate destroys surfactant, which causes alveolar collapse, leading to hypoxia. Other factors to identify are the type of material aspirated and the amount. Syrup of Ipecac is used for ingestions. ABGs would be considered more of a diagnostic tool.

41. **Correct answer: D**
PEEP is useful in ARDS (acute respiratory distress syndrome) because PEEP can open collapsed alveoli. Barotrauma and decreased cardiac output and venous return are complications of PEEP. PEEP must be regulated so as not to cause barotraumas, but still keep alveoli from collapsing during expiration.

42. **Correct answer: B**
Because PEEP raises intrathoracic pressure and PVR, blood backs up and can cause hepatic congestion. The increased intrathoracic pressure also can compress blood vessels, cause or exacerbate hypovolemia, and cause low cardiac output.

43. **Correct answer: A**

    Increased PEEP may cause barotrauma. Any pressure in the thorax decreases preload, cardiac output, and blood pressure. Forward blood flow is impeded by increased pressure in the pulmonary vasculature. A pulmonary air leak could occur from the increased pressure caused by PEEP.

44. **Correct answer: A**

    An indication for the use of PEEP is to help reduce the need for FiO_2. PEEP helps keep alveoli open, raising PaO_2, so it decreases the need for FiO_2.

45. **Correct answer: B**

    Signs and symptoms of a pulmonary embolus can include pleuritic chest pain and decreased cardiac output. An acute pulmonary embolism can be associated with right heart failure. The PAS and PVR will be elevated. The patient may suffer from nonspecific chest pain, dyspnea, tachycardia, hypotension, shock, and possibly coma.

46. **Correct answer: C**

    A normal D-dimer rules out a pulmonary embolism. If the D-dimer is elevated, it may be caused by multiple other conditions. Hyperventilation occurs subsequent to hypoxemia, so respiratory alkalosis will be present. Heparin does not dissolve existing clots.

47. **Correct answer: A**

    Use Moses' sign to assess for deep venous thrombosis (DVT). Moses' sign is elicited by pressing the calf toward the tibia. This may also elicit pain. These results are not exclusive to DVT but may complement a diagnosis. Traditionally, we were taught to assess Homan's sign: dorsiflexion of the ankle while bending the knee. If that elicited pain, the patient had a problem with circulation and possibly DVT.

48. **Correct answer: C**

    A very common and significant finding in a patient with a pneumomediastinum is Hamman's sign. Hamman's sign is a "crunching" sound or a slight clicking sound with each heart sound auscultated over the apex of the heart.

49. **Correct answer: B**

    Not placing the ABG sample on ice will cause the $PaCO_2$ to rise approximately 3–10 mmHg per hour and invalidate the sample. The PaO_2 and the pH will decrease. Even with the advent of new technology, there are still facilities where samples have to be manually transported to a central testing site.

50. **Correct answer: B**

    Methylxanthines are an important classification of drugs. In addition to theophylline, caffeine and theobromine are also methylxanthines. Methylxanthines can be found in coffee, tea, and cocoa. Low doses of drugs in this classification can stimulate cortical arousal and in higher doses cause insomnia. They can cause tachycardias and increase production of gastric acid and digestive enzymes. Methylxanthines also inhibit histamine release.

51. **Correct answer: A**

    Jack is probably hypochloremic. Chronic hypoxia leads to chronic respiratory acidosis. The kidneys then retain bicarbonate in the form of sodium bicarbonate. The bicarbonate is exchanged for sodium chloride. Ammonia is an acid, and excess amounts must be removed from the body. This is done by releasing ammonium chloride. In chronic hypoxia there is an increase in bicarbonate levels and a decrease in chloride levels. Other causes of hypochloremia are NG suction, vomiting, and diarrhea.

52. **Correct answer: D**
    Hypoxemia is a decreased oxygen level in the arterial blood or a $PaO_2 < 80$ mmHg. Hypoxia is a decreased oxygen level at the cellular level.

53. **Correct answer: C**
    At higher altitudes there is decreasing atmospheric pressure to force oxygen into the lungs, and therefore the O_2 saturation would decrease. To compensate, the person must breathe faster. The percentage of oxygen remains the same and the partial pressure of the oxygen decreases. Arterial PaO_2 decreases and the O_2 saturation decreases as well. The rapid breathing will result in hyperventilation, raising the pH and lowering the $PaCO_2$ levels.

54. **Correct answer: C**
    Hyperventilating causes respiratory alkalosis because the patient is unable to get enough oxygen due to bronchial constriction. Hypoventilation causes a buildup of CO_2, causing respiratory acidosis.

55. **Correct answer: B**
    Neostigmine counteracts the effects of Pavulon. Neostigmine is an enzyme that prevents acetylcholine breakdown into its enzyme. It improves impulse transmission. Sometimes the neostigmine causes bradycardia and increases bronchial secretions, so atropine may be used with the neostigmine to mitigate the effects. Narcan is an opioid antagonist.

56. **Correct answer: B**
    Airflow in a patient with status asthmaticus may be improved by the use of heliox. Heliox is a helium–oxygen mixture that can help with delivery of inhaled medications to decrease the work of breathing. The PEEP must be carefully regulated so as not to cause barotrauma or a dynamic hyperinflation and it might improve airflow. Norepinephrine is a vasoconstrictor. Nebulizers may also work, but if the patient is compromised the effectiveness is minimal at best

57. **Correct answer: D**
    If you hear faint breath sounds on the left side of the chest and normal sounds on the right side immediately after your patient has been intubated, most likely the right mainstem bronchus has been intubated. The right mainstem bronchus is somewhat wider and has less of an angle off the mainstem bronchus, so it is much more readily intubated.

58. **Correct answer: C**
    Inhaled nitric oxide (iNO) is a selective pulmonary vasodilator to treat pulmonary hypertension. iNO reduces death or the need for extracorporeal membrane oxygenation (ECMO), but the positive effect is in reducing the ECMO requirement. Do not use iNO on patients who are dependent on a right-to-left shunt.

59. **Correct answer: A**
    An action of nitric oxide is to cause vascular smooth muscle relaxation. Nitric oxide is the molecule released from the endothelium that enables smooth muscle relaxation. Nitric oxide inhibits platelet aggregation and adherence and is thought to alter

vascular permeability. Nitric oxide may also participate in nonspecific immunity because it is generated when macrophages are activated.

60. **Correct answer: D**

    CPAP, or continuous positive airway pressure, may be delivered by nasal prongs, nasopharyngeal tubes, or endotracheal tubes. CPAP provides increased pressure to the posterior pharynx and increases transpulmonary pressure. CPAP can prevent alveolar collapse and helps prevent obstructive apnea.

61. **Correct answer: B**

    Excessive CPAP may increase intrathoracic pressure to the point of compressing the right atrium and vena cava. The preload will be decreased and cardiac output will be reduced.

62. **Correct answer: C**

    If positive inspiratory pressure (PIP) is increased on a mechanical ventilator, the result is a decrease in the $PaCO_2$ and an increase in the PaO_2.

63. **Correct answer: C**

    If a patient is retaining pCO_2, it is possible to help wash it out by increasing the respiratory rate (the ventilator rate in this case) or increasing the tidal volume.

64. **Correct answer: B**

    A disadvantage of using a pressure ventilator is possible overdistention. Lung compliance can change fairly quickly. Compliance can be likened to the elasticity of the lung. If it is less compliant, it can be described as stiffer. If it is more compliant, it can be said to be easier to inflate and deflate. If a pressure ventilator is used and the lung becomes more compliant, the alveoli and lung may overdistend. If the lung is less compliant, less tidal volume will be delivered because the ventilator only delivers to a preset volume.

65. **Correct answer: B**

    In a volume-limited ventilator, it is possible to increase ventilation by increasing the delivered tidal volume or increasing the ventilator rate. Oxygenation can be increased by increasing the PEEP, FiO_2, or tidal volume.

66. **Correct answer: B**

    High-frequency ventilators have the advantage of transporting CO_2 out of the lungs with smaller pressure and volume fluctuations than are required during conventional mechanical ventilation. Originally, it was thought that adequate gas exchange could be obtained at relatively low mean airway pressures, but now it is known that recruiting lung volume is essential in not only optimizing oxygenation but also in minimizing lung injury.

67. **Correct answer: B**

    High-frequency jet ventilators (HFJV) deliver high-flow, short-duration pulses of pressurized gas directly into the upper airway through a specially made endotracheal lumen. The pulses are delivered to the upper airway and are superimposed on gas flow from a conventional ventilator that provides positive end-expiratory pressure (PEEP). In addition, conventional breaths may be delivered in conjunction with the jet ventilation. The systems operate at rates of 150–600 breaths per minute and exhalation is passive.

68. **Correct answer: B**
    On a high-frequency ventilator, the sigh setting is a backup rate that provides a set number of ventilations per minute that recruit additional alveoli and minimize microatelectasis while high-frequency ventilation is utilized.

69. **Correct answer: C**
    This result is uncompensated respiratory alkalosis. The pH is greater than 7.45 so the value is an uncompensated alkalosis. To determine whether the alkalosis is respiratory or metabolic, find the value that represents alkalosis. In this case, the CO_2 at < 35 mmHg.

70. **Correct answer: A**
    This result is compensated metabolic acidosis. The pH is between 7.35 and 7.45, so the value is compensated, but because it is closer to 7.35, the value is considered acidotic. To determine whether the acidosis is respiratory or metabolic, find the value that represents acidosis. In this case, the HCO_3 at < 22 mEq/L.

71. **Correct answer: C**
    The pH is between 7.35 and 7.45, the CO_2 is between 35 and 45 mmHg, and the HCO_3 is between 22 and 26 mEq/L. All the results are within normal ranges, so this ABG is considered normal.

72. **Correct answer: A**
    This result is an uncompensated (mixed) respiratory/metabolic alkalosis. The pH is greater than 7.45 so the value is uncompensated. To determine whether the acidosis is respiratory or metabolic, find the value that represents alkalosis. This would be both the HCO_3 at > 26 mEq/L and the CO_2 < 35 mmHg, meaning the cause of the alkalosis is both respiratory and metabolic in nature.

73. **Correct answer: B**
    This ABG result indicates a compensated respiratory acidosis. The pH is between 7.35 and 7.45, so the value is compensated, but because it is closer to 7.35 the value is considered acidotic. To determine whether the acidosis is respiratory or metabolic, find the value that represents acidosis. In this case, the CO_2 at > 45 mmHg.

74. **Correct answer: D**
    The result of this blood gas analysis is an uncompensated metabolic acidosis. The pH is less than 7.35, so the value is uncompensated acidosis. To determine whether the acidosis is respiratory or metabolic, find the value that represents acidosis. In this case, the HCO_3 < 22 mEq/L.

75. **Correct answer: C**
    This blood gas result indicates an uncompensated respiratory acidosis. The pH is < 7.35 so the value indicates an uncompensated acidosis. Next, determine which respiratory or metabolic value represents acidosis. In this case, the CO_2 at > 45 mmHg.

76. **Correct answer: A**
    This result is an uncompensated metabolic alkalosis. The pH is greater than 7.45, so the value is uncompensated. To determine whether the alkalosis is respiratory or metabolic, find the value that represents alkalosis. In this case, the HCO_3 at > 26 mEq/L.

77. **Correct answer: B**

    The pH is between 7.35 and 7.45, the CO_2 is between 35 and 45 mmHg, and the HCO_3 is between 22 and 26 mEq/L. All the results are within normal ranges, so this ABG is considered normal.

78. **Correct answer: D**

    This is an uncompensated (mixed) respiratory/metabolic acidosis. The pH is less than 7.35, so the value is uncompensated acidosis. To determine whether the acidosis is respiratory or metabolic, find the value that represents acidosis. This would be both the HCO_3 at < 22 mEq/L and the CO_2 > 45 mmHg, meaning the cause of the acidosis is both respiratory and metabolic in nature.

79. **Correct answer: B**

    This blood gas result indicates a compensated metabolic acidosis. The pH is between 7.35 and 7.45, so the gas is compensated, but the value is closer to acidosis, making the value compensated acidosis. Determine which respiratory or metabolic value is acidotic. In this case, the HCO_3 at < 22 mEq/L.

80. **Correct answer: A**

    This result signifies an uncompensated respiratory alkalosis. The pH is greater than 7.45, so the value is uncompensated alkalosis. To determine whether the alkalosis is respiratory or metabolic, find the value that represents alkalosis. In this case, the CO_2 at < 35 mmHg.

81. **Correct answer: C**

    This result demonstrates a compensated respiratory alkalosis. The pH is between 7.35 and 7.45, so the value is compensated, but because it is closer to 7.45, the value is considered alkalotic. To determine whether the alkalosis is respiratory or metabolic, find the value that represents alkalosis. In this case, the CO_2 at < 35 mmHg.

82. **Correct answer: B**

    This result is an uncompensated respiratory acidosis. The pH is less than 7.35, so the value is uncompensated. To determine whether the acidosis is respiratory or metabolic, find the value that represents acidosis. In this case, the CO_2 at > 45 mmHg.

83. **Correct answer: A**

    The pH (between 7.35 and 7.45), the CO_2 (between 35 and 45 mmHg), and the HCO_3 (22 and 26 mEq/L) are within normal ranges, so the ABG is considered normal.

84. **Correct answer: B**

    This result is an uncompensated (mixed) respiratory/metabolic acidosis. The pH is less than 7.35, so the value is uncompensated acidosis. To determine whether the acidosis is respiratory or metabolic, find the value that represents acidosis. This would be both the HCO_3 at < 22 mEq/L and the CO_2 > 45 mmHg, meaning the cause of the acidosis is both respiratory and metabolic in nature.

85. **Correct answer: D**

    The guidelines from the Centers for Disease Control and Prevention (CDC) recommend that any equipment that comes in direct contact with patient mucosal membranes must undergo wet-heat pasteurization at > 158°F for at least 30 minutes and be packaged in sterile wrapping for the next use. An autoclave may also be used for reusable equipment. Any single-use equipment is recommended for resterilization per FDA guidelines by a third-party agency prior to use with another patient. If equipment must be washed after sterilization, the CDC recommends the use of sterile water, not normal saline. Many emergency departments utilize the respiratory therapy department to maintain and sterilize all respiratory equipment. As a patient advocate, the nurse should be aware of and ensure equipment is properly sterilized prior to use on his or her patient.

86. **Correct answer: D**
Fluid therapy in ARDS is directed toward maintaining a low circulating fluid volume. The fluid volume is kept low to keep the PAOP (PCWP) at minimal levels. If too much fluid is present, there may be leakage through damaged capillaries into the interstitial space.

87. **Correct answer: C**
Normal saline use in tracheal suctioning research has proven that normal saline causes anxiety, increased risk for hospital-acquired pneumonia, and bronchoconstriction. Current recommendations focus on dry suctioning, frequent oral care, balanced hydration, and position changes prevent complications associated with intubation and mechanical ventilation.

88. **Correct answer: B**
SIMV, or synchronized intermittent mandatory ventilation, still provides a set frequency of breaths and either volume or pressure. The patient is permitted to breathe spontaneously at their own volume between mandatory ventilations. If the spontaneous breath occurs at the same time as a mandatory breath, the ventilator will synchronize with the patient, thus preventing "stacked" breaths. The other modes of ventilation listed (CMV, HFV, and oscillation) represent full control of setting by an operator and not the patient's responses.

89. **Correct answer: A**
This is a very advanced question. The topic discussed here is more for your awareness, rather than test content. The plateau or alveolar pressure should be limited to 30 cm H_2O, maximum. If a higher pressure is maintained, microvascular permeability is increased. The high pressure may also cause a stress fracture of capillary endothelium, epithelium, and basement membranes. This may cause the lung to completely rupture. If this happens, blood, fluids, proteins, and exudates will leak into the air spaces and the tissue. The reverse is also true, and air may leak into the tissues. If the pressure can be maintained at 30 cm H_2O, CO_2 may rise and cause a rise in intracranial pressure and a respiratory acidosis results. By slowly reducing tidal volume, the kidneys will be able to compensate for the respiratory acidosis.

90. **Correct answer: A**
One cause of decreased SvO_2 is an increased metabolic rate. An increased metabolic rate would increase the O_2 uptake by tissues resulting in a lower value measured by venous blood gases. The other answers result in a lower tissue oxygen requirement, and thus higher values of oxygen remain in the bloodstream.

91. **Correct answer: B**
When a closed system is used, there is extra weight that can increase tension on the catheter or tubing. This may cause the ET to move. Lack of available oxygen and cost effectiveness are characteristics of open catheter suctioning. The inline system is

multiuse and is cost effective. Many manufacturers make the inline tubing for both ET tubes and tracheostomy tubes. Nurses must make certain they are using the correct tube for suctioning. Another problem with the inline catheters is the extra tubing that hangs out when the catheter is not in use. Patients may easily reach this tubing and extubate themselves or push the catheter down the airway and obstruct airflow.

92. Correct answer: A

A disadvantage of using a tracheostomy tube is subcutaneous emphysema. There are a large number of potential complications with the use of a tracheostomy tube. Some of these complications include tracheal stenosis, tracheal malacia, aspiration, infection, hemorrhage, subcutaneous emphysema, and pneumothorax.

93. Correct answer: D

The function of a stoma stent is to keep the stoma tract open. The stents can be manufactured in either the straight or curved configuration. The stent rests against the anterior wall of the trachea and allows for freer passage of air and the patient can breathe spontaneously around the tube. Because of the differing nature of air passages, the stents are made straight and curved.

94. Correct answer: B

Silicone or plastic tracheostomy tubes contain wires. The magnet in the MRI will attract the wires in the tube. The silicone or plastic tubes cannot tolerate repeated cleanings. Use of a one-way speaking valve is contraindicated when using a foam cuff because the cuff may lie at an angle to the valve due to its orientation in the airway. Cost is actually higher to facilities because the tubes are difficult to keep clean and are labor intensive.

95. Correct answer: D

Ella is exhibiting signs and symptoms of oxygen toxicity after 5 days of oxygen therapy at > 50% FiO_2. Nonrebreather masks provide a minimum of 60% FiO_2 at 6 Lpm. An arterial blood gas would show an increased PaO_2 > 100 mmHg, ruling out respiratory failure (PaO_2 < 60) that would require intubation. The dry hacking cough rules out pulmonary edema and the need for Lasix. Numbness in the extremities is from the oxygen radicals in the blood, not a neurologic impairment that would indicate the need for a CT scan with possible tPA administration.

96. Correct answer: D

Four days of high FiO_2 has resulted in a nitrogen wash-out resulting in atelectasis. Nitrogen's high partial pressure is necessary to maintain alveolar inflation. It is important to titrate FiO_2 to maintain saturations within a prescribed range when oxygen therapy is utilized. Pulmonary edema results in coarse breath sounds. With a unilateral pneumothorax there would be tracheal deviation. Sepsis would not necessarily present with diminished breath sound, but with additional findings of increased purulent secretions, coarse breath sounds and altered laboratory diagnostic results.

97. Correct answer: C

From birth, chest wall compliance decreases. Much of the decrease is due to degeneration and calcification of the costal cartilage; the elasticity decreases as well. Vertebrae develop osteoporosis and a degree of kyphosis can occur. Weight gain is common and posture is affected. Children are more commonly suffering from obesity and frequently develop back problems early in life. The chest wall compliance decreases as does vital capacity. Residual volume increases, PaO_2 decreases, and $PaCO_2$ increases.

98. **Correct answer: A**
The oxyhemoglobin dissociation curve is a curve that reflects the relationship between dissolved oxygen and the affinity for oxygen by the hemoglobin molecule.

99. **Correct answer: D**
Mesothelioma is a cancer of the mesothelium. Most cases begin in the pleura or peritoneum. Mesothelioma is a relatively rare cancer, with approximately 2,000 new cases diagnosed in the United States each year. It occurs more often in men than in women, and the risk of developing this disease increases with age. Symptoms of mesothelioma may not appear until 30 to 50 years after exposure to asbestos. An increased risk of developing mesothelioma has been found among shipyard workers, people who work in asbestos mines and mills, producers of asbestos products, workers in the heating and construction industries, and other trades people.

Symptoms of mesothelioma include dyspnea, pleural effusions, weight loss, and abdominal pain and swelling due to an excess of fluid in the abdomen. Other symptoms of peritoneal mesothelioma may include bowel obstruction, clotting disorders, anemia, and fever. Symptoms with metastases may include pain, dysphagia, or swelling of the neck or face.

Asbestos has been widely used in many industrial products, including cement, duct linings, sound insulation, brake linings, roof shingles, flooring products, textiles, and thermal insulation. If tiny asbestos particles float in the air, especially during the manufacturing process, they may be inhaled or swallowed and can cause serious health problems. In addition to mesothelioma, exposure to asbestos increases the risk of lung cancer, asbestosis, and cancers of the trachea, larynx, and kidney. Smoking does not appear to increase the risk of mesothelioma, but the combination of smoking and exposure increases a person's risk of developing bronchial cancer.

While researching this topic I discovered a sobering piece of information: More than 110,000 schools in the United States still contain some form of asbestos.

100. **Correct answer: A**
Generally, the time it took for the intubator to complete the task is not documented. However, if there was an unusual occurrence or a complication, it should be properly documented. The depth of the tube is important to chart because it gives a reference point for any questions about tube migration. The size of the tube may be too small or large, so it would have to be adjusted to the next appropriate size. A CXR is done to confirm tube placement, and the time it is done should be documented. Any medications given during the procedure should be documented as to reason for administration, patient response, and follow-up, such as vital sign measurements or untoward reactions.

101. **Correct answer: B**
CPAP should be used with caution in patients with basilar skull fractures. Research has shown that pneumocephalus may occur if a basilar skull fracture exists. CPAP helps by increasing the functional residual capacity by helping to reexpand the alveoli. Patients who have acute cardiogenic pulmonary edema may also benefit from the use of CPAP.

102. **Correct answer: C**

Sildenafil is given orally to inhibit rapid rise in pulmonary artery pressure secondary to hypoxia.

103. **Correct answer: D**

Ketamine is both an analgesic and an amnestic.

104. **Correct answer: B**

Fingertip clubbing is an indication of chronic hypoxia.

105. **Correct answer: C**

The normal value is 35–40 mmHg, so perfusion is adequate. The mixed venous sample is a way of assessing ventilation and circulation. If the mixed venous PaO_2 is low, this means the tissues extract a normal amount of oxygen and return deoxygenated blood to the heart. The sample is drawn from the distal port of the pulmonary artery catheter.

106. **Correct answer: D**

A wider endotracheal tube is necessary. Pressures that exceed 60 mmHg usually mean only one side of the tube is sealed. The trachea is somewhat oval and the tube and cuff are circular. If there was a cuff leak, pressure would be lower and the patient might be able to speak or make noise with the tube in place.

107. **Correct answer: D**

A semireclining or upright position promotes upper lobe drainage. Fluid or secretions will collect if the patient is flat.

108. **Correct answer: C**

To evacuate hemothorax, the tube is placed in the fifth intercostal space, midaxillary line. The chest tube will be low in the thoracic cavity and uses gravity to help clear the fluid. If a hemothorax is not completely removed, there is a possibility an infection will result, which can lead to empyema. When assessing a patient, it is a good idea to ask (if possible) the origin of any small scars on the thoracic area. It may take years to develop a problem leading to this condition.

109. **Correct answer: B**

ARDS is a type of hypoxemic respiratory failure; the $PaCO_2$ may be decreased or normal. There may be a ventilation/perfusion mismatch (pneumonia, atelectasis) due to an intrapulmonary shunt. Or, there is increased alveolar dead space (shock, pulmonary embolism). Pulmonary fibrosis may reduce diffusion capacity (COPD, ARDS).

110. **Correct answer: C**

The patient will have a sudden decrease in the $PetCO_2$ due to loss of blood flow in the pulmonary vasculature. The decrease in blood flow increases dead space with a resultant decrease in the $PetCO_2$.

111. **Correct answer: C**

Sometimes balloons are old and weakened and rupture easily. The balloons are made of rubber and will disintegrate in the presence of circulating lipoproteins. If the balloon does rupture, it will not wedge, and you can attempt to aspirate blood through the inflation port. If you cannot aspirate the blood, the balloon is probably ruptured. Immediately place a piece of tape with a notation that the balloon is ruptured so the next nurse will not attempt to use the port and inject air into the pulmonary circulation. Sometimes the balloon shatters into small parts and these become emboli. Another precaution (before insertion) is to determine if the patient has a preexisting rubber allergy.

112. **Correct answer: B**
The hypoxemic drive to breathe originates in the aortic and carotid arteries. In the bifurcation of the internal and external carotid arteries, carotid bodies and aortic bodies (in the carotid arch) are chemoreceptors. When the supply of oxygen decreases, stimulation of the aortic and/or carotid bodies occurs and, in turn, stimulates cortical activity. The result is adrenal gland secretions (epinephrine, norepinephrine), tachycardia, tachypnea, increased respiratory rate, and increased blood pressure.

113. **Correct answer: A**
The functional residual capacity is defined as the amount of air in lungs after normal expiration. The formula for functional residual capacity is FRC = ERV (expired residual volume) + the RV (residual volume). The normal FRC in healthy lungs is about 2,000–3,000 ml.

114. **Correct answer: B**
Severe carbon monoxide poisoning occurs when carboxyhemoglobin levels are higher than 20–40%. If carbon monoxide levels are above 60%, the patient will be comatose and probably die.
   Smokers often have levels of 5–10%. Normal levels in nonsmokers are less than 2%.

115. **Correct answer: D**
Elimination of carbon monoxide from the body is via the lungs. In cases of severe carbon monoxide (CO) poisoning, hyperbaric therapy must be utilized to force the CO molecule off the hemoglobin, but it is eliminated by the lungs.

116. **Correct answer: D**
Subcutaneous emphysema usually occurs in the thorax as a result of a pulmonary air leak. This air leak may be secondary to the patient receiving positive pressure ventilation or from alveolar rupture from a pneumothorax. The air travels along under the skin and may be easily palpated and may feel like a crackling sensation. Patients who have chest tubes often have at least a small amount of subcutaneous emphysema at the tube insertion site. Sometimes the patient feels pain when palpation is performed because the air tears the tissue. The free air must be reabsorbed, and this may take several days.

117. **Correct answer: B**
Pulse oximetry should never be used during a cardiac arrest. During resuscitation, blood pressure and blood flow may vary. The pharmacologic effects of medications such as vasoactive drugs used during resuscitation will compromise SpO_2 values.

118. **Correct answer: B**
Pulse oximetry values do not directly correlate with PaO_2. You must use ABGs to determine PaO_2, the amount of oxygen available to the tissues. SpO_2 only measures the number of hemoglobin binding sites that are occupied compared with the number of hemoglobin binding sites available. The columns listed below show the probable correlation.

Values of Pulse Oximetry	Probable PaO$_2$
97	100
95	80
94	70
90	60
85	50
75	40
57	30
32	20
10	10

119. **Correct answer: C**

    To prevent complications with chest tube drainage systems, the suction level should not be higher than −40 cm/H$_2$O. Maintaining suction levels at higher than −40 cm/H$_2$O may cause re-expansion pulmonary edema, pleural air leaks, and lung tissue entrapment. The lung may not be able to expand properly.

120. **Correct answer: B**

    Chest tube drainage tubing should be placed horizontally on the bed and down to the collection chamber. If a mediastinal chest tube is in place, bubbling in the water seal chamber may indicate a communication between the mediastinal space and the pleural space. The physician should be notified immediately. However, some sporadic bubbling will occur when suction is first turned on because fluid has to displace air in the collection chamber. Chest tube tubing that is dependent or coiled will allow for the accumulation of drainage. This obstruction may increase pressure in the lung.

121. **Correct answer: C**

    Acetyl-cysteine is considered to be a mucolytic agent. Acetyl-cysteine has a sulfide group that effectively splits disulfine bonds in mucin molecules. The viscosity of the mucus is reduced. Atropine is an anticholinergic. Terbutaline and albuterol are B$_2$ agonists.

122. **Correct answer: D**

    Side effects of acetyl-cysteine include bronchospasms. Thinning the mucus may promote excessive coughing with resultant brochospasms. Additional side effects include rhinorrhea, stomatitus, nausea, and vomiting.

123. **Correct answer: D**

    Emphysema actually increases lung compliance. Pulmonary edema, pleural effusions, and obesity decrease lung compliance. Other factors that decrease compliance are atelectasis, fibrotic changes, abdominal distension, pain (causes splinting), and flail chest (pain and loss of structure).

124. **Correct answer: C**

    Prior to insertion of an LMA, the patient must have an absent gag reflex. The laryngeal mask airway cannot be inserted by nurses unless they have specialized training. The LMA does not usually cause hoarseness because it does not pass through the vocal cords. There is a high risk of aspiration with LMA usage.

125. **Correct answer: D**
One of the most effective ways to relieve bronchospasms is to use a B_2 receptor agonist. The B_2 receptor agonists lower cellular calcium levels and relax bronchial smooth muscle. The selective B_2 receptor agonists do not produce cardiac stimulation. The cardiac stimulation can result in tachycardia and reduced cardiac output.

126. **Correct answer: C**
Symptoms from aspirated gastric contents have a gradual onset. The patient may develop ARDS, but not always. If the pH is > 2.5, very little necrosis will occur. If the pH is < 2.5, there is probability of pulmonary edema, necrosis, bleeding, and atelectasis.

127. **Correct answer: C**
The best position to place this patient to minimize the venous air embolism is Trendelenburg with left decubitus tilt. This position minimizes any air from migrating through the heart and into the lungs.

128. **Correct answer: A**
A venous air embolism may be caused by hemodialysis. Other potential causes are central and pulmonary artery catheters, endoscopy, and automatic pressure-driven injectors.

129. **Correct answer: B**
A risk factor for thrombolic emboli includes carcinoma. Neoplasms, obesity, trauma, dysrhythmias, congestive heart failure (CHF), and prolonged immobility are also factors.

130. **Correct answer: C**
The definitive study for determination of thrombolic emboli is a pulmonary angiography.
This study involves catheterization of the right ventricle and then injective dye into the pulmonary artery. The pulmonary vasculature is easily seen. The location of the embolus is easily found because the dye trail comes to a sudden end.

131. **Correct answer: B**
Blood gas results you would expect to see for a patient with thrombotic emboli are pH 7.50, PaO_2 74, $PaCO_2$ 52, HCO_3 24. These blood gases indicate respiratory acidosis with hypoxemia.

132. **Correct answer: A**
Blood gases in a pregnant woman with complications indicate compensated respiratory alkalosis. Progesterone levels increase the respiratory rate and decrease the $PaCO_2$. The kidneys will increase bicarbonate production. The patient will hyperventilate, blowing off excess bicarbonate and raising the pH.

133. **Correct answer: A**
Prone positioning is the best position to promote drainage and oxygenation for a patient with ARDS. It is often the most difficult position to achieve without proper lifting and safety devices.

134. **Correct answer: C**
Pulmonary hypertension is generally defined as a mean pulmonary artery pressure of ≥ 25 mmHg. The increase in pressure may be related to increased blood flow or obstruction of blood flow through the lungs.

135. **Correct answer: C**

Patients with pulmonary hypertension present with dyspnea during exertion, right-sided heart failure, increased respiratory and heart rates, and a prominent S_2. Additional signs of pulmonary hypertension include fatigue and lethargy, enlarged liver, and pulmonary congestion. Cyanosis is a late sign of pulmonary hypertension.

136. **Correct answer: B**

Calcium channel blockers are used to treat primary pulmonary hypertension. Patients treated with nitric oxide improve faster when treated with calcium channel blockers due to abnormalities in the membrane function.

137. **Correct answer: D**

Without initial, aggressive treatment of pulmonary hypertension, the medial smooth muscles in arterioles irreversibly thicken. This is due to development of high right-sided ventricular pressures and heart failure.

138. **Correct answer: C**

Pulmonary hypertension results in hypoxia and hypoxemia, leading to vasoconstriction. As vasoconstriction continues, the vessel walls begin to alter with increase in elastin and collagen. Prolonged vasoconstriction leads to increased shunting and blood pooling. Serum testing for abnormalities further increases the risks and progression of irreversible epithelial changes.

139. **Correct answer: A**

An absolute contraindication for use of rapid sequence intubation (RSI) is a total loss of facial and/or oropharyngeal landmarks, which requires a surgical airway. Another absolute contraindication is a total upper airway obstruction that requires surgical intervention. Relative contraindications for RSI include an airway where intubation may not be successful or an arrest "crash" intubation when there is no time for pre-oxygenation, pretreatment, or induction and paralysis.

140. **Correct answer: D**

Rapid sequence intubation (RSI) is not necessary to use for all cervical spine–injured patients. It would be appropriate for use if there is edema and loss of airway patency. Prolonged respiratory effort that results in fatigue or failure, a stab wound to neck with an expanding hematoma, and an uncooperative trauma patient with life-threatening injuries are indications for use of RSI.

141. **Correct answer: C**

During rapid sequence intubation cricoid cartilage pressure is often used to help prevent vomiting and aspiration of gastric contents. The esophagus is obstructed by the pressure to the anterior neck. This maneuver is known as the Sellick maneuver.

142. **Correct answer: C**

Sternocleodomastoid retractions indicate that an asthmatic patient is using accessory muscles to facilitate ventilation. Air is trapped in the air passages, so the patient has to create a higher negative pleural pressure by elevating the rib cage.

143. **Correct answer: C**

Your patient ceased wheezing during his asthma attack. This change in his condition means respiratory failure and intubation are imminent. If the patient is wheezing, that means air is at least traveling through air passages. When the lumen in the bronchioles is totally closed from swelling or an obstruction, wheezing ceases.

144. **Correct answer: B**
Wheezing would not be present if the patient had pneumonia. There is an old mnemonic for asthma that can assist the ED nurse with determining a possible cause of a patient's distress. This mnemonic is ASTHMATIC:

A	Asthma	Precipitating factor or event
S	Stasis	DVT, pulmonary embolus
T	Toxins	Smoke, chemical irritants, insecticides, perfumes, cleaning agents
H	Heart	CHF, noncardiogenic pulmonary edema
M	Mechanical	Foreign body aspiration
A	Allergy	Anaphylaxis, aspiration (gastric contents), near drowning
T	Trauma	Upper airway, possible lower airway
I	Infection	Bronchitis, bronchiolitis, croup, pneumonia
C	Congenital	Cystic fibrosis
	Chronic	COPD

145. **Correct answer: D**
Slo-BID is a form of theophylline. Side effects of theophylline include muscle cramps, jitteryness, headache, nausea, vomiting, dysrhythmias, and gastrointestinal issues.

146. **Correct answer: A**
Long-acting forms of B_2 agonists used in the treatment of asthma include salmeterol (Serevent®) and formoterol (Foradil®). Short-acting beta$_2$ agonists used for emergency treatment of asthma include albuterol (Proventil® HFA, Ventolin® HFA, Accuneb®, ProAir®), metaproterenol (Alupent®), levalbuterol (Xoponex® HFA, Xoponex® nebulizer solution), and pirbuterol (Maxair®).

147. **Correct answer: B**
This patient probably has a pneumomediastinum. The crunching sound is known as Hamman's sign. The sound varies with the heartbeat and is more pronounced in the left lateral decubitus position at the apex.

148. **Correct answer: B**
The most common symptoms seen with active TB are night sweats, fever, fatigue, hemoptysis, weight loss, and chest pain. The cough would not be dry, and there would not be wheezing.

149. **Correct answer: A**
The patient has a positive PPD. Until a chest x-ray and AFB sputum culture are done, this patient is highly suspicious for TB. It is important to find out if the patient received BCG if they were born outside the United States. Once TB is confirmed, treatment should start right away for this patient and he should be placed in a room with a laminar airflow system.

150. **Correct answer: C**
Rimantadine is used to shorten the length and severity of influenza. Isoniazid, rifampin, and pyrazidamide are all medications used to treat latent TB infections.

SECTION 4: PULMONARY REFERENCES

Abman, S. (2008). The dysmorphic pulmonary circulation in bronchopulmonary dysplasia: A growing story. *American Journal of Respiratory and Critical Care Medicine, 178*(2), 114–115.

Agbaht, K., Lisboa, T., Pobo, A., Rodriguez. A., Sandiumenge, A., Diaz, E., & Rello, J. (2007). Management of ventilator-associated pneumonia in a multidisciplinary intensive care unit: Does trauma make a difference? *Intensive Care Medicine, 33*(8), 1387–1395.

Ahrens, T., & Sona, C. (2003). Capnography application in acute and critical care. *AACN Clinical Issues, 14,* 123–132.

American Heart Association. (2010). Guidelines 2010 for cardiopulmonary resuscitation and emergency cardiovascular care. Retrieved October 18, 2010, from www.americanheart.org

Antonelli, M., Azoulay, E., Bonten, M., Chastre, J., Citerio, G., Conti, G., . . . De Backer, D. (2010). Year in review in intensive care medicine 2009. Part III: Mechanical ventilation, acute lung injury and respiratory distress syndrome, pediatrics, ethics and miscellanea. *Intensive Care Medicine, 36*(4), 567–584.

Baltacioğlu, F., Çimşit, N., Bostanci, K., Yüksel, M., & Kodalli, N. (2010). Transarterial microcatheter glue embolization of the bronchial artery for life-threatening hemoptysis: Technical and clinical results. *European Journal of Radiology, 73*(2), 380–384.

Bashore, T. M., Granger, C. B., Hranitzky, P., & Patel, M. R. (2010). Heart disease. In S. J. McPhee & M. A. Papadakis (Eds.), *Lange 2010 current medical diagnosis and treatment* (49th ed., pp. 358–366). New York: McGraw-Hill Medical.

Bhandari, V., Choo-Wing, R., Lee, C., Yusuf, K., Nedrelow, J. H., Ambalavanan, N., . . . Elias, J. A. (2008). Developmental regulation of NO-mediated VEGF-induced effects in the lung. *American Journal of Respiratory Cell and Molecular Biology, 39*(4), 420–430.

Bigatello, L. M., Davidson, K. R., & Stelfox, H. T. (2005). Respiratory mechanics and ventilatory waveforms in the patient with acute lung injury. *Respiratory Care, 50*(2), 235–245.

Caruana, J. A., Anain, P. M., & Pham, D. T. (2009). The pulmonary embolism risk score system reduces the incidence and mortality of pulmonary embolism after gastric bypass. *Surgery, 146*(4), 678–685.

Centers for Disease Control and Prevention. (2002). Guideline for hand hygiene in health-care settings: Recommendations of the healthcare infection control practices advisory committee and the HICPAC/SHEA/APIC/IDSA hand hygiene task force. *Morbidity and Mortality Weekly Report, 51*(RR16), 1–44.

Centers for Disease Control and Prevention. (2004). Guidelines for preventing health-care associated pneumonia: 2003 recommendations of the CDC and the healthcare infection control practices advisory committee. *Morbidity and Mortality Weekly Report, 53*(RR03), 1–36.

Chernecky, C., & Berger, B. (2004). *Laboratory tests and diagnostic procedures* (4th ed.). Philadelphia: Saunders.

Chun, J-Y., & Belli, A-M. (2010). Immediate and long-term outcomes of bronchial and non-bronchial systemic artery embolisation for the management of haemoptysis. *European Radiology, 20*(3), 558–565.

Church, D. G., Matthay, M. A., Liu, K., Milet, M., & Flori, H. (2009). Blood product transfusions and clinical outcomes in pediatric patients with acute lung injury. *Pediatric Critical Care Medicine, 10*(3), 297–302.

Cosentini, R., Aliberti, S., Bignamini, A., Piffer, F., & Brambilla, A. M. (2009). Mortality in acute cardiogenic pulmonary edema treated with continuous positive airway pressure. *Intensive Care Medicine, 35*(2), 299–305.

Dellamonica, J., Louis, B., Lyazidi, A., Vargas, F., & Brochard, L. (2008). Intrapulmonary percussive ventilation superimposed on conventional ventilation: bench study of humidity and ventilator behaviour. *Intensive Care Medicine, 34*(11), 2035–2043.

Dueker, C. W. (2004). Immersion in fresh water and survival. *Chest, 126*(6), 2027–2028.

Durbin, C. G. (2005). Applied respiratory physiology: Uses of ventilator waveforms and mechanics in the management of critically ill patients. *Respiratory Care, 50,* 287–293.

Emergency Nurses Association, Newberry, L., & Criddle, L. M. (2007). *Sheehy's manual of emergency care* (6th ed.). St. Louis, MO: Mosby.

Eppert, H. D. (2010). Disease prevention update: Tetanus toxoid, reduced diphtheria toxoid, and acellular pertussis—who, what, when, why, and how? *JEN: Journal of Emergency Nursing, 36*(2), 122–124.

Frankel, S. K., & Schwarz, M. (2009). Update in idiopathic pulmonary fibrosis. *Current Opinion in Pulmonary Medicine, 15*(5), 463–469

Fung, Y. L., & Silliman, C. C. (2009). The role of neurophils in the pathogenesis of transfusion-related acute lung injury. *Transfusion Medicine Reviews, 23*(4), 266–283.

Gasparis Vonfrolio, L., & Noone, J. (1997). *Emergency nursing examination review* (3rd ed.). Staten Island, NY: Power Publications.

Grewal, S., Ali, S., McConnell, D. W., Vandermeer, B., & Klassen, T. P. (2009). A randomized trial of nebulized 3% hypertonic saline with epinephrine in the treatment of acute bronchiolitis in the emergency department. *Archives of Pediatrics and Adolescent Medicine, 163*(11), 1007–1012.

Guyton, A. C., & Hall, J. E. (2005). *Textbook of medical physiology* (11th ed.). Philadelphia, PA: Saunders.

Halliday, H. (2008). Surfactants: past, present and future. *Journal of Perinatology, 28*(S1), S47–S56.

Hardin, S. R., & Kaplow, R. (2010). *Cardiac surgery essentials for critical care nursing*. Sudbury, MA: Jones & Bartlett Learning.

Hickey, J. V. (2008). *The clinical practice of neurological and neurosurgical nursing* (6th ed.). Philadelphia, PA: Lippincott Williams & Wilkins.

Holleran, R. S. (2005). *Emergency transport nursing* (4th ed.). St. Louis, MO: Mosby.

Hoshino, T., Kato, S., Oka, N., Imaoka, H., Kinoshita, T., Takei, S., . . . Aizawa, H. (2007). Pulmonary inflammation and emphysema: Role of the cytokines IL-18 and IL-13. *American Journal of Respiratory and Critical Care Medicine, 176*(1), 49–62.

Hwang, J. H., Misumi, S., Sahin, H., Brown, K. K., Newell, J. D., & Lynch, D. A. (2009). Computed tomographic features of idiopathic fibrosing interstitial pneumonia: Comparison with *pulmonary* fibrosis related to collagen vascular disease. *Journal of Computer Assisted Tomography, 33*(3), 410–415.

Inal, M. T. (2007). Laryngospasm-induced pulmonary edema. *Internet Journal of Anesthesiology, 15*(1), 5.

Iyer, V., Joshi, A., & Ryu, J. (2009). Spontaneous pneumomediastinum: Analysis of 62 consecutive adult patients. *Mayo Clinic Proceedings, 84*(5), 417–421.

Jacobs, B. B., and Hoyt, K. S. (2007). *Trauma nursing core course provider manual* (6th ed.). Bedford, IL: Emergency Nurses Association.

Johnson, J. M. (2009). Management of acute cardiogenic pulmonary edema: A literature review. *Advanced Emergency Nursing Journal, 31*(1), 36–43.

Jones & Bartlett Learning (2011). *2011 nurse's drug handbook* (10th ed.). Sudbury, MA: Jones & Bartlett Learning.

Jones, K. L. (2006). *Smith's recognizable patterns of human malformation* (6th ed.). Philadelphia, PA: Elsevier.

Kealey, G. P. (2009). Carbon monoxide toxicity. *Journal of Burn Care and Research, 30*(1), 146–147.

Lippincott. (2010). *Professional guide to signs and symptoms* (6th ed.). Philadelphia, PA: Lippincott.

Maggiorini, M. (2010). Prevention and treatment of high-altitude pulmonary edema. *Progress in Cardiovascular Diseases, 52*(6), 500–506.

Martin, B. (2010). Family presence during resuscitation and invasive procedures: AACN practice alert. Retrieved from http://www.aacn.org

Medina, J., & Puntillo, K. (2006). *AACN protocols for practice: Palliative care and end-of-life issues in critical care*. Sudbury, MA: Jones and Bartlett.

Mireku, N., Wang, Y., Ager, J., Reddy, R. C., & Baptist, A. P. (2009). Changes in weather and the effects on pediatric asthma exacerbations. *Annals of Allergy, Asthma & Immunology, 103*(3), 220–224.

Mohsen, T., Zeid, A. A., & Haj-Yahia, S. (2007). Lobectomy or pneumonectomy for multidrug-resistant pulmonary tuberculosis can be performed with acceptable morbidity and mortality: A seven-year review of a single institution's experience. *Journal of Thoracic and Cardiovascular Surgery, 134*(1), 194–198.

Mulkey, Z., Yarbrough, S., Guerra, D., Roongsritong, C., Nugent, K., & Phy, M. P. (2008). Postextubation *pulmonary* edema: A case series and review. *Respiratory Medicine, 102*(11), 1659–1662.

Prescribing Reference. (2009, Summer). *NPPR: Nurse Practitioner's Prescribing Reference, 16*(2).

Proehl, J. A. (2008). *Emergency nursing procedures* (4th ed.). St. Louis, MO: Saunders.

Roch, A., Blayac, D., Ramiara, P., Chetaille, B., Marin, V., Michelet, P., . . . Carpentier, J. P. (2007). Comparison of lung injury after normal or small volume optimized resuscitation in a model of hemorrhagic shock. *Intensive Care Medicine, 33*(9), 1645–1654.

Spooner, L. M., & Liu, E. (2009). Tuberculosis, CNS. In F. J. Domino, R. A. Baldor, A. M. Erlich, & J. Golding (Eds.), *The 5-minute clinical consult 2010* (18th ed., pp. 1358–1359). Philadelphia, PA: Lippincott Williams & Wilkins.

Stenmark, K. R., & Rabinovitch, M. (2010). Emerging therapies for the treatment of pulmonary hypertension. *Pediatric Critical Care Medicine, 11*(2 suppl), S85–S90.

Suntharalingam, J., Treacy, C. M., Doughty, N. J., Goldsmith, K., Soon, E., Toshner, M. R., & Pepke-Zaba, J. (2008). Long-term use of sildenafil in inoperable chronic thromboembolic pulmonary hypertension. *Chest, 134*(2), 229–236.

Tsangaris, I., Galiatsou, E., Kostanti, E., & Nakos, G. (2007). The effect of exogenous surfactant in patients with lung contusions and acute lung injury. *Intensive Care Medicine, 33*(5), 851–855.

Urdem, L. D., Stacy, K. M., & Lough, M. E. (2005). *Thelan's critical care nursing* (5th ed.). St. Louis, MO: Mosby.

Varpula, M., Tallgren, M., Saukkonen, K., Voipio-Pulkki, L., & Pettilä, V. (2005). Hemodynamic variables related to outcome in septic shock. *Intensive Care Medicine, 31*(8), 1066–1071.

Watson, S., & Gorski, K. A. (2011). *Invasive cardiology* (3rd ed.). Sudbury, MA: Jones & Bartlett Learning.

Wing, R., Lee, C., Yusuf, K., Nedrelow, J., Ambalavanan, N., Malkus, H., Homer, R., & Elias, J. (2008). Developmental regulation of NO-mediated VEGF-induced effects in the lung. *American Journal of Respiratory Cell and Molecular Biology, 39*(4), 420–430.

Yiming, M., Lederer, D., Sun, L., Huertas, A., Issekutz, A., & Bhattacharya, S. (2008). Platelets enhance endothelial adhesiveness in high tidal volume ventilation. *American Journal of Respiratory Cell and Molecular Biology, 39*(5), 569–575.

SECTION 5:

Orthopedic and Musculoskeletal

1. Which of the following statements about splints is true?
   A. An air splint is inflatable and provides soft padding to an extremity
   B. Hard splints increase angulation
   C. Traction splints decrease angulation
   D. A traction splint may be soft and nonrigid

2. A third-degree strain is distinguished by
   A. Point tenderness, localized pain
   B. Spasm
   C. Loss of muscle function
   D. Ecchymosis

3. A fracture at the junction of the proximal and middle thirds of the ulna is known as
   A. A Volkmann's fracture
   B. A Monteggia's fracture
   C. An intercondylar fracture
   D. A Colles' fracture

4. Your patient was climbing a ladder in an attempt to hang Christmas lights. He slipped and fell on his outstretched arm. He sustained a fracture to the distal ends of the radius and ulna. This type of fracture is known as a
   A. Colles' fracture
   B. Navicular fracture
   C. Scaphoid fracture
   D. Volkmann's fracture

5. Which of the following statements about a stable pelvic fracture is true?
   A. A stable pelvic fracture results when the posterior elements of the ring are disrupted
   B. Stable pelvic fractures are only caused by direct trauma and crush injuries
   C. Stable fractures cause large amounts of bleeding
   D. Stable fractures do not transect the pelvic ring

6. The type of knee injury most likely to be caused by hyperextension trauma is
   A. A medial meniscus injury
   B. Severe muscle injury
   C. Anterior and posterior cruciate ligament injury
   D. A patellar dislocation

7. A distinguishing characteristic of a patellar fracture is
   A. Patient inability to abduct the leg
   B. Patient inability to actively extend the knee
   C. The examiner's inability to adduct the leg
   D. The examiner's inability to aspirate fluid from the knee area

8. Your patient was running to first base during a baseball game. When he placed his foot on the bag he heard a loud sound and could not apply weight on that leg. He is in moderate pain and cannot bear weight on the affected leg. You suspect
   A. A patellar fracture
   B. A severe quadriceps tear
   C. An Achilles tendon rupture
   D. An anterior cruciate ligament tear

9. Which of the following actions should not be performed initially in the ED when a patient has sustained a pelvic fracture?
   A. A FAST examination
   B. Placement of a urinary catheter
   C. Administration of analgesia
   D. Administration of a neuromuscular blockade

10. If a patient has truncal obesity and has sustained a pelvic fracture, it is possible to initially stabilize the fracture via
    A. Internal rotation of lower extremities and taping the knees together
    B. Closing the fracture under fluoroscopy
    C. Surgery only
    D. Fluoroscopy

11. Which of the following medications is not appropriate for initial treatment of a patient with a pelvic fracture?
    A. Hydrocodone bitartrate
    B. Oxycodone and acetaminophen
    C. Fentanyl
    D. NSAIDs

12. Pelvic fractures are usually classified as stable or unstable. The definition of an unstable pelvic fracture is
    A. A fracture where the pelvic ring is broken in one section and no rotational displacement exists
    B. A fracture with external rotation, vertical compression, and without shear
    C. The pelvic ring is fractured in more than one place with two displacements on the ring
    D. A fracture that involves moderate displacement of the ring

13. Your patient has sustained an ulnar fracture. Which of the following types of splints would be appropriate for this type of injury?
    A. A spade splint
    B. A gutter splint
    C. A spica splint
    D. A Hare splint

14. The most common forearm fracture is a
    A. Colles' fracture
    B. Homan's fracture
    C. Volkmann's fracture
    D. Distal radius fracture

15. Humerus stress fractures are likely to occur from unconditioned or immature bones and muscles when engaged in
    A. Playing ice hockey
    B. Catching a football
    C. Bowling
    D. Pitching a baseball overhand

16. An example of a pathologic cause of a proximal humerus fracture is
    A. An automobile accident
    B. Bone cancer
    C. A fall
    D. Sports injuries

17. The nerve most commonly injured in a proximal humerus fracture is
    A. The axillary nerve
    B. The radial nerve
    C. The suprascapular nerve
    D. The musculocutaneous nerve

18. Your patient has sustained a proximal humerus fracture and damage to the radial nerve. Which of the following observations validates this type of injury?
    A. Swelling at the wrist
    B. Extension of the forefinger and middle finger
    C. Wrist drop
    D. The patient guarding his shoulder

19. Your patient is a 40 year old woman who presents with complaints of inability to sleep, an ache in the right shoulder, pain on palpation of the right deltoid, and pain when attempting to internally rotate the right arm. The most probable cause of these symptoms is
    A. A fractured proximal humerus
    B. A shoulder separation
    C. A chronic rotator cuff tear
    D. A shoulder dislocation

20. Which of the following muscles is not part of the rotator cuff?
    A. Deltoid
    B. Supraspinatus
    C. Subscapularis
    D. Teres minor

21. The retroperitoneal space may accumulate as much as _____ liter(s) of blood before venous tamponade occurs.
    A. One
    B. Two
    C. Four
    D. Five

22. Which of the following statements is true about an acute rotator cuff tear?
    A. Symptoms appear slowly and result in moderate diffuse pain in the arm
    B. The patient is unable to adduct the arm and there is severe pain
    C. The patient experiences pain in the affected arm for about 6 hours
    D. The patient may feel a tearing sensation and exhibit point tenderness over the site

23. The type of amputation that has the greatest chance of reimplantation is
    A. Shearing
    B. Guillotine
    C. Avulsive
    D. Crush

24. The most serious complication of casting and splinting is
    A. Decreased circulation
    B. Paresthesias
    C. Pain
    D. Compartment syndrome

25. Which of the following statements about splints is not correct?
    A. Splints are easier to apply than casts
    B. Splints are easily removed for inspection of an injured area
    C. Splints allow for swelling during the acute phase of an injury
    D. Splints are circumferential

26. Which of the following conditions is usually not a consideration when deciding whether to apply a splint or a cast?
    A. The potential for instability
    B. The risk of complications
    C. The severity of a sprain
    D. The patient's functional requirements

27. A 28 year old male presents with peristernal pain that worsens on inspiration and movement. The patient states the pain began during a tennis match. On inspection no visual swelling, deformity, or ecchymosis is seen. On palpation the skin temperature is noted to be normal and there is point tenderness over the area. It is likely this patient is suffering from
    A. Pericarditis
    B. A pleural effusion
    C. Costochondritis
    D. A fractured rib

28. A closed wound that occurs when a blood vessel ruptures and bleeds into surrounding tissue is known as a(n)
    A. Hematoma
    B. Contusion
    C. Abrasion
    D. Lacunar stroke

29. At 5 to 7 days after a contusion is sustained, the contusion changes color from the periphery to the inside and becomes
    A. Reddish blue
    B. Yellow
    C. Brown
    D. Green

30. If a patient presents with contusions that are yellow tinged, the contusion is probably about _____ days old.
    A. 1–5
    B. 5–7
    C. 7–10
    D. 10–14

31. Your patient was a restrained passenger in a rollover accident and sustained only multiple contusions on both legs. Appropriate patient teaching about RICE therapy includes
    A. Keeping feet and legs dependent to increase the blood flow to the area
    B. Do not wrap or splint the extremities
    C. Do not take analgesics for 48 hours
    D. Apply cold packs ×20 minutes, four times a day for 48–72 hours

32. The ED physician is evaluating a patient for carpal tunnel syndrome. The physician will attempt to elicit Tinel's sign. Tinel's sign is considered positive when
    A. Pain is felt in the ring finger of the affected arm
    B. Pain and paresthesia worsen when the medial nerve is tapped
    C. Numbness occurs when the back of the hands are pressed together for 1 minute
    D. The thumb can be adducted

33. When performing a peripheral nerve assessment for ulnar nerve impairment, normal findings include
    A. The ability to fan the fingers and have feeling on top of the small finger
    B. Feeling on the dorsum of the thumb and the ability to extend the thumb
    C. The ability to oppose the thumb to base of small finger and to feel on the tip of the index finger
    D. Feeling on the palm and ability to clench the fist

34. A deformity of the distal portion of a joint that is angulated away from the midline of the body is called a
    A. Sprain
    B. Valgus
    C. Varus
    D. Strain

35. A C-reactive protein level would be negative in a patient with
    A. Pneumonia
    B. Rheumatoid arthritis
    C. Widespread metastases
    D. Acute inflammation

36. The type of fracture caused by an angulation force of direct trauma is known as
    A. An oblique fracture
    B. A spiral fracture
    C. A transverse fracture
    D. A depressed fracture

37. A complete joint disruption with the articular surfaces no longer in contact is known as a(n)
    A. Strain
    B. Dislocation
    C. Avulsion
    D. Subluxation

38. A posterior dislocation of the glenohumeral joint in the shoulder may be caused by
    A. Falls from bicycles or motorcycles
    B. An athletic injury, usually a recurrent injury
    C. A direct blow to the point of the shoulder
    D. Seizures

39. Which of the following statements is true regarding management of a severed part after a traumatic amputation?
    A. Leave all foreign matter intact so it can be removed in the operating room
    B. Place the part in ice water for transport
    C. Scrub the severed part gently
    D. Rinse the part with a sterile isotonic solution

40. A contraindication to the use of a vacuum splint is
    A. All jewelry must be removed
    B. Open wounds must be covered prior to application
    C. Traction must be applied to the limb before the splint may be applied
    D. The splint is nontransparent

41. Which of the following statements is true regarding the use of air splints?
    A. Air splints are not suitable for angulated fractures
    B. Overinflation may not provide adequate support to a fracture
    C. Air splints are effective for fractures of the femur or humerus
    D. Once inflated, air splints maintain rigidity and require little maintenance

42. Which statement does not represent a complication of air splinting?
    A. Talcum powder or cornstarch causes breakdown of the skin
    B. Excessive pressure variations may exist
    C. Compression of nerves may occur
    D. Removal may be difficult

43. When applying an air splint to an elderly patient, the ED nurse should consider
    A. Elevating the limb to aid blood flow to the heart
    B. Placing a thin layer of smooth padding under the splint
    C. Adducting the limb to ease stress
    D. Twisting the valve counterclockwise to even pressures and prevent skin breakdown

44. The preferred splint for a femur fracture is
    A. Kirschner wire
    B. A fiberglass spica splint
    C. A traction splint
    D. A posterior long leg splint

45. Which of the following types of traction splints is classified as a unipolar traction splint?
    A. Hare
    B. Fernotrac
    C. Kendrick
    D. Thomas

46. Traction splints are used for
    A. Distal fibula fractures
    B. Distal tibia fractures
    C. Upper extremity fractures
    D. Femur fractures

47. Which of the following splints can be applied by one person?
    A. Hare splint
    B. Thomas splint
    C. Kendrick splint
    D. Sager splint

48. The _____ traction splint does not require anterior padding in the anterior groin area.
    A. Kendrick
    B. Hare
    C. Sager
    D. Thomas

49. You are assisting with the fitting of a patient for a walker. Your patient should have his or her elbow bent at
    A. 20 degrees
    B. 30 degrees
    C. 40 degrees
    D. 45 degrees

50. Forrest fractured his humerus in a car accident 3 weeks ago. Yesterday he developed a fever and now has a temperature of 101.7°F. He complains of pain in the upper arm, his capillary refill is 9 seconds, his distal pulses are moderate to poor, and his fingers are cold. There are small areas just distal of the cast that are swollen and look like bubbles. There is a foul odor emanating from the cast. As an ED nurse, you suspect Forrest is suffering from
    A. Compartment syndrome
    B. *Clostridium tetani*
    C. Gangrene
    D. Tetany

51. While assisting a patient with fitting for a cane, the cane should be placed next to the heel on the _____ side and the elbow flexed at _____ degrees.
    A. Injured, 45
    B. Uninjured, 20
    C. Injured, 15
    D. Uninjured, 30

52. Sara joined a parachuting club. On her first jump with the instructor, their parachute failed to open completely, and they both forcefully struck the ground with their feet. The type of fractures Sara would probably incur would be
    A. Calcaneus and thoracic
    B. Cervical and thoracic compression
    C. Lumbosacral compression and calcaneus
    D. Pelvic and thoracic

53. A possible complication with the administration of a Thomas splint is
    A. Flexion and outward rotation of the proximal femur
    B. Improvement of a muscle spasm
    C. Displacement of the distal third of the fractured femur
    D. Compression of the medial nerve

54. When using a battery-powered ring cutter, it is important for the nurse to
    A. Use the diamond disk for a gold ring
    B. Use the carbide blade for a steel ring
    C. Place the cutting guard over the ring
    D. Cover the area with a water-soluble lubricating jelly

55. Piercings and use of body jewelry are increasingly common. Which of the following statements is false regarding body jewelry?
   A. Body jewelry should be removed prior to defibrillation
   B. Jewelry that is removed should be considered contaminated with body fluid
   C. Removal may allow healing and development of abscess formation
   D. Most jewelry is magnetic and requires removal for an MRI

56. A complication that would not occur when removing an oral piercing is
   A. Abscess formation at the piercing site
   B. Aspiration
   C. Tooth breakage
   D. Edema

57. Your patient requires application of a long leg fiberglass splint. The patient should be positioned
   A. Upright
   B. Supine
   C. Flat on the abdomen
   D. In semi-Fowler's

58. If a patient has sustained an unstable ankle fracture, which position would not be appropriate for splinting?
   A. Supine
   B. Prone
   C. Upright
   D. Lateral

59. If your patient is obese and has sustained a lower leg or unstable ankle fracture, which position would be inappropriate for splinting?
   A. Upright
   B. Supine
   C. Prone
   D. Semi-Fowlers

60. A posterior short leg splint should be applied
   A. From the metatarsal 1 inch below the popliteal area to 1 inch beyond the toes
   B. From 1.5 inches beyond the toes to 1.5 inches below the popliteal area
   C. From 2 inches below the popliteal area to 2 inches beyond the toes
   D. From 1 inch below the popliteal area to 2 inches beyond the toes

61. Normal tissue pressure is approximately 10 mmHg. When a patient has compartment syndrome, a pressure exceeding _____ indicates the need for a fasciotomy.
   A. 15–25 mmHg
   B. 20–30 mmHg
   C. 25–35 mmHg
   D. 30–40 mmHg

62. When patients require wound cleansing, a solution that effectively kills gram-negative and gram-positive rods, viruses, and fungi is
    A. Sterile water
    B. Hydrogen peroxide
    C. A povidone-iodine solution
    D. Tap water and soap

63. Epinephrine is frequently used in the treatment of
    A. Patients with known peripheral vascular disease
    B. Lip lacerations that extend through the lip border
    C. The face and scalp to slow absorption
    D. Cartilaginous areas of the ear and nares

64. All types of local anesthetics are vasodilators and cause relaxation of smooth muscles except
    A. Cocaine
    B. Lidocaine
    C. Tetracaine
    D. Pramosone

65. An example of an ester compound is
    A. Procaine
    B. Lidocaine
    C. Mepivacaine
    D. Bupivacaine

66. Your patient requires suturing of a laceration. The patient has a history of malignant hyperthermia. An appropriate local anesthetic agent for this patient is
    A. Lidocaine
    B. Procaine
    C. Mepivacaine
    D. Bupivacaine

67. Which of the following local anesthetics may cause methemoglobinemia?
    A. Lidocaine
    B. Procaine
    C. Mepivacaine
    D. Prilocaine

68. Your patient is to undergo a digital block for a reduction of an interphalangeal joint dislocation. The anesthetic of choice is
    A. Epinephrine
    B. Buffered lidocaine
    C. Prilocaine
    D. Benzocaine

69. Zack's father was driving his car through an intersection when his vehicle was T-boned by another car. Zack suffered a fractured pelvis and left femur and was stabilized in the ED. Zack is awaiting surgical fixation of the fractures. When auscultating lung sounds, you hear what you believe to be bowel sounds in his chest. Zack also states he has moderate shoulder pain on the left side and he is mildly tachypneic. Zack will probably be diagnosed with
    A. A fractured scapula
    B. A hemothorax
    C. Diaphragmatic rupture
    D. Bowel rupture

70. Courtney fell down a flight of stairs, breaking ribs and suffering internal injuries. Which of the following injuries would mandate the use of pain control?
    A. Flail chest
    B. ARDS
    C. A splenectomy
    D. Hemothorax

71. Barbara was admitted to the ED for multiple fractures and contusions after a motor vehicle accident this evening. She complains of dyspnea and petechiae are noted. Barbara is probably suffering from
    A. A pulmonary embolus
    B. Thrombocytopenia
    C. A venous air embolus
    D. A fat embolus

72. Your patient has sustained a laceration on the forehead. Which of the following statements is true about wounds in this area?
    A. Do not shave the eyebrows
    B. Only cleanse the skin with a mild antiseptic solution
    C. Observe for redness, swelling, heat, and discharge
    D. Use sunblock over the wound for at least 6 months

73. Which of the following statements about abrasions is false?
    A. Abrasions are full thickness denudations
    B. Dirt and debris must be removed from the face within 8 hours
    C. Avoid direct sunlight for at least 6 months
    D. Abrasions are quite painful

74. If the full thickness of skin is peeled away from a digit, hand, foot, or limb resulting in devascularization of the skin, this type of injury is known as
    A. An amputation
    B. A laceration
    C. A degloving injury
    D. A Petersen avulsion

75. The patient you are caring for impaled his forearm on a wood fence. Which of the following statements about this type of injury is false?
    A. Any remaining particles of wood may be difficult to visualize on X-ray
    B. Vegetative foreign bodies are highly reactive and easily lead to infection
    C. Vegetative foreign bodies may require anesthetic for removal
    D. Soak the affected area for at least 30 minutes to facilitate removal

76. Fibroblast activity maximizes about 1 week after a patient has sustained a laceration. The ED nurse knows the next probable step in the care of this patient is
    A. Have the patient return to the ED and administer tetanus toxoid
    B. Continue observation of this wound for another week
    C. Culture the wound and obtain a WBC count
    D. Remove the sutures and use tape on the wound

77. Which of the following wounds is at greatest risk of contamination from a *Pseudomonas* infection?
    A. A laceration from a pocket knife
    B. A plantar puncture wound through a shoe
    C. A degloved finger
    D. A paper cut

78. Which of the following statements accurately describes a gunshot wound?
    A. The exit wound is generally smaller than the entrance wound
    B. The entrance wound is smaller than the bullet diameter
    C. A perforating wound is one where the bullet remains inside the patient
    D. A penetrating wound is one where the bullet passes through the patient

79. The police dispatcher has notified the ED that one of their officers has been shot with a Black Talon round from a handgun. This information is important for the patient's care because
    A. Minor injury will exist because of mushrooming
    B. Severe burned tissue will be present at the entrance wound site
    C. The round will have a great amount of kinetic energy
    D. The round is a nonpenetrating round used on movie sets

80. A necrotizing infection associated with animal bites is likely caused by which of the following organisms?
    A. *Clostridium tetani*
    B. *Pasteurella multocida*
    C. *Staphylococcus*
    D. *Pseudomonas*

81. Gas gangrene is most frequently associated with
    A. *Staphylococcus aureus*
    B. Duck embryo vaccine
    C. *Clostridium perfringens*
    D. A virus

82. Your patient has been diagnosed with gas gangrene. Of the following choices, which is the probable cause of his condition?
    A. Ingestion of improperly canned beans
    B. An arm scratch from a cat
    C. A herpes simplex infection
    D. An insulin injection

83. Which of the following actions must be performed when preparing a patient for fixed wing air transport?
    A. Always use a pneumatic antishock garment (PASG)
    B. Bivalve a circumferential plaster cast
    C. Try to use air splints whenever possible
    D. Splint forearms with an anterior gutter splint

84. Localized areas of bone destruction that are replaced with overdeveloped, light porous bone and associated with deformities are known as
    A. Paget's disease
    B. Osteoporosis
    C. Osteoneogenesis
    D. Osteoma

85. The best diagnostic method for soft tissue disorders such as tendon ruptures and muscle tears is
    A. Plain X-ray films
    B. Magnetic resonance imaging
    C. Arthroscopy
    D. Technetium bone scans

86. Your patient has suffered a stress fracture. Which of the following is the best method to diagnose this condition?
    A. Computerized tomography
    B. Angiography
    C. Magnetic resonance imaging
    D. Technetium bone scan

87. Which of the following laboratory tests would you expect the physician to order to help determine if your patient has muscular dystrophy?
    A. Serum glutamic-oxaloacetic transaminase level
    B. Uric acid level
    C. Calcium level
    D. Amylase level

88. Which of the following is not an expected age-related change in an elderly patient?
    A. A longer contraction time in muscles
    B. An increase in bone minerals
    C. Loss of vertebral height
    D. Inability to regenerate muscle fibers

89. A boxer's fracture is a fracture involving the
    A. Proximal second phalanx
    B. Distal fifth metacarpal
    C. Proximal third metacarpal
    D. Distal fourth phalanx

90. Your patient was riding his motorcycle in traffic when he had to swerve suddenly to avoid a crash. The motorcycle went out from under the patient and he skidded on the pavement. The type of injury you would expect to see is
    A. A laceration
    B. A fracture
    C. An avulsion
    D. Tattooing

91. In general, sutures that have been placed on the eyelids should be removed within
    A. 1 to 3 days
    B. 3 to 5 days
    C. 4 to 7 days
    D. 7 to 10 days

92. Ian sustained a crush injury to his ankle about a week ago. He now is complaining of weakness, inability to sleep, difficulty speaking and swallowing, progressive muscle paralysis, and blurred vision. On examination you notice dilated, fixed pupils and dry mucous membranes. Ian is probably suffering from
    A. Guillain-Barré syndrome
    B. Gas gangrene
    C. Hyperemia
    D. Wound botulism

93. Which of the following animal bites is most likely to result in the need for antirabies prophylaxis?
    A. Dog
    B. Raccoon
    C. Rabbit
    D. Mouse

94. Sutures placed in an upper or lower extremity and not over a joint should be removed within
    A. 1 to 3 days
    B. 3 to 5 days
    C. 4 to 7 days
    D. 7 to 10 days

95. Individuals at risk for osteoporosis are
    A. Hunters
    B. Chronic alcohol abusers
    C. Obese individuals
    D. Athletes

96. Which of the following individuals is at high risk of developing an infection from *Clostridium tetani*?
    A. A farmer cutting himself on a tractor blade
    B. A women cutting herself with a kitchen knife
    C. A man cutting himself with a bagel slicer
    D. A resident puncturing himself with a sterile IV catheter

97. Ecchymotic splotches sometimes seen on labia, scrotum, and perineum secondary to pelvic fractures are known as
    A. Cullen's sign
    B. Coopernail's sign
    C. Mose's sign
    D. Grey-Turner's sign

98. Your patient sustained a cervical injury. When he flexed his neck, he complained of sudden electric-like shocks going down his spine. This phenomenon is known as
    A. Cullen's sign
    B. Kernig's sign
    C. Lhermitte's sign
    D. Tresilian's sign

99. Which of the following bacteria is the most common cause of skin infections?
    A. *Pseudomonas aeruginosa*
    B. *Staphylococcus aureus*
    C. Streptococcal A infections
    D. Clostridium infections

100. What is the treatment of choice for a *Staphylococcus aureus* skin infection?
    A. A single intramuscular injection of ceftriaxone
    B. Surgical incision and drainage of all *S. aureus* infections
    C. Dual oral antibiotic therapy for 14 days
    D. Dual intravenous antibiotic therapy for 14 days

101. The type of vertebral fracture that results from the mechanism of injury known as axial loading is
    A. A simple fracture
    B. A compression fracture
    C. A teardrop fracture
    D. A burst fracture

102. The type of vertebral fracture that results from the mechanism of injury known as hyperflexion is called a
    A. Wedge fracture
    B. Compression fracture
    C. Simple fracture
    D. Teardrop fracture

103. Joe fell from a 10-foot ladder. His hip is dislocated. How would you determine if the hip is anteriorly or posteriorly dislocated?
   A. Anterior hip dislocations present with internal rotation
   B. Anterior hip dislocations present with adduction
   C. Posterior hip dislocations present without any rotation
   D. Posterior hip dislocations present with internal rotation and adduction

104. What is a Bennet's fracture?
   A. A fracture of the forefinger metacarpal
   B. A fracture plus dislocation of the metacarpal bone at the base of the thumb
   C. A comminuted intra-articular fracture of the thumb and CMC joint
   D. An open fracture of the middle finger

SECTION 5: ORTHOPEDIC AND MUSCULOSKELETAL ANSWERS

1. **Correct answer: C**
   Traction splints decrease angulation, support fractures, and provide traction. Splints, in general, should decrease pain, provide support, and help limit further soft tissue and bone involvement. Splints also help minimize injury to arteries, veins, and nerves.

2. **Correct answer: C**
   A third-degree strain is distinguished by loss of muscle function (at time of injury), discoloration, hematoma, swelling, and a "snapping" or "popping" noise at the time of the injury.

3. **Correct answer: B**
   A fracture at the junction of the proximal and middle thirds of the ulna is known as a Monteggia's fracture. If the patient has sustained this type of fracture, there is often a dislocation of the radial head. Neurovascular function may be compromised. If the fracture is due to a direct blow, it is sometimes called a "nightstick fracture." Patients usually demonstrate swelling, pain on ROM, crepitus, and deformity.

4. **Correct answer: A**
   Fractures to the distal ends of the radius and ulna are known as Colles' or, occasionally, "silver fork" fractures. It is incumbent on the nurse to consider shoulder, humeral, or hand fractures as well. The lumbar area of the spine may have been injured and the patient may have a compression fracture and possible calcaneal fractures.

5. **Correct answer: D**
   Stable fractures do not transect the pelvic ring and usually do not cause excessive bleeding. A large percentage of patients with a pelvic injury also have trauma to other areas of the body.

6. **Correct answer: C**
   The type of knee injury most likely to be caused by hyperextension trauma is an anterior and posterior cruciate ligament injury.

7. **Correct answer: B**
   A distinguishing characteristic of a patellar fracture is the patient's inability to actively extend the knee. Patellar fractures are usually associated with trauma or indirectly from quadriceps contractions or severe pulls. The patient will have severe pain and hemiarthrosis.

8. **Correct answer: C**
   This patient probably stepped on his forefoot when he crossed the base. The knee was probably hyperextended and an Achilles tendon rupture occurred. The nurse should be able to see some deformity along the normal course of the tendon. The patient may require surgical repair. If the patient requires a walking cast, the nurse needs to provide crutches and splint the foot in plantar flexion.

9. **Correct answer: B**
   When a patient has sustained a pelvic fracture, a urinary catheter should not be placed immediately. Urethral injury should be ruled out either by examination or urethrography. If a urologist is unable to see the patient and a catheter must be placed, consider the use of a suprapubic catheter.

If the nurse obtains vascular access, analgesia and fluids may be given. In addition to a FAST exam, a chest X-ray should be obtained to locate potential injuries and bleeding sites. If the patient is to receive a neuromuscular blockade, it is crucial to stabilize the pelvis first because the muscles may be the only thing maintaining pelvic stability.

10. **Correct answer: A**

    If a patient has truncal obesity and has sustained a pelvic fracture, it is possible to initially stabilize the fracture via internal rotation of lower extremities and taping the knees together.

11. **Correct answer: D**

    NSAIDs are not appropriate initial treatment for a patient with a pelvic fracture because of the high risk of bleeding. It is also a good idea to avoid NSAIDs until the patient has been ruled out for other injuries, hypertension, bleeding disorders, or if they are taking anticoagulants.

12. **Correct answer: C**

    The definition of an unstable pelvic fracture is when the pelvic ring is fractured in more than one place with two displacements on the ring. A rotational displacement is always present and bleeding is likely.

13. **Correct answer: B**

    An ulnar gutter splint is appropriate for this type of injury. This splint extends along the ulna, partially covering the forearm from below the elbow to the palm of the hand.

14. **Correct answer: D**

    The most common forearm fracture is a distal radius fracture. This type of fracture is commonly caused by falls on an outstretched hand. This fracture may also be caused by direct injury. The nurse should observe and assess for radial shortening, ulnar nerve involvement, carpal tunnel syndrome, tendon rupture, and reflex sympathetic dystrophy.

15. **Correct answer: D**

    Stress fractures of the humerus are likely to occur from unconditioned or immature bones and muscles when engaged in pitching a baseball overhand. The rotator cuff, pectoralis major, and deltoid muscles may be weakened. An additional cause of this type of fracture is violent muscle contractions, such as those seen in seizures and electrical shock.

16. **Correct answer: B**

    A pathologic cause of a proximal humerus fracture is an existing condition such as bone cancer, bone cysts, osteoporosis, or Paget's disease.

17. **Correct answer: A**

    The nerve most commonly injured in a proximal humerus fracture is the axillary nerve. The patient may suffer loss of sensation over the lateral deltoid area. Vascular injuries are rare, but the nurse should carefully assess for neurovascular status because peripheral pulses may still be obtained because of collateral circulation around the scapula. The shoulder girdle may develop a mass that can be palpated and that may indicate an arterial rupture. An angiogram may be indicated.

18. **Correct answer: C**

    A proximal humerus fracture with damage to the radial nerve results in wrist drop. The radial nerve innervates dorsal extrinsic muscles of the forearm. Damage to the nerve may be assessed by having the patient abduct and extend the thumb and attempt to extend the wrist. If the nerve is damaged, the fingers will be flexed at the MCP joints and the thumb will be adducted.

19. **Correct answer: C**

    This patient most likely has a chronic rotator cuff tear. The pain in the deltoid, inability to sleep, and inability to internally rotate the arm with pain are classic signs of this condition. The patient will also have pain when attempting to lift the arm (abduct) to the side. Pain gradually worsens, and the patient may not be able to lift his or her arm to the level of the shoulder to the front and side.

20. **Correct answer: A**

    The deltoid muscle is not considered to be a part of the rotator cuff. The four muscles considered part of the rotator cuff are the supraspinatus, teres minor, subscapularis, and the infraspinatus. The supraspinatus and the infraspinatus muscles are the most commonly injured muscles in the rotator cuff.

21. **Correct answer: D**

    The retroperitoneal space may accumulate as much as 5 liters of blood before venous tamponade occurs. If the pubic symphysis diastasis is spread > 3 cm, venous tamponade may not occur until several units of blood have accumulated. If a posterior instability has occurred, it may result in a blood loss of more than 15 units.

22. **Correct answer: D**

    With an acute rotator cuff tear, the patient may feel a tearing sensation and exhibit point tenderness over the injury site. Pain is usually intense and will last a few days secondary to spasm and bleeding. The patient will not be able to abduct their arm without assistance.

23. **Correct answer: B**

    The type of amputation that has the greatest chance of reimplantation is the guillotine. The edges are more easily approximated. Reimplantations of the upper extremities are more successful than those of the lower extremities.

24. **Correct answer: D**

    The most serious complication of casting and splinting is compartment syndrome. Compartment syndrome occurs when pressures in a closed space compromise blood flow and tissue perfusion. Ischemia results and potentially causes edema and impairment of vascular and neurological tissue.

    Patients should be taught that increased pain, numbness, tingling, swelling, color change, or delayed capillary refill in the immobilized area is serious and requires an immediate visit to an ED or urgent care facility. The cast or splint will probably be removed.

25. **Correct answer: D**

    Splints are not circumferential. Splints are not only noncircumferential but usually held in place by an elastic bandage. Splints allow for easy access to an injury site, are fast and easy to apply, and allow for swelling during the acute inflammatory phase of injury. Circumferential casts may cause pressure-related complications. These complications include skin breakdown, necrosis, compartment syndrome, and thermal injury.

26. **Correct answer: C**
    The severity of a sprain usually would not be considered if trying to determine treatment for a sprain. Sprains, tendon injuries, soft tissue injuries in general, and stable fractures are usually splinted. Casts are used for complex or unstable fractures.

27. **Correct answer: C**
    Costochondritis is often found in persons who engage in repetitive activities such as tennis. This patient likely has costochondritis, but the ED nurse should anticipate the patient being evaluated for possible cardiac pathology.

28. **Correct answer: B**
    A closed wound that occurs when a blood vessel ruptures and bleeds into surrounding tissue is known as a contusion. A hematoma may form secondary to a contusion. Patients need to be evaluated as to potential causes: abuse, anticoagulant use (including diet, use of power drinks), bleeding/clotting disorders, type of activity, medications (including vitamins as many now contain herbal anticoagulants).

29. **Correct answer: D**
    At 5 to 6 days after a contusion is sustained, the periphery of the contusion changes color from the periphery to the inside and becomes green tinged. The ED nurse needs to take color into consideration to help evaluate the history of the injury.

30. **Correct answer: C**
    If a patient presents with contusions that are yellow tinged, the contusion is probably about 7–10 days old. From 1 to 5 days the contusion is usually purple or reddish-blue, green from 5 to 7 days, yellow from 7 to 10 days, and brown at 10–14 days.

31. **Correct answer: D**
    Appropriate patient teaching about RICE therapy includes application of cold packs ×20 minutes, four times a day for 48–72 hours. Wrap the cold source to prevent thermal injury. Additional teaching should also include resting extremities and elevating as close to level of the heart as possible during the first 24 hours. Compression bandages with an elastic bandage should be used and analgesics taken as ordered.

32. **Correct answer: B**
    Tinel's sign is considered positive when pain and paresthesia worsen when the medial nerve is tapped along its course in the wrist.

33. **Correct answer: A**
    When performing a peripheral nerve assessment for ulnar nerve impairment, normal motor and sensory findings include the ability to fan the fingers and have feeling on top of the small finger. Feeling on the dorsum of the thumb and the ability to extend the thumb is an indication of normal motor and sensory function of the radial nerve. The ability to oppose the thumb to base of small finger and to feel on the tip of the index finger is the expected result when testing the medial nerve.

34. **Correct answer: B**
    A deformity of the distal portion of a joint that is angulated away from the midline of the body is called a valgus. An example is a patient with "knock knees."

35. **Correct answer: A**
    A C-reactive protein level is negative in a patient with pneumonia. The C-reactive protein is positive in cases of rheumatoid arthritis, widespread metastases, and acute inflammation.

36. **Correct answer: C**
    The type of fracture caused by an angulation force of direct trauma is known as a transverse fracture. An oblique fracture is usually caused by a twisting force. A spiral fracture is often caused by a twisting force when the foot is firmly planted. A depressed fracture is caused by blunt force on a flat bone.

37. **Correct answer: B**
    A complete joint disruption with the articular surfaces no longer in contact is known as a dislocation. Dislocations may damage or impinge on surrounding tissue and need to be reduced as soon as possible. Muscle spasm around the joint can be severe and require muscle relaxants. On rare occasions the patient may require general anesthesia to successfully reduce the dislocation.

38. **Correct answer: D**
    A posterior dislocation of the glenohumeral joint in the shoulder may be caused by a tonic-clonic seizure. This type of rare injury occurs from an extended arm forcefully abducted and internally rotated.

39. **Correct answer: D**
    The amputated part should be rinsed with sterile normal saline or lactated Ringer's. No tap water or other solutions should be used. The part should be placed in a plastic bag and then sealed shut. That bag should be placed in another container with ice and water or refrigerated to 4°C. The bag should be labeled with the patient's name, date, and time per hospital protocol.

40. **Correct answer: D**
    A contraindication to the use of a vacuum splint is that the splint is nontransparent and may prevent reassessment after it is applied to a distal limb. After the splint is applied, make certain the valve is closed securely or air will leak out and the rigidity of the splint will be lost.

41. **Correct answer: A**
    Air splints are not suitable for angulated fractures or fractures that involve joints. Air splints leak and must be watched carefully because support for the fracture will be lost. Air splints are not effective for fractures of the humerus or femur.

42. **Correct answer: A**
    Talcum powder and cornstarch help prevent the air splint from adhering to skin and makes removal easier. Excessive pressure variations exist and pressure may cause compartment syndrome, nerve compression, and soft tissue damage. Loss of inflation may result in inadequate stabilization of the fracture.

43. **Correct answer: B**
    When applying an air splint to an elderly patient, the ED nurse should consider placing smooth padding under the splint. Adducting the limb may cause further injury and pain as would elevating the limb. Turning the valve counterclockwise will open the valve and let air out.

44. Correct answer: C
The preferred splint for a femur fracture is a traction splint.

45. Correct answer: C
Kendrick splints are classified as unipolar splints. The Sager comes in both models. The unipolar splints use one metal rod to stabilize the leg. The bipolar splints, Hare, Thomas, and Fernotrac, have two metal rods, one for each side of the leg.

46. Correct answer: D
Traction splints are specific for femur fractures. They cannot be used on foot, ankle, upper extremity, distal tibia, or distal fibula fractures.

47. Correct answer: D
The Sager splint may be applied by one person.

48. Correct answer: C
The Sager traction splint does not require anterior padding in the anterior groin area.

49. Correct answer: B
Your patient should have his or her elbow bent at 30 degrees while being fitted for a walker.

50. Correct answer: C
Forrest is suffering from gangrene.

51. Correct answer: D
While assisting a patient with fitting for a cane, the cane should be placed next to the heel on the uninjured side and the elbow flexed at 30 degrees.

52. Correct answer: C
Sara landed on her feet and most likely sustained calcaneus and lumbosacral compression fractures.

53. Correct answer: A
A possible complication with the administration of a Thomas splint is flexion and outward rotation of the proximal femur. A goal is to improve muscle spasm. Displacement would involve the proximal third of the fractured femur. The medial nerve is in the arm, so it would not be affected by the femur splint.

54. Correct answer: D
When using a battery-powered ring cutter, it is important for the nurse to cover the area with a water-soluble lubricating jelly to dissipate heat generated by the cutter. The patient can be easily burned during ring removal. It is also possible to place ice directly on the ring. Diamond disks are for cutting steel, iron, brass, and platinum. Carbide disks are for cutting gold, silver, copper, aluminum, and plastic.

55. Correct answer: D
Most jewelry is nonmagnetic and does not require removal for an MRI unless it covers the body part being examined. Body jewelry should be removed prior to defibrillation to prevent burns and arcing. Jewelry that is removed should be considered contaminated with body fluid. Removal of body jewelry may heal over the piercing site and promote development of an abscess.

Orthopedic and Musculoskeletal | 125

56. **Correct answer: A**

    A complication that would not occur when removing an oral piercing is abscess formation at the piercing site. The abscess may form after the removal, not during the removal.

57. **Correct answer: B**

    Your patient requires application of a long leg fiberglass splint. The patient should be positioned supine.

58. **Correct answer: B**

    Patients who have sustained unstable ankle fractures should not be placed in the prone position. The calf might be flexed and the splint may be improperly fitted, causing tissue damage or lack of support.

59. **Correct answer: C**

    Obese patients placed in the prone position for splinting may have difficulty breathing.

60. **Correct answer: C**

    A posterior short leg splint should be applied from 2 inches below the popliteal area to 2 inches beyond the toes. The nurse should ensure the patient's foot is at 90 degrees to the leg and that circulation and knee flexion is not compromised.

61. **Correct answer: D**

    When a patient has compartment syndrome, a pressure exceeding 30–40 mmHg indicates the need for a fasciotomy.

62. **Correct answer: C**

    Povidone-iodine solutions effectively kill gram-negative and gram-positive rods, viruses, and fungi. The nurse should always ask about patient sensitivity or allergies to iodine or shellfish prior to its use.

63. **Correct answer: C**

    Epinephrine is used in the treatment of the face and scalp to slow absorption and lower peak blood levels.

64. **Correct answer: A**

    Cocaine is a vasoconstrictor. It is used frequently for patients with epistaxis. Cocaine should not be given to patients with a history of abuse or who are allergic to exogenous catecholamines.

65. **Correct answer: A**

    An example of an ester compound is procaine. Esters are hydrolyzed by pseudocholinesterase in the serum. Cocaine is an ester but is excreted unchanged in urine. Esters usually cause more allergic reactions than other compounds.

66. **Correct answer: B**

    An appropriate local anesthetic agent for a patient with a history of malignant hyperthermia is procaine.

67. **Correct answer: D**

    Methemoglobinemia may be caused by prilocaine. This condition may also be caused by benzocaine and xylocaine. Methemoglobinemia may also be caused by benzene, antibiotics (including dapsone and chloroquine), and nitrites. Some of the symptoms include headache, fatigue, dyspnea, and cyanosis.

68. **Correct answer: B**

    For a reduction of an interphalangeal joint dislocation, the anesthetic of choice (from this selection) is buffered lidocaine. This procedure should be relatively short and the buffered lidocaine reduces pain from a digital block.

69. **Correct answer: C**

    Zack's abdominal contents have probably entered the thoracic cavity secondary to a diaphragmatic tear. If air also enters the thoracic cavity, it will increase intrathoracic pressure and help to transmit sound. It is usually the left side of the diaphragm that ruptures, and Zack was injured on the left. It is postulated that perhaps the liver, because it is large, protects the right side of the diaphragm. A fractured pelvis usually also results in almost a 50% increased probability of a ruptured diaphragm.

70. **Correct answer: A**

    Pain control is absolutely necessary with a flail chest. A flail chest results when two or more adjacent ribs are broken in two or more places. The chest wall is unstable. Usually, during inspiration the chest wall moves outward with an increase in negative intrathoracic pressure. In cases of flail chest, the opposite movement of the chest wall is seen. This is known as a "paradoxical" movement. Eventually, the result will be atelectasis and alveolar collapse, with possible development of ARDS. To adequately stabilize the fracture, sometimes neuromuscular blockade is used. The patient must be given pain medication and sedation. Also, pain is the priority because the work of breathing (WOB) needs to be reduced. Just think about any time you have ever had a pain in your side and how difficult it was to take a full breath.

71. **Correct answer: D**

    Fractures, usually long bone fractures, can release free fatty acids, which cause fatty emboli. Fat globules float around and obstruct the pulmonary vasculature.

72. **Correct answer: A**

    Do not shave eyebrows because the eyebrows may not regrow normally and will look distorted.

73. **Correct answer: A**

    Abrasions are partial thickness denudations, not full thickness denudations, of skin. An abrasion may be quite painful because of exposed nerve endings. Avoid direct sunlight for at least 6 months because pigmentary changes may take place. Dirt and debris should be removed from the face within 8 hours and should be removed from extremities within 4 to 6 hours.

74. **Correct answer: C**

    If the full thickness of skin is peeled away from a digit, hand, foot, or limb resulting in devascularization of the skin, this type of injury is known as a degloving injury.

75. **Correct answer: D**

    Wounds that may have wood splinters should not be soaked because the wood absorbs liquid and swells, causing further pain and tissue damage. In addition, the wood may disintegrate during removal.

76. **Correct answer: D**

    Fibroblast activity maximizes about 1 week after a patient has sustained a laceration. The wound may not have enough tensile strength to maintain the approximation of the wound, so using tape to maintain wound adhesion may be necessary.

77. **Correct answer: B**

    The type of injury at greatest risk of contamination from a *Pseudomonas* infection is a plantar puncture wound through a shoe.

78. **Correct answer: B**

    The entrance wound from a bullet is generally smaller than the bullet diameter. This is due to the elasticity of the skin. Exit wounds are larger than entrance wounds.

79. **Correct answer: C**

    Black Talon, Hydra-Shok, or Golden Saber rounds are designed to ensure complete transference of the kinetic energy to the target. The energy of a projectile may be incompletely transferred to the target if the round is not stopped by the tissue. This patient is at risk for catastrophic injury.

80. **Correct answer: B**

    A necrotizing infection associated with animal bites is likely caused by *Pasteurella multocida*. This infection may progress to cellulitis, osteomyelitis, and pleuritis. The disease itself is called pasteurellosis.

81. **Correct answer: C**

    Gas gangrene is most frequently associated with *Clostridium perfringens*. This pathogen is an anaerobic, gram-positive, spore-forming bacillus. Other bacteria are also capable of producing gas, and nonclostridial organisms have been isolated in 60–85% of cases of gas gangrene. The most frequently identified aerobic gram-negative bacteria were *Escherichia coli*, *Proteus* species, *Pseudomonas aeruginosa*, and *Klebsiella pneumoniae*.

82. **Correct answer: D**

    Posttraumatic causes of gas gangrene can include intramuscular or subcutaneous injections with insulin, epinephrine, quinine, or cocaine. Most cases involve automobile collisions, crush injuries, thermal injuries, gunshot wounds, farm or industrial injuries, and compound fractures.

    Postoperative clostridial infections are frequently caused from colon resections, ruptured appendix, bowel perforation, GI surgery, cholecystectomy, colonoscopy, and abortions.

83. **Correct answer: B**

    Prior to fixed wing air transport it is necessary to bivalve a plaster cast if it is circumferential. Changes in atmospheric pressure will cause the extremity to expand. Air splints are dangerous because they may impede circulation due to gas expansion.

84. **Correct answer: A**

    Paget's disease is when localized areas of bone destruction are replaced with overdeveloped, light porous bone and associated with deformities. In this condition the skull often thickens and weight-bearing bones may bend. Middle-aged and elderly males are usually affected.

85. **Correct answer: B**

    The best diagnostic method for soft tissue disorders such as tendon ruptures and muscle tears is magnetic resonance imaging. The MRI is also useful to help diagnose meniscal damage, tumors, degenerative disorders, and spinal structures.

86. **Correct answer: D**

    The technetium bone scan is the best method to diagnose stress fractures and metastatic disease.

87. **Correct answer: A**

    A serum glutamic-oxaloacetic transaminase level is helpful in the diagnosis of muscular dystrophy.

88. **Correct answer: B**

    Elderly individuals lose bone minerals and bone mass. A longer contraction time in muscles, loss of vertebral height, and inability to regenerate muscle fibers are normal processes of aging.

89. **Correct answer: B**

    A boxer's fracture is a fracture involving the distal fifth metacarpal. This type of fracture occasionally involves the head of the metacarpal but is known as a fracture of the fourth or fifth metacarpal neck.

90. **Correct answer: D**

    The type of injury you would expect to see when a motorcycle rider skids on pavement is tattooing. This injury is caused by sideways (tangential) dermal and epidermal trauma. It is a form of abrasion. Nerve endings are exposed, and the wound is very painful. This wound requires meticulous care, debridement, and possible antibiotic prophylaxis.

91. **Correct answer: B**

    In general, sutures that have been placed on the eyelids should be removed within 3 to 5 days. Sutures placed on the face or lips should also be removed within 3 to 5 days.

92. **Correct answer: D**

    Ian is probably suffering from wound botulism. His symptoms of weakness, inability to sleep, difficulty speaking and swallowing, progressive muscle paralysis, and blurred vision with dilated, fixed pupils are classic for this condition. Botulinum toxin blocks motor nerves' ability to release acetylcholine, the neurotransmitter that relays nerve signals to muscles. Eventually, the muscles of respiration will be affected and death will occur from respiratory failure.

93. **Correct answer: B**

    Antirabies prophylaxis is administered as a matter of course to individuals who have been bitten by raccoons, bats, skunks, and foxes. Generally, patients bitten by rodents rarely require postexposure antirabies prophylaxis.

94. **Correct answer: D**

    Sutures placed in an upper or lower extremity and not over a joint should be removed within 7 to 10 days.

95. **Correct answer: B**
Individuals at risk for osteoporosis are chronic alcohol abusers, long-term steroid users, tall thin people, and postmenopausal women. Additional risk factors are a family history of osteoporosis and a history of previous fractures.

96. **Correct answer: A**
The farmer is at the highest risk for a *Clostridium tetani* infection because the organism lives in soil.

97. **Correct answer: B**
Ecchymotic splotches sometimes seen on labia, scrotum, and perineum secondary to pelvic fractures are known as Coopernail's sign.

98. **Correct answer: C**
When a patient's neck is flexed and sudden shocks travel down the spine and into the limbs, it is known as Lhermitte's sign. Lhermitte's sign, sometimes called the barber chair phenomenon, indicates involvement of the posterior columns and is often seen in patients with multiple sclerosis. This condition may also occur with myelopathy, vitamin B12 deficiency, and cancer radiation therapy.

99. **Correct answer: B**
Staphylococcus aureus is the most common cause of most skin and nosocomial infections. It can cause carbuncles, furuncles, mastitis, cellulitis, impetigo, osteomyelitis, and endocarditis to name a few. Part of the virulence of *S. aureus* is that it is a component of the normal skin flora and is also present in the nasal passages.

100. **Correct answer: C**
For the patient who is not immunocompromised it is safe to use dual oral antibiotic therapy for 14 days. Oral antibiotics used may include cephalexin, Septra DS, doxycycline, levofloxacin, or ciprofloxacin. Rifampin is sometimes added as a synergist to other antibiotics especially when MRSA is a consideration.

101. **Correct answer: D**
The type of vertebral fracture that results from the mechanism of injury known as axial loading is a burst fracture. This type of fracture may result in spinal cord compression and/or a comminuted fracture of a vertebral body.

102. **Correct answer: D**
The type of vertebral fracture that results from the mechanism of injury known as hyperflexion is called a teardrop fracture. A small anterior edge of a vertebrae breaks and may impinge on the spinal cord. Sometimes the patient will also have a posterior malalignment of the vertebrae.

103. **Correct answer: D**
Posterior hip dislocations present with internal rotation and adduction. Anterior hip dislocations present with external rotation and abduction.

104. **Correct answer: B**
A Bennett's fracture is a fracture plus dislocation of the metacarpal bone at the base of the thumb. If the force of the injury is severe and the bone breaks into several pieces, it is known as a Rolando fracture.

SECTION 5: ORTHOPEDIC AND MUSCULOSKELETAL REFERENCES

Abman, S. (2008). The dysmorphic pulmonary circulation in bronchopulmonary dysplasia: A growing story. *American Journal of Respiratory and Critical Care Medicine, 178*(2), 114–115.

Agbaht, K., Lisboa, T., Pobo, A., Rodriguez, A., Sandiumenge, A., Diaz, E., & Rello, J. (2007). Management of ventilator-associated pneumonia in a multidisciplinary intensive care unit: Does trauma make a difference? *Intensive Care Medicine, 33*(8), 1387–1395.

Ahrens, T., & Sona, C. (2003). Capnography application in acute and critical care. *AACN Clinical Issues, 14*(2), 123–132.

American Heart Association. (2010). Guidelines 2010 for cardiopulmonary resuscitation and emergency cardiovascular care. Retrieved October 18, 2010, from www.americanheart.org

Anonymous. (2010). Endoscopic compartment release for chronic exertional compartment syndrome: Surgical technique and results. *American Journal of Sports Medicine, 38*(8), 1661–1666.

Antonelli, M., Azoulay, E., Bonten, M., Chastre, J., Citerio, G., Conti, G., . . . Zhang, H. (2010). Year in review in intensive care medicine 2009. Part III: Mechanical ventilation, acute lung injury and respiratory distress syndrome, pediatrics, ethics and miscellanea. *Intensive Care Medicine, 36*(4), 567–584.

Balogh, Z. J., van Wessem, K., Yoshino, O., & Moore, F. A. (2009). Postinjury abdominal compartment syndrome: Are we winning the battle? *World Journal of Surgery, 33*(6), 1134–1141.

Baltacioğlu, F., Çimşit, N., Bostanci, K., Yüksel, M., & Kodalli, N. (2010). Transarterial microcatheter glue embolization of the bronchial artery for life-threatening hemoptysis: Technical and clinical results. *European Journal of Radiology, 73*(2), 380–384.

Bashore, T. M., Granger, C. B., Hranitzky, P., & Patel, M. R. (2010). Heart disease. In S. J. McPhee & M. A. Papadakis (Eds.), *Lange 2010 current medical diagnosis and treatment* (49th ed., pp. 358–366). New York: McGraw-Hill Medical.

Bhandari, V., Choo-Wing, R., Lee, C., Yusuf, K., Nedrelow, J. H., Ambalavanan, N., . . . Elias, J. A. (2008). Developmental regulation of NO-mediated VEGF-induced effects in the lung. *American Journal of Respiratory Cell and Molecular Biology, 39*(4), 420–430.

Bigatello, L. M., Davidson, K. R., & Stelfox, H. T. (2005). Respiratory mechanics and ventilatory waveforms in the patient with acute lung injury. *Respiratory Care, 50,* 235–245.

Boland, M. R., & Heck, C. (2009). Acute exercise-induced bilateral thigh compartment syndrome. *Orthopedics, 32*(3), 218.

Burghardt, R. D., Siebenlist, S., Döbele, S., Lucke, M., & Stöckle, U. (2010). Compartment syndrome of the thigh. A case report with delayed onset after stable pelvic ring fracture and chronic anticoagulation therapie. *BMC Geriatrics, 10,* 51.

Caruana, J. A., Anain, P. M., & Pham, D. T. (2009). The pulmonary embolism risk score system reduces the incidence and mortality of pulmonary embolism after gastric bypass. *Surgery, 146*(4), 678–685.

Castro-Garcia, J., Davis, B. R., & Pirela-Cruz, M. A. (2010). Bilateral gluteal compartment syndrome: A rare but potentially morbid entity. *American Surgeon, 76*(7), 752–754.

Centers for Disease Control and Prevention. (2002). Guideline for hand hygiene in health-care settings: Recommendations of the Healthcare Infection Control Practices Advisory Committee and the HICPAC/SHEA/APIC/IDSA Hand Hygiene Task Force. *Morbidity and Mortality Weekly Report, 51*(RR16), 1–44.

Centers for Disease Control and Prevention. (2004). Guidelines for preventing health-care associated pneumonia: 2003 recommendations of the CDC and the Healthcare Infection Control Practices Advisory Committee. *Morbidity and Mortality Weekly Report, 53*(RR03), 1–36.

Chernecky, C., & Berger, B. (2004). *Laboratory tests and diagnostic procedures* (4th ed.). Philadelphia: Saunders.

Chun, J.-Y., & Belli, A.-M. (2010). Immediate and long-term outcomes of bronchial and non-bronchial systemic artery embolisation for the management of haemoptysis. *European Radiology, 20*(3), 558–565.

Church, D. G., Matthay, M. A., Liu, K., Milet, M., & Flori, H. (2009). Blood product transfusions and clinical outcomes in pediatric patients with acute lung injury. *Pediatric Critical Care Medicine, 10*(3), 297–302.

Cosentini, R., Aliberti, S., Bignamini, A., Piffer, F., & Brambilla, A. M. (2009). Mortality in acute cardiogenic pulmonary edema treated with continuous positive airway pressure. *Intensive Care Medicine, 35*(2), 299–305.

Crawford, B., & Comstock, S. (2010). Acute compartment syndrome of the dorsal forearm following noncontact injury. *Canadian Journal of Emergency Medical Care, 12*(5), 453–456.

D'Asero, G., Tati, E., Petrocelli, M., Brinci, L., Palla, L., Cerulli, P., & Cervelli, V. (2010). Compartment syndrome of the hand with acute bullous eruption due to extravasation of computed tomography contrast material. *European Review for Medical And Pharmacological Sciences, 14*(7), 643–646.

Dellamonica, J., Louis, B., Lyazidi, A., Vargas, F., & Brochard, L. (2008). Intrapulmonary percussive ventilation superimposed on conventional ventilation: Bench study of humidity and ventilator behaviour. *Intensive Care Medicine, 34*(11), 2035–2043.

Di Stazio, C., Guadagni, I., Pellino, G., De Rosa, M., Selvaggi, F., & Sciaudone, G. (2010). Compartment syndrome of the leg after pelvic surgery: Can it always be avoided? *American Surgeon, 75*(12), 1260–1262.

Dueker, C. W. (2004). Immersion in fresh water and survival. *Chest, 126*(6), 2027–2028.

Durbin, C. G. (2005). Applied respiratory physiology: Uses of ventilator waveforms and mechanics in the management of critically ill patients. *Respiratory Care, 50*, 287–293.

Emergency Nurses Association, Newberry, L., & Criddle, L. M. (2007). *Sheehy's manual of emergency care* (6th ed.). St. Louis, MO: Mosby.

Eppert, H. D. (2010). Disease prevention update: Tetanus toxoid, reduced diphtheria toxoid, and acellular pertussis—who, what, when, why, and how? *JEN: Journal of Emergency Nursing, 36*(2), 122–124.

Frankel, S. K., & Schwarz, M. (2009). Update in idiopathic pulmonary fibrosis. *Current Opinion in Pulmonary Medicine, 15*(5), 463–469

Fung, Y. L., & Silliman, C. C. (2009). The role of neurophils in the pathogenesis of transfusion-related acute lung injury. *Transfusion Medicine Reviews, 23*(4), 266–283.

Gasparis Vonfrolio, L., & Noone, J. (1997). *Emergency nursing examination review* (3rd ed.). Staten Island, NY: Power Publications.

Grewal, S., Ali, S., McConnell, D. W., Vandermeer, B., & Klassen, T. P. (2009). A randomized trial of nebulized 3% hypertonic saline with epinephrine in the treatment of acute bronchiolitis in the emergency department. *Archives of Pediatrics and Adolescent Medicine, 163*(11), 1007–1012.

Guyton, A. C., & Hall, J. E. (2005). *Textbook of medical physiology* (11th ed.). Philadelphia: Saunders.

Halliday, H. (2008). Surfactants: Past, present and future. *Journal of Perinatology, 28*(S1), S47–S56.

Hardin, S. R., & Kaplow, R. (2010). *Cardiac surgery essentials for critical care nursing*. Sudbury, MA: Jones & Bartlett Learning.

Hickey, J. V. (2008). *The clinical practice of neurological and neurosurgical nursing* (6th ed.). Philadelphia: Lippincott Williams & Wilkins.

Holleran, R. S. (2005). *Emergency transport nursing* (4th ed.). St. Louis, MO: Mosby.

Hoshino, T., Kato, S., Oka, N., Imaoka, H., Kinoshita, T., Takei, S., . . . Aizawa, H. (2007). Pulmonary inflammation and emphysema: Role of the cytokines IL-18 and IL-13. *American Journal of Respiratory and Critical Care Medicine, 176*(1), 49–62.

Hwang, J. H., Misumi, S., Sahin, H., Brown, K. K., Newell, J. D., & Lynch, D. A. (2009). Computed tomographic features of idiopathic fibrosing interstitial pneumonia: Comparison with *pulmonary* fibrosis related to collagen vascular disease. *Journal of Computer Assisted Tomography, 33*(3), 410–415.

Inal, M. T. (2007). Laryngospasm-induced pulmonary edema. *Internet Journal of Anesthesiology, 15*(1), 5.

Iyer, V., Joshi, A., & Ryu, J. (2009). Spontaneous pneumomediastinum: Analysis of 62 consecutive adult patients. *Mayo Clinic Proceedings, 84*(5), 417–421.

Jacobs, B. B., & Hoyt, K. S. (2007). *Trauma nursing core course provider manual* (6th ed.). Bedford, IL: Emergency Nurses Association.

Jobin, C. M., Ludwig, S. C., Zahiri, H., Cushman, J., & Paryavi, E. (2010). Acute exertional lumbar paraspinal compartment syndrome. *Spine, 35*(25), E1529–E153.

Johnson, J. M. (2009). Management of acute cardiogenic pulmonary edema: A literature review. *Advanced Emergency Nursing Journal, 31*(1), 36–43.

Jones & Bartlett Learning (2011). *2011 nurse's drug handbook* (10th ed.). Sudbury, MA: Jones & Bartlett Learning.

Jones, K. L. (2006). *Smith's recognizable patterns of human malformation* (6th ed.). Philadelphia: Elsevier.

Kanlic, E. M., Pinski, S. E., Verwiebe, E. G., Saller, J., & Smith, W. R. (2010). Acute morbidity and complications of thigh compartment syndrome: A report of 26 cases. *Patient Safety in Surgery, 4*(1), 13.

Kealey, G. P. (2009). Carbon monoxide toxicity. *Journal of Burn Care and Research, 30*(1), 146–147.

Lippincott. (2010). *Professional guide to signs and symptoms* (6th ed.). Philadelphia: Lippincott.

Maggiorini, M. (2010). Prevention and treatment of high-altitude pulmonary edema. *Progress in Cardiovascular Diseases, 52*(6), 500–506.

Malik, A. A., Khan, W. S., Chaudhry, A., Ihsan, M., & Cullen, N. P. (2009). Acute compartment syndrome—A life and limb threatening surgical emergency. *Journal of Perioperative Practice, 19*(5), 137–142.

Mallo, G. C., Stanat, S. J., Al-Humadi, M., & Divaris, N. (2009). Posterior thigh compartment syndrome as a result of a basketball injury. *Orthopedics, 32*(12), 923–925.

Martin, B. (2010). Family presence during resuscitation and invasive procedures: AACN practice alert. Retrieved November 2, 2010, from http://www.aacn.org

McKellop, J. A., & Mukherji, S. K. (2010). Emergency head and neck radiology: neck infections. *Applied Radiology, 39*(7), 23–24, 26–29.

Medina, J., & Puntillo, K. (2006). *AACN protocols for practice: Palliative care and end-of-life issues in critical care.* Sudbury, MA: Jones and Bartlett.

Mireku, N., Wang, Y., Ager, J., Reddy, R. C., & Baptist, A. P. (2009). Changes in weather and the effects on pediatric asthma exacerbations. *Annals of Allergy, Asthma & Immunology, 103*(3), 220–224.

Mohsen, T., Zeid, A. A., & Haj-Yahia, S. (2007). Lobectomy or pneumonectomy for multidrug-resistant pulmonary tuberculosis can be performed with acceptable morbidity and mortality: A seven-year review of a single institution's experience. *Journal of Thoracic and Cardiovascular Surgery, 134*(1), 194–198.

Mulkey, Z., Yarbrough, S., Guerra, D., Roongsritong, C., Nugent, K., & Phy, M. P. (2008). Postextubation *pulmonary* edema: A case series and review. *Respiratory Medicine, 102*(11), 1659–1662.

Oprel, P. P., Eversdijk, M. G., Vlot, J., Tuinebreijer, W. E., & den Hartog, D. (2010). The acute compartment syndrome of the lower leg: A difficult diagnosis? *Open Orthopaedics Journal, 4*, 115–119.

Perry, J., Balasubramanian, S., & Imray, C. (2009). Systemic capillary leak syndrome resulting in compartment syndrome and the requirement for a surgical airway. *Anaesthesia, 64*(6), 679–682.

Pirela-Cruz, M. A., & Scher, D. L. (2010). Exposure of distal radius fractures using a direct radial approach with mobilization of the superficial branch of the radial nerve. *Techniques in Hand & Upper Extremity Surgery, 14*(4), 218–221.

Ploumis, A., Casnellie, M., Graber, J. N., & Dykes, D. C. (2010). Acute tibial compartment syndrome following spine surgery. *Orthopedics, 33*(6), 447.

Prescribing Reference. (2009, Summer). *NPPR: Nurse Practitioner's Prescribing Reference, 16*(2).

Proehl, J. A. (2008). *Emergency nursing procedures* (4th ed.). St. Louis, MO: Saunders.

Rajic, N., Savic, A., Popovic, S., Urosevic, I., & Savic, I. (2009). Successful control of bleeding during supracondylar amputation caused by severe compartment syndrome in patient with haemophilia A and high titre of inhibitor. *Official Journal of the World Federation of Hemophilia, 15*(2), 601–602.

Rehman, S., & Joglekar, S. B. (2009). Acute isolated lateral compartment syndrome of the leg after a noncontact sports injury. *Orthopedics, 32*(7), 523.

Roch, A., Blayac, D., Ramiara, P., Chetaille, B., Marin, V., Michelet, P., . . . Carpentier, J. P. (2007). Comparison of lung injury after normal or small volume optimized resuscitation in a model of hemorrhagic shock. *Intensive Care Medicine, 33*(9), 1645–1654.

Shadgan, B., Menon, M., Sanders, D., Berry, G., Martin, C., Duffy, P., . . . O'Brien, P. J. (2010). Current thinking about acute compartment syndrome of the lower extremity. *Canadian Journal of Surgery, 53*(5), 329–334.

Shah, N. (2009). Acute exercise-induced compartment syndrome of the lower leg: A case report. *Current Sports Medicine Reports, 8*(6), 288–290.

Shaikh, N. (2010). Common complication of crush injury, but a rare compartment syndrome. *Journal of Emergencies, Trauma and Shock, 3*(2), 177–181.

Spooner, L. M., & Liu, E. (2009). Tuberculosis, CNS. In F. J. Domino, R. A. Baldor, A. M. Erlich, & J. Golding (Eds.), *The 5-minute clinical consult 2010* (18th ed., pp. 1358–1359). Philadelphia: Lippincott Williams & Wilkins.

Stenmark, K. R., & Rabinovitch, M. (2010). Emerging therapies for the treatment of pulmonary hypertension. *Pediatric Critical Care Medicine, 11*(2 suppl), S85–S90.

Suntharalingam, J., Treacy, C. M., Doughty, N. J., Goldsmith, K., Soon, E., Toshner, M. R., & Pepke-Zaba, J. (2008). Long-term use of sildenafil in inoperable chronic thromboembolic pulmonary hypertension. *Chest, 134*(2), 229–236.

Tsangaris, I., Galiatsou, E., Kostanti, E., & Nakos, G. (2007). The effect of exogenous surfactant in patients with lung contusions and acute lung injury. *Intensive Care Medicine, 33*(5), 851–855.

Urdem, L. D., Stacy, K. M., & Lough, M. E. (2005). *Thelan's critical care nursing* (5th ed.). St. Louis, MO: Mosby.

Varpula, M., Tallgren, M., Saukkonen, K., Voipio-Pulkki, L.-M., & Pettilä, V. (2005). Hemodynamic variables related to outcome in septic shock. *Intensive Care Medicine, 31*(8), 1066–1071.

Verwiebe, E. G., Kanlic, E. M., Saller, J., & Abdelgawad, A. (2009). Thigh compartment syndrome, presentation and complications. *Bosnian Journal of Basic Medical Sciences, 9*(suppl 1), 28–33.

Watson, S., & Gorski, K. A. (2011). *Invasive cardiology* (3rd ed.). Sudbury, MA: Jones & Bartlett Learning.

Wing, R., Lee, C., Yusuf, K., Nedrelow, J., Ambalavanan, N., Malkus, H., Homer, R., & Elias, J. (2008). Developmental regulation of NO-mediated VEGF-induced effects in the lung. *American Journal of Respiratory Cell and Molecular Biology, 39*(4), 420–430.

Yiming, M., Lederer, D., Sun, L., Huertas, A., Issekutz, A., & Bhattacharya, S. (2008). Platelets enhance endothelial adhesiveness in high tidal volume ventilation. *American Journal of Respiratory Cell and Molecular Biology, 39*(5), 569–575.

SECTION 6:

Maxillofacial and Ocular

1. A LeFort I fracture is a fracture of the
   A. Maxilla
   B. Zygomatic arch
   C. Mandible
   D. Frontal bone

2. Which of the following statements is true about alveolar fractures?
   A. Alveolar fractures are the result of high-energy trauma
   B. Alveolar fractures can occur in isolation
   C. Alveolar fractures occur bilaterally at sites away from direct trauma
   D. Alveolar fractures occur at the condylar neck in the mandible

3. The physician is assessing your patient for a possible facial fracture. He places one hand on the maxillary teeth and the other on the bridge of the nose. Only the teeth move. This result indicates
   A. A probable LeFort I fracture
   B. A nasal fracture
   C. A zygomatic arch fracture
   D. A mandibular fracture

4. The cranial nerve responsible for movement of the eyeball and innervation of the lateral rectus muscle is
   A. CN III
   B. CN VIII
   C. CN II
   D. CN VI

5. The cranial nerve responsible for movement of the eyeball and innervation of the superior oblique muscle is
   A. CN II
   B. CN III
   C. CN IV
   D. CN VIII

6. If a bone fragment from the zygomatic arch impinges on the temporalis muscle and the coronoid process, tonic contractions of the muscles of mastication may result. This is known as
   A. Palsy
   B. Masseteritis
   C. Trismus
   D. Chvostek's sign

7. Your elderly patient slipped and fell against the curb of a sidewalk, causing a blowout fracture. The patient has extraocular muscle nerve palsy and diplopia. The cranial nerves affected in the case are
   A. Cranial nerves II, III, and IV
   B. Cranial nerves III, IX, and X
   C. Cranial nerves IV, X, and VIII
   D. Cranial nerves III, IV, and VI

8. The three main branches of the trigeminal nerve are the
   A. Facial, abducens, and trochlear
   B. Supraorbital, supratrochlear, and infratrochlear
   C. Ophthalmic, maxillary, and mandibular
   D. Zygomatic, buccal, and cervical

9. All the muscles of facial expression are supplied by the _____ nerve.
   A. Oculomotor
   B. Facial
   C. Spinal accessory
   D. Cervical plexus

10. Your patient was kicked in the face while practicing Taekwondo 2 days ago. She awoke this morning with a headache and flashes of light in her peripheral vision. She also states she has floaters in her eyes and that her vision is "murky" in some areas. Your priority for treatment is to
    A. Turn on all the lights
    B. Shield the eyes
    C. Check the ocular pH
    D. Arrange an ophthalmology consult

11. Frank was playing volleyball and was struck in the face by the ball when it was spiked. Two of Frank's teeth were avulsed. Which of the following is the best medium for transporting Frank's teeth?
    A. Diet Coke
    B. Water
    C. Hank's solution
    D. Milk

12. Your patient has acute angle glaucoma. The physician orders Diamox to be administered. As an ED nurse, you know it is important to monitor serum levels for
    A. Hypercalcemia
    B. Hypokalemia
    C. Hypernatremia
    D. Hypoglycemia

13. The gold standard for airway management in the patient with maxillofacial injuries is via
    A. Nasotracheal intubation
    B. Tracheostomy
    C. Oral intubation
    D. A King airway

14. Your patient was skiing and struck a tree. He sustained a concussion and trauma to his jaw and nose. He has malocclusion of the upper incisors and chipped lower incisors. The priority for nursing care is
    A. Relief of pain
    B. Airway management
    C. Administration of antibiotics
    D. Obtaining a CT scan

15. Your patient is a 30 year old man who stated he was struck on the right side of his face with a fist during an attempted robbery. He had negative LOC, is alert and oriented ×4. He has cervical tenderness, periorbital ecchymosis with tactile crepitus with facial swelling, and mild dysphagia. His chest X-ray showed mediastinal air. This finding is indicative of
    A. A pneumomediastinum
    B. A pneumothorax
    C. Cardiac tamponade
    D. A pleural effusion

16. Which of the following statements is false regarding maxillofacial injuries?
    A. Care of the patient with facial fractures should follow the same standardized approach to initial assessment as is provided for every trauma patient
    B. Oral placement of gastric tubes, airways, and endotracheal tubes for trauma patients with suspected facial fractures is preferred
    C. Up to 70% of patients with maxillary fractures will have a severe injury to the cranial base, cervical spine, or thorax
    D. Patients with basilar skull fractures should be intubated via the nasotracheal route

17. Your patient was playing paintball when he removed his goggles to clean them. At that moment he was struck near the left eye by a paintball. He presented to the ED with complaints of burning in the eye. The physician elects to irrigate the eye to try and remove the paint. The best solution for irrigation is
    A. Lactated Ringer's
    B. D5 Isolyte M
    C. D5W
    D. Sterile water

18. Your patient has sinusitis. Which type of X-ray is most commonly ordered to show a view of the paranasal sinuses?
    A. Cranial vault view
    B. Ludwig's view
    C. Anterior view
    D. Water's view

19. While assessing a patient with a basilar skull fracture, the nurse notices a stain on the patient's pillow. The stain is a small amount of blood encircled by a pale yellow stain. This stain is called
    A. Halo sign
    B. Battle's sign
    C. Grey-Turner's sign
    D. Ludwig's sign

20. Which of the cranial nerves (CN) are affected by a basilar skull fracture?
    A. I, VII, VIII
    B. I, II, III
    C. I, V, VIII
    D. II, III, VIII

21. Which cranial nerve is affected in a patient with Bell's palsy?
    A. Cranial nerve V
    B. Cranial nerve VIII
    C. Cranial nerve VII
    D. Cranial nerve VI

22. What is the treatment of choice for Bell's palsy?
    A. There is no known treatment
    B. Steroids and antiviral medications such as acyclovir
    C. Azithromycin only
    D. High doses of steroids for 6 months

23. Patients with Bell's palsy are unable to perform which of the following activities?
    A. Whistle or puff out both cheeks
    B. Extraocular eye movements
    C. Move the arm on the affected side
    D. Smell strong odors

24. Which of the following are symptoms of Ménière's disease?
    A. Fullness in the ear and sneezing
    B. Recurrent ear infections
    C. Tinnitus, hearing loss, and vertigo
    D. Vertigo only

25. Janet, a 53 year old woman, presents to the ED with 4 days of severe vertigo. She reports a high-pitched buzzing sound in her left ear. As the ED nurse you suspect Janet has which of the following conditions?
    A. An inner ear infection
    B. A ruptured tympanic membrane
    C. Ménière's disease
    D. Von Ludwig's syndrome

26. Your patient was admitted with midface trauma and will require an otoscope for an intranasal examination. The physician will be assessing for
    A. A LeFort II fracture
    B. Avulsed teeth
    C. Ocular injuries
    D. A septal hematoma

27. Tiffany presents to your ED complaining about bilateral eye pain, conjunctival erythema, and swollen eyelids. Tiffany also states that when she blinks, her eyes feel as if they have sand in them. She also states the symptoms started about 4 hours after she completed a session in a tanning bed. You suspect Tiffany has
    A. Cataracts
    B. A corneal abrasion
    C. Photokeratitis
    D. Cornea

28. Your 54 year old male patient is complaining of loss of hearing in his left ear after a cold. Today he has been very dizzy with violent vertigo at times with vomiting. He keeps complaining about the loud noise in his left ear. When you do your initial assessment you notice he has nystagmus toward the affected ear. What illness do you suspect?
    A. Otorrhea
    B. Ataxia
    C. Labyrinthitis
    D. Otitis externa

29. What is the treatment of choice for labyrinthitis with hearing loss?
    A. High-dose steroids, vestibular suppressants, and antibiotics if there is a bacterial infection
    B. Antihistamines, vestibular suppressants, and ciprofloxacin
    C. Surgical consult to drain affected ear of infection
    D. Afrin nasal spray, ibuprofen, and penicillin

30. What patient teaching should be performed before discharge of a patient with labyrinthitis?
    A. There are no special precautions for discharge teaching
    B. No alcohol, avoid salt, avoid rapid head movement
    C. There are no dietary restrictions with labyrinthitis
    D. Diet as tolerated, antibiotic therapy

31. Your patient is a 30 year old woman admitted to the ED with fever of 101°F and a severe sore throat with dysphagia. Her only history is a mild sore throat 3 days ago. From which of the following conditions is the patient probably suffering?
    A. Streptococcal infection
    B. Mononucleosis
    C. Thrush
    D. Peritonsilar abscess

32. What is the treatment of choice for a peritonsilar abscess?
    A. Incision and drainage of abscess and antibiotics
    B. Antibiotics alone
    C. High-dose steroids only
    D. Pain and fever control

33. Snow blindness can occur under which of the following circumstances?
    A. Arc welding, tanning beds, highly reflective snow fields
    B. Tanning booths, any snowy day, bright headlights at night
    C. Arc welding, headlights, flashlights
    D. Flashlights, headlights, any snowy day

SECTION 6: MAXILLOFACIAL AND OCULAR ANSWERS

1. **Correct answer: A**
   A LeFort I fracture involves a horizontal maxillary fracture that transverses the inferior maxilla and separates the hard palate and alveolar process from the remaining maxilla.

2. **Correct answer: B**
   Alveolar fractures can occur in isolation from direct low-energy force or through an extension of the fracture line into the alveolar area of the mandible or maxilla.

3. **Correct answer: A**
   Placing one hand on the anterior maxillary teeth and the other on the bridge of the nose with movement of only the teeth indicates a LeFort I fracture. Movement near the bridge of the nose indicates a Le Fort II or III fracture.

4. **Correct answer: D**
   The cranial nerve responsible for eyeball movement and innervation of the lateral rectus muscle is the abducens nerve, CN VI.

5. **Correct answer: C**
   The cranial nerve responsible for movement of the eyeball and innervation of the superior oblique muscle is the trochlear nerve, CN IV.

6. **Correct answer: C**
   Tonic contractions of the muscles of mastication are known as trismus. This condition may also be caused by tetanus or pericoronitis.

7. **Correct answer: D**
   The extraocular muscle nerve palsy and diplopia are caused by injury to cranial nerves III, IV, and VI.

8. **Correct answer: C**
   The three main branches of the trigeminal nerve are the ophthalmic, maxillary, and mandibular.

9. **Correct answer: B**
   All the muscles of facial expression are supplied by the facial nerve.

10. **Correct answer: B**
    This patient is probably suffering from a detached retina. The eyes must be shielded immediately to prevent further injury. The patient is probably anxious because of the vision changes, so it is important to minimize external stimuli and eye movement. Arranging the ophthalmology consult is important but can be done after measures are taken to save the patient's vision.

11. **Correct answer: C**
    Hank's solution contains all the metabolites, such as Ca, PO_4, K^+, and glucose, necessary to maintain normal cell metabolism for several hours. Diet Coke is too acidic and will damage the teeth. Water is hypotonic and will cause the cells to lyse. Milk is occasionally used to transport teeth, but cells on knocked-out teeth roots in milk don't

die immediately. However, they are unable to replicate (mitose) and are less able to reform new cells when reimplanted.

12. **Correct answer: B**
    When Diamox is administered, it is important to monitor potassium levels for hypokalemia. Hydrogen ion excretion in the renal tubules is inhibited and the low potassium levels may cause dysrhythmias.

13. **Correct answer: C**
    The gold standard for airway management in the patient with maxillofacial injuries is via oral intubation and is often performed with rapid sequence induction. Airway management modalities should be utilized based on the severity of the maxillofacial distortion, debris present, edema, and potential for compromise.

14. **Correct answer: B**
    This patient has a concussion and may have an altered level of consciousness. Facial trauma may also impinge on the airway. Both conditions warrant airway management as the priority of nursing care.

15. **Correct answer: A**
    This patient has a pneumomediastinum secondary to facial trauma that leads to subcutaneous cervicofacial emphysema and tracking of air into the mediastinum along lines of fascia. Granted this would be extremely rare, but it is important for the ED nurse to consider even the remotest possibilities.

16. **Correct answer: D**
    Patients with basilar skull fractures should be intubated via the oral tracheal route to avoid inadvertent cranial intubation.

17. **Correct answer: A**
    The best solution for irrigating the eye is lactated Ringer's solution because it has approximately the same pH (6 to 7.5) as tears (7.1). Paintball guns now are so advanced they shoot the paintball at the same velocities as pellet guns, but have 10 times the mass. The paintball is smaller than the orbit, so it has the potential for blowout fractures and complete disruption of the globe.

18. **Correct answer: D**
    The Water's view, or occipitomental view, is the most commonly ordered view to show the paranasal sinuses. In this view the maxillary, frontal, anterior ethmoidal, and sphenoid sinuses can be seen.

19. **Correct answer: A**
    The halo sign, a stain with a small amount of blood encircled by a pale yellow stain, is indicative of a basilar skull fracture. This can be a dangerous sign for the patient as meningitis can easily develop.

20. **Correct answer: A**
    CN I is the frequently affected cranial nerve in a basilar skull fracture and leads to a loss of sense of smell. CN VII and CN VIII are less likely to be affected unless it is a severe head injury.

21. **Correct answer: C**
   In Bell's palsy or facial paralysis the seventh cranial nerve (VII) is affected. The cause is thought to be related to the herpes simplex virus that can cause cold sores. The patient presents with a unilateral facial droop, flat affect on the affected side, inability to close the eye, and inability to smile. Drooling may also be present. This disorder often runs in families.

22. **Correct answer: B**
   Bell's palsy is best treated with tapering steroids and antiviral medications in the acute phase. Artificial tears and eye patches may be needed if the affected eye does not close. Aspiration may occur if the palsy is severe.

23. **Correct answer: A**
   The patient with Bell's palsy has a paralysis of the facial muscles and therefore cannot move the affected side of the mouth to whistle or puff out both cheeks.

24. **Correct answer: C**
   Ménière's disease is characterized by unilateral tinnitus, vertigo, and hearing loss. Nystagmus may also be present. The symptoms may present to varying degrees.

25. **Correct answer: C**
   Patients with Ménière's disease often present to the ED when the vertigo becomes intolerable. The eighth cranial nerve (vestibulocochlear or auditory nerve) may be affected in both the vestibular and cochlear branches. Another name for this disease is labyrinth hydrops, or accumulation of fluid in the inner ear. It is treated with diuretics and a low-sodium diet.

26. **Correct answer: D**
   Patients admitted with midface trauma should be assessed for septal hematoma with an otoscope for intranasal examination. A septal hematoma is blood collecting under the septum. If not treated it may deteriorate into an abscess or avascular necrosis. There is also the possibility that cerebrospinal fluid may be found, indicating an ethmoid bone fracture.

27. **Correct answer: C**
   Bilateral eye pain, conjunctival erythema, swollen eyelids, and a feeling that something is in the eye is usually indicative of ultraviolet photokeratitis. Exposure to the ultraviolet light in the tanning booth may cause permanent injury such as cataracts.

28. **Correct answer: C**
   This patient's symptoms are classic for labyrinthitis. Other symptoms include ataxia, fever, salivation, malaise, otalgia, otorrhea, and fullness in the affected ear. Diagnosis includes an audiogram and cultures of the affected ear if there is otorrhea. Other diagnoses to consider include idiopathic hearing loss, ototoxicity, brainstem infarct, syphilis, benign paroxysmal positional vertigo, or Ménière's disease.

29. **Correct answer: A**
   The treatment of choice for labyrinthitis with hearing loss is high-dose steroids, vestibular suppressants, and antibiotics if there is a bacterial infection. The high-dose steroids reduce the risk of permanent hearing loss. Vestibular suppressants are drugs like meclizine that reduce vertigo; tricyclic antidepressants like diazepam may also be

helpful. Antibiotics should only be used if there is evidence of infection. Antiviral drugs like acyclovir may be used for suspected viral cause. Surgery is very rarely used to treat labyrinthitis.

30. **Correct answer: B**
    When teaching a patient with labyrinthitis, it is important to mention that alcohol and salt can cause symptoms to return and increase tinnitus. Rapid head movement can stimulate the return of severe vertigo.

31. **Correct answer: D**
    Peritonsilar abscess is often seen after a mild sore throat or tonsillitis. The symptoms worsen and the patient may exhibit a fever > 100.4°F, dysphagia, and enlarged tonsils with collection of pus between the tonsillar pillars. There may be drooling or excessive saliva and clenching of the masseter muscle, as well.

32. **Correct answer: A**
    Incision and drainage of the peritonsilar abscess is the highest priority. Some studies suggest that a single high dose of steroids helps reduce the pain and swelling in the area. Depending on the causative organism, antibiotics that may be used to treat this condition include penicillin G or penicillin V, amoxicillin-clavulanate, erythromycin, cephalexin, and metronidazole.

33. **Correct answer: A**
    Snow blindness, also known as radiation keratitis, can be caused by exposure to any UVB rays. Injury to the eyes caused by highly reflective snowy fields, especially in high altitudes, is where the term snow blindness originated. Today, exposure to UVB rays from welder's arcs, tanning booths, carbon arcs, photographic flood lamps, lightning, electric sparks, and halogen desk lamps are additional causes of this type of injury.

SECTION 6: MAXILLOFACIAL AND OCULAR REFERENCES

Blacker, D. J., & Wijdicks, E. F. M. (2004). Clinical characteristics and mechanisms of stroke after polytrauma. *Mayo Clinic Proceedings, 79*(5), 630–635.

Brown, J. B., Stassen, N. A., Bankey, P. E., Sangosanya, A. T., Cheng, J. D., & Gestring, M. L. (2011). Mechanism of injury and special consideration criteria still matter: An evaluation of the National Trauma Triage Protocol. *Journal of Trauma-Injury Infection & Critical Care, 70*(1), 38–45.

Cavallini, G., Martini, A., Campi, L., & Forlini, M. (2009). Bottle cork and cap injury to the eye: A review of 34 cases. *Graefe's Archive for Clinical and Experimental Ophthalmology, 247*(4), 445–450.

Chau, J., Lee, D., & Lo, S. (2010). Eye irrigation for patients with ocular chemical burns: A systematic review. *Systematic Reviews - Joanna Briggs Institute*, 470–519.

Cockerham, G., Goodrich, G., Weichel, E., Orcutt, J., Rizzo, J., Bower, K., & Schuchard, R. (2009). Eye and visual function in traumatic brain injury. *Journal of Rehabilitation Research and Development, 46*(6), 811–818.

Cole, P., Kaufman, Y., & Hollier, L. (2009). Principles of facial trauma: Orbital fracture management. *Journal of Craniofacial Surgery, 20*(1), 101–104.

Emergency Nurses Association, Newberry, L., & Criddle, L. M. (2005). *Sheehy's manual of emergency care* (6th ed.). St. Louis, MO: Mosby.

Frakes, M., & Evans, T. (2004). Evaluation and management of the patient with LeFort facial fractures. *Journal of Trauma Nursing, 11*(3), 95–101; quiz 102.

Fréchède, B., Mcintosh, A., Grzebieta, R., & Bambach, M. (2009). Hybrid III ATD in inverted impacts: Influence of impact angle on neck injury risk assessment. *Annals of Biomedical Engineering, 37*(7), 1403–1414.

Gasparis Vonfrolio, L., & Noone, J. (1997). *Emergency nursing examination review* (3rd ed.). Staten Island, NY: Power Publications.

Gassner, H. G., Brissett, A. E., Otley, C. C., Boahene, D. K., Boggust, A. J., Weaver, A. L., & Sherris, D. A. (2006). Botulinum toxin to improve facial wound healing: A prospective, blinded, placebo-controlled study. *Mayo Clinic Proceedings, 81*(8), 1023–1028.

Haan, J., Glassman, E., Hartsock, R., Radcliffe, J., & Scalea, T. (2009). Isolated rollover mechanism does not warrant trauma center evaluation. *American Surgeon, 75*(11), 1109–1111.

Hardin, S. R., & Kaplow, R. (2010). *Cardiac surgery essentials for critical care nursing*. Sudbury, MA: Jones & Bartlett Learning.

Holleran, R. S. (2005). *Emergency transport nursing* (4th ed.). St. Louis, MO: Mosby.

Jacobs, B. B., & Hoyt, K. S. (2007). *Trauma nursing core course provider manual* (6th ed.). Bedford, IL: Emergency Nurses Association.

Jones & Bartlett Learning (2011). *2011 nurse's drug handbook* (10th ed.). Sudbury, MA: Jones & Bartlett Learning.

Kloss, F. R., Tuli, T., Haechland, O., & Gassner, R. (2006). Trauma injuries sustained by cyclists. *Trauma, 8*(2), 77–84

Kohn, M. A., Hammel, J. M., Bretz, S. W., & Stangby, A. (2004). Trauma team activation criteria as predictors of patient disposition from the emergency department. *Academy of Emergency Medicine, 11*(1), 1–9.

Kükner, A., Yilmaz, T., Çelebi, S., Karslioglu, S., Alagöz, G., Serin, D., Acar, M., & Özveren, M. (2009). Characteristics of pellet injuries to the orbit. *Ophthalmologica, 223*(6), 390–395.

LeBlanc, J. M., Haas, C. E., Vicente, G., & Colon, L. A. (2005). Evaluation of lacrimal fluid as an alternative for monitoring glucose in critically ill patients. *Intensive Care Medicine, 31*(10), 1442–1445.

Lee, J., Kwon, S., Chai, S., & Kim, H. (2009). A case of transient myopia after blunt eye trauma. *Japanese Journal of Ophthalmology, 53*(6), 665–667.

Lippincott. (2010). *Professional guide to signs and symptoms* (6th ed.). Philadelphia: Lippincott.

Lystad, R., Pollard, H., & Graham, P. (2009). Epidemiology of injuries in competition taekwondo: A meta-analysis of observational studies. *Journal of Science and Medicine in Sport, 12*(6), 614–621.

Militsakh, O., & Kriet, J. D. (2008). Masticatory diplopia. *Ear, Nose & Throat Journal, 87*(1), 39–40.

Mitchener, T., & Hauret, K. (2009). Air medical evacuations of soldiers for oral-facial disease and injuries, 2005, Operations Enduring Freedom/Iraqi Freedom. *Military Medicine, 174*(4), 376–381.

Monksfield, P., Whiteside, O., Jaffé, S., Steventon, N., & Milford, C. (2005). Pneumomediastinum, an unusual complication of facial trauma. *Ear, Nose & Throat Journal, 84*(5), 298–301.

Nersesyan, H., & Kattah, J. (2009). Monocular paralysis of vertical ductions after facial trauma. *New England Journal of Medicine, 360*(e1).

Olateju, O. S., Oginni, F. O., Fatusi, O. A., Faponle, F., & Akinpelu, O. (2007). Multiple midface degloving injury in an elderly man: Challenges and management outcome. *Journal of the National Medical Association, 99*(7), 810–813.

Philippens, M., Wismans, J., Forbes, P., Yoganandan, N., Pintar, F., & Soltis, S. (2009). ES2 neck injury assessment reference values for lateral loading in side facing seats. *Stapp Car Crash Journal, 53*(1), 421–441.

Proehl, J. A. (2008). *Emergency nursing procedures* (4th ed.). St. Louis, MO: Saunders.

Ram, J., Sukhija, J., Behera, D., & Gupta, A. (2010). Ocular and systemic morbidity profile in mass formic acid injuries. *Ophthalmic Surgery, Lasers and Imaging, 41*(1), 123–127.

Salonen, E. M., Koivikko, M. P., & Koskinen, S. K. (2008). Acute facial trauma in falling accidents: MDCT analysis of 500 patients. *Emergency Radiology, 15*(4), 241–247.

Shahim, F., Cameron, P., & McNeil, J. (2006). Maxillofacial trauma in major trauma patients. *Australian Dental Journal, 51*(3), 225–230.

Sheerin, F., & de Frein, R. (2007). The occipital and sacral pressures experienced by healthy volunteers under spinal immobilization: A trial of three surfaces. *Journal of Emergency Nursing, 33*(5), 447.

Simms, C., Madden, B., FitzPatrick, D., & Tiernan, J. (2009). Rear-impact neck protection devices for adult wheelchair users. *Journal of Rehabilitation Research and Development, 46*(4), 499–514.

Urdern, L. D., Stacy, K. M., & Lough, M. E. (2005). *Thelan's critical care nursing* (5th ed.). St. Louis, MO: Mosby.

Warrier, S., Wells, J., Prabhakaran, V., & Selva, D. (2010). Traumatic rupture of the superior oblique muscle tendon resulting in acquired Brown's syndrome. *Journal of Pediatric Ophthalmology and Strabismus, 47*(3), 168–170.

Watson, S., & Gorski, K. A. (2011). *Invasive cardiology* (3rd ed.). Sudbury, MA: Jones & Bartlett Learning.

Yano, H., Suzuki, Y., Yoshimoto, H., Mimasu, R., & Hirano, A. (2010). Linear-type orbital floor fracture with or without muscle involvement. *Journal of Craniofacial Surgery, 21*(4), 1072–1078.

SECTION 7:
Neurology

1. What patient parameters does the Glasgow Coma Scale measure?
   A. Verbal response, orientation, and activity
   B. Eye opening, motor response, and verbal response
   C. Eye opening, orientation, and motor response
   D. Verbal response, orientation, and eye opening

2. What Glasgow Coma Scale score indicates coma?
   A. 8–10
   B. 6–7
   C. 5–6
   D. 4–5

3. A 69 year old man comes to the ED complaining of left chest pain that radiates to his back. He thinks he somehow burned himself. When you remove his shirt there are erythematous blisters from the spine to the sternum. The blisters are most likely which of the following disorders?
   A. Herpes zoster infection (shingles)
   B. Sjögren's syndrome
   C. Stevens-Johnson syndrome
   D. A second-degree burn

4. Your patient has been diagnosed with sine shingles. What lab test(s) do you anticipate?
   A. CBC, CMP, sedimentation rate
   B. Varicella-zoster virus culture
   C. CBC, CMP, varicella titer
   D. Blood cultures

5. Under which of the following circumstances is a lumbar puncture contraindicated?
   A. Signs of increased intracranial pressure of unknown origin
   B. Signs of an intracranial hemorrhage
   C. Signs of Guillain-Barré syndrome
   D. Obtaining a specimen for laboratory study

6. What results do you anticipate from a lumbar puncture in a patient with suspected Guillain-Barré syndrome?
   A. The cerebrospinal fluid (CSF) is normal
   B. The glucose level is down but the CSF is otherwise normal
   C. There is a high red blood cell count in the CSF
   D. The CSF protein level is elevated but the cell count is normal

7. A 24 year old female with a fever of 105.7°F is brought to the ED by paramedics. The ED physician does a lumbar puncture for evaluation of this patient's cerebrospinal fluid. Which of the following results would you expect to see if this patient has bacterial meningitis?
   A. Xanthochromia, elevated CSF glucose, decreased protein
   B. Decreased CSF specific gravity, increased protein levels, normal cell count
   C. Elevated specific gravity, cloudy CSF, decreased glucose, elevated WBCs
   D. Increased protein levels, elevated cell count and CSF glucose

8. In a patient with a complete transection of the spinal cord at the C2-3 level you expect which of the following findings?
   A. Full sensation of the face, intermittent breathing, shoulder shrug
   B. Some sensation on the occiput, face, and ears, no diaphragm movement
   C. Complete loss of sensory and motor function below the level of the injury
   D. No movement of the diaphragm, shoulder shrug

9. Your patient has an old injury to C5. He has a blood pressure of 215/129 and his pulse is 175. What is the cause of his symptoms?
   A. Autonomic dysreflexia
   B. Hypertension
   C. Spinal shock
   D. Neurogenic shock

10. At what highest level of cervical spinal cord injury can a patient survive without ventilator assistance?
    A. C3-4
    B. C7-8
    C. C5-6
    D. All cervical spinal cord–injured patients require ventilator assistance

11. Where does the dermatome for the fifth thoracic spinal nerve cross the anterior portion of a patient's body?
    A. At the level of the axilla
    B. At the level of the xyphoid process
    C. At the level of the clavicular line
    D. At the nipple line

12. Cerebral aneurysms are most often found in the
    A. Internal carotid arteries
    B. Bifurcations of the anterior-posterior Circle of Willis
    C. Temporal artery
    D. Vertebral arteries

13. The most common first symptom of a rupturing cerebral aneurysm is
    A. Fever
    B. Nuchal rigidity
    C. Nausea and vomiting
    D. An explosive headache, often "worst headache of my life"

14. Nursing management of a patient with a cerebral aneurysm includes
    A. Ambulation, monitoring of vital and neurologic signs
    B. Glasgow Coma Scale assessments and monitoring for cerebral vascular spasm
    C. Maintaining normal intracranial pressure
    D. Maintaining systolic blood pressure less than 120 mmHg

15. What is the formula for cerebral perfusion pressure (CPP)?
    A. CPP = SBP – MAP – ICP
    B. CPP = MAP – ICP
    C. CPP = ICP – MAP
    D. CPP = MAP – CVP – ICP

16. The goal for cerebral perfusion pressure (CPP) is a pressure of
    A. 50–80 mmHg
    B. 20–40 mmHg
    C. 10–20 mmHg
    D. 40-60 mmHg

17. Your head-injured patient has developed nystagmus. Nystagmus may be defined as
    A. Eyes deviated to the side of the injury
    B. A convergent gaze
    C. Rhythmic tremor or shaking of the eyes
    D. Divergent gaze

18. Spinal reflexes indicate
    A. Functional upper motor neurons
    B. Nonfunctional lower motor neurons
    C. Nonfunctional upper motor neurons
    D. Functional lower motor neurons

19. Spinal shock is defined as a(n)
    A. Areflexia at or below the spinal cord injury
    B. Hyperreflexia and spasticity after spinal cord injury
    C. Areflexia that rises above the site of injury
    D. Spasticity below injury site

20. Neurogenic shock differs from spinal shock in which of the following ways?
    A. It is a less severe form of shock with spinal cord injury that causes a brief decrease in blood pressure
    B. It is a more severe form of shock that causes cardiovascular collapse in patients with a spinal cord injury above T6
    C. It is a more severe shock that increases paralysis and death
    D. It is a more severe form of shock that occurs within hours after a spinal cord injury and causes increased sympathetic outflow

21. Arteriovenous malformations (AVMs) are
    A. Commonly found misshapen blood vessels
    B. More common in women than in men
    C. A complex tangle of misshapen blood vessels susceptible to hemorrhage
    D. Never seen in children

22. The hallmark symptom of encephalopathy from any cause is
    A. An altered mental state
    B. Liver failure
    C. Renal failure
    D. Infection

23. Treatment of encephalopathy includes
    A. Antibiotics
    B. High-dose steroids
    C. Treating the underlying cause
    D. Electrolyte replacement

24. Diagnostic tests for a patient with encephalopathy could include
    A. BMP, CRP, and CXR
    B. Blood tests, CSF evaluation, and EEG
    C. EEG and Dilantin levels
    D. Lumbar puncture and cervical ultrasound

25. A sympathetic response to a stimulus results in
    A. Heightened awareness, increased blood pressure, bronchial dilation, and increased glucogenosis
    B. Dilated pupils, bronchial relaxation, increased gastric motility, normal urine output
    C. Vasodilatation, increased blood pressure, decreased gastric secretions, pupils at 3 mm
    D. Increased respiratory depth, increased heart rate, decreased gastric motility, sphincter dilation

26. Tyler was injured while skateboarding and has a T8 spinal cord injury. He has been diagnosed with spinal shock. The ED nurse knows the symptoms of spinal shock include
    A. Areflexia, autonomic dysfunction, loss of sensation, eliminatory dysfunction
    B. Areflexia, peripheral vasodilatation, decreased SVR, loss of sensation
    C. Areflexia, heightened sensation, cardiovascular shock
    D. Areflexia, bowel and bladder dysfunction, bradycardia

27. The most accurate method of measuring intracranial pressure is
    A. A subarachnoid bolt
    B. Intraventriculostomy
    C. An epidural catheter
    D. A subdural catheter

28. Normal intracranial pressure is in the range of
    A. 0–5 mmHg
    B. 4–15 mmHg
    C. 16–20 mmHg
    D. 20–40 mmHg

29. Where should the transducer for any type of intracranial pressure monitoring system be placed?
    A. Foramen ovale
    B. Aqueduct of Sylvius
    C. Foramen of Monro
    D. Fourth ventricle

30. What is the effect of Cushing syndrome in a patient with increased intracranial pressure?
    A. Increased systolic blood pressure, widening pulse pressure, bradycardia
    B. Elevated blood pressure, narrow pulse pressure, tachycardia
    C. Bradycardia, low blood pressure, narrow pulse pressure
    D. Tachycardia, increased systolic blood pressure, widening pulse pressure

31. Which of the following mechanisms decreases intracranial pressure?
    A. CO_2 retention
    B. PaO_2 less than 50 mmHg
    C. Increased cerebrospinal fluid absorption
    D. Increased metabolic activity

32. Mrs. P., a patient with a closed head injury, has a Foley catheter. In 1 hour her urine output increased from 30 ml/hour to 1000 ml of very pale, clear urine. The ED nurse knows the increase in urine output is probably due to
    A. A volume shift from the third space
    B. Syndrome of inappropriate antidiuretic hormone
    C. Diabetes insipidus
    D. Diuresis from steroids

33. As an emergency department nurse you know the treatment of diabetes insipidus includes which of the following interventions?
    A. Fluid restriction
    B. Intravenous replacement to cover the increased urine output
    C. Diuretics
    D. Demeclocycline

34. In what manner is the spinothalamic tract tested?
    A. Deep tendon reflexes
    B. Babinski reflex
    C. Pinprick or monofilament testing
    D. Patellar tendon reflex

35. What is one cause of autonomic hyperreflexia?
    A. Diarrhea
    B. Suctioning
    C. Constipation
    D. Warm breeze

36. What is autonomic hyperreflexia?
    A. Malfunction of the autonomic nervous system seen with head injury
    B. Malfunction of the autonomic nervous system seen with spinal cord injury
    C. Malfunction of the autonomic nervous system seen with pituitary tumor removal
    D. Malfunction of the autonomic nervous system seen with epidural bleeds

37. Felix is a patient with a gunshot wound to his T11-12 spine. Upon assessment you find motor paralysis on the same side as the gunshot wound but loss of pain and temperature sensation on the opposite side. This phenomenon is known as
    A. Grey–Turner syndrome
    B. Cushing syndrome
    C. Syndrome X
    D. Brown Sequard syndrome

38. What is the most common etiology of meningococcal meningitis?
    A. *Streptococcus pneumonia*
    B. *Neisseria meningitidis*
    C. *Staphylococcus aureus*
    D. *Haemophilius influenza*

39. What is the hallmark symptom of meningococcal meningitis?
    A. Headache
    B. Petechiae
    C. Malaise
    D. Vomiting

40. A positive Babinski or plantar reflex indicates
    A. A reflex elicited with a reflex hammer to the Achilles tendon
    B. Normal neurologic functioning
    C. Upper motor neuron lesion of the pyramidal tract
    D. Lower motor neuron lesion of the pyramidal tract

41. What is the proper technique for eliciting a Babinski response?
    A. Stroke the sole of the foot from side to side
    B. Stroke the sole of the foot along the lateral sole from the heel up toward toes and across the ball of the foot
    C. Strike the heel and the ball of the foot
    D. Strike the Achilles tendon with a reflex hammer

42. What effect is seen with a normal response to the Doll's eyes maneuver?
    A. Disconjugate gaze with head turn
    B. Conjugate gaze in the opposite direction as the head is turned
    C. Conjugate gaze in the same direction as the head is turned
    D. Nystagmus with head turning

43. Susan P., a 21 year old woman, was injured in a motor vehicle accident. It is now about 40 minutes after the accident and she is demonstrating decerebrate posturing. As the ED nurse, you know decerebrate posturing displays as
    A. One arm flexed, one flaccid, legs flaccid
    B. Both arms fully extended and internally rotated, legs flaccid
    C. Both arms fully extended and internally rotated, legs fully extended with toes pointed
    D. Flaccid arms and legs extended

44. Your patient suddenly develops right pupil dilation. What significance does this change indicate?
    A. Basilar skull fracture
    B. Uncal herniation
    C. Brainstem herniation
    D. Cerebral vascular accident

45. Cerebrospinal fluid is formed in which of the following locations in the brain?
    A. Lateral ventricles
    B. Choroid plexus
    C. Subarachnoid space
    D. Arachnoid villi

46. What volume of cerebrospinal fluid is produced each day?
    A. 1000–1200 ml
    B. 600–700 ml
    C. 400–800 ml
    D. 800–900 ml

47. George C., a 55 year man with meningitis, is having a lumbar puncture. As the ED nurse you know the cerebrospinal fluid (CSF) should be
    A. Hazy with a glucose level of 85
    B. Clear with RBCs present
    C. Clear and colorless with less than 45 mg/dl of protein
    D. Clear and colorless with a white blood cell count greater than 150 cells/mm2

48. When performing a neurologic examination, the six cardinal eye directions for eye movement are controlled by which of the following cranial nerves?
    A. CN II, III, IV
    B. CN III, IV, VI
    C. CN II, V, VII
    D. CN V, VI, VII

49. Your patient was an unrestrained driver in a motor vehicle crash where he struck and fractured the windshield. He has a left frontal lobe injury. Which of the following symptoms would you expect in this patient?
    A. Hearing and balance impairment
    B. Sensory and memory problems
    C. Personality changes, poor short-term memory
    D. Loss of motor function, hearing problems

50. What does the acronym RIND represent?
    A. Recurrent ischemic neurologic default
    B. Reversible intracerebral neurologic deficit
    C. Recurrent intracerebral neurologic default
    D. Reversible ischemic neurologic deficit

51. What differentiates a transient ischemic attack (TIA) from a reversible ischemic neurologic deficit (RIND)?
    A. TIA lasts less than 24 hours, a RIND lasts more than 24 hours
    B. TIA lasts less than 6 hours, a RIND lasts more than 48 hours
    C. TIA lasts more than 24 hours, a RIND lasts less than 24 hours
    D. TIA lasts less than 24 hours, a RIND less than 6 hours

52. You are educating your patient and his family about stroke. Part of your talk involves modifiable risk factors for stroke. Which of the following are modifiable risk factors for stroke?
    A. Alcohol use, obesity, family history
    B. Alcohol use, smoking, obesity
    C. Alcohol use, family history, smoking
    D. Alcohol use, family history, hypertension

53. Your patient has had a major left-sided stroke. What is the most common cause of stroke in the United States?
    A. Uncontrolled diabetes mellitus
    B. Cocaine abuse
    C. Uncontrolled hypertension
    D. Tobacco addiction

54. What are the two major types of stroke?
    A. Ischemic and lacunar
    B. Ischemic and hemorrhagic
    C. Hemorrhagic and transient ischemic attack
    D. Hemorrhagic and reversible ischemic neurologic deficit

55. Why does diabetes mellitus increase the risk of stroke?
    A. Increased risk of hypertension
    B. Decreased neuroreceptor response in cerebral circulation
    C. Accelerated atherosclerosis of the large arteries
    D. Increased risk of clot formation

56. Your patient with uncontrolled hypertension is most likely to have which of the following types of stroke?
    A. Ischemic
    B. Lacunar
    C. Transient ischemic attack
    D. Reversible neurologic deficit

57. You are caring for a 72 year old man with a left-sided cerebrovascular accident. Which symptoms do you expect to see?
    A. Hearing deficits, left vision problems, left facial droop
    B. Speech deficits, loss of right visual field, right facial droop
    C. Loss of right visual field, receptive aphasia, left facial droop
    D. Speech deficits, left visual field loss, left facial droop

58. Which hemisphere, cerebral or cerebellar, is more likely to be affected by stroke?
    A. Right cerebellar hemisphere
    B. Right cerebral hemisphere
    C. Left cerebral hemisphere
    D. Left cerebellar hemisphere

59. Your priority in caring for a patient with a cerebrovascular accident is
    A. Prevention of decubitus ulcers
    B. Prevention of aspiration of food or fluid
    C. Prevention of contractures
    D. Prevention of depression

60. Which area in the cerebrum controls verbal expression?
    A. Wernicke's area
    B. Broca's area
    C. Limbic area
    D. Pontine area

61. Fred F., an 80 year old African American man, has had a left temporal cerebrovascular accident due to uncontrolled hypertension. As his nurse, you know that Fred is likely to have which of the following deficits?
    A. Motor deficits
    B. Expressive aphasia
    C. Receptive aphasia
    D. Balance deficits

62. Pam, a 35 year old woman, has Guillain-Barré syndrome. What is the most important diagnostic parameter for this patient?
    A. Blood pressure
    B. Negative inspiratory force (NIF)
    C. Pain level
    D. Cerebrospinal fluid study results

63. Which results would you expect in the evaluation of the cerebrospinal fluid in a patient with Guillain-Barré syndrome?
    A. Increased white blood cells
    B. Increased protein levels
    C. Increased glucose levels
    D. Anaerobic bacteria

64. Which of the following descriptions would be the most appropriate for the patient with Guillain-Barré syndrome?
    A. Impaired motor weakness, impaired respiratory function, acute pain
    B. Impaired respiratory function, impaired nutrition, acute pain
    C. Impaired motor weakness, impaired bowel function, acute pain
    D. Impaired respiratory function, impaired bowel function, acute pain

65. Your patient with Guillain-Barré syndrome is experiencing a great deal of pain. Why is this occurring?
    A. Parasympathetic function
    B. Sympathetic inactivity
    C. Autonomic dysfunction
    D. Sympathetic function

66. Nursing management of a patient with Guillain-Barré includes which of the following actions?
    A. Monitoring labs and neurologic signs
    B. Monitoring respiratory status and neurologic signs
    C. Monitoring respiratory status and lab results
    D. Monitoring labs results and urinary output

67. A nursing diagnosis for the patient with Guillain-Barré includes
    A. Impaired nutrition
    B. Risk for impaired respiratory function
    C. Impaired fluid balance
    D. Impaired body image

68. Tyrell has three large aneurysms in his Circle of Willis. What methods are used to treat these types of aneurysms?
    A. Clipping the aneurysms and endovascular coiling
    B. Clipping of the aneurysms and tPA administration
    C. Medical management of blood pressure and Amicar infusion
    D. Amicar infusion and tPa administration

69. Death from status epilepticus is usually caused by which of the following mechanisms?
    A. Airway blockage leads to severe cerebral hypoxia
    B. A hypermetabolic state within the brain
    C. Falls from seizure causing head trauma
    D. Aspiration pneumonia

70. Beth is a patient with new onset grand mal seizures. While moving her to the gurney you witness a seizure. What is the first action you should take to protect this patient?
    A. Hold the patient down to prevent injury
    B. Roll Beth to her right side and protect the airway
    C. Insert an oral airway and call for help
    D. Hit the Code Blue button

71. Mike had a grand mal seizure lasting 70 seconds. As soon as the seizure passed, he was fully awake and asking for food. Given the patient's reaction to his seizure, you should
    A. Tell the patient you know he faked the seizure
    B. Feed the patient
    C. Notify the attending physician and anticipate a psychological evaluation
    D. Give Dilantin 1 gram slowly

72. John Doe is admitted to the ED for seizure activity. The nurse should anticipate which of the following laboratory tests?
    A. CBC, lipid panel, toxicology screen
    B. CBC, toxicology screen, LFTs
    C. CBC, CMP, lipid panel
    D. CBC, CMP, sedimentation rate, CRP, RPR, toxicology screen

73. Which diagnoses should be considered as the cause of any patient's seizures?
    A. Alcohol abuse and hypertension
    B. Panic attack and psychological illness
    C. Panic attack and transient ischemic attack
    D. Cardiac arrhythmias and hypertension

74. Aggrenox is commonly used to treat
    A. Myocardial infarction
    B. Cerebrovascular accident
    C. Pulmonary embolism
    D. Deep vein thrombosis

75. Fran has been diagnosed with multiple sclerosis (MS). She was admitted to the emergency department after an acute exacerbation during which she experienced left-side weakness. You know that multiple sclerosis is classified as which of the following types of disease?
    A. Motor disorder of the spinal cord
    B. Demyelinating disorder of the brain and spinal cord
    C. Motor disorder of the brain and spinal cord
    D. Demyelinating disease of the spinal cord

76. Fran is very depressed. She states, "I don't want to die like my mother did with MS." She is exhibiting behavior consistent with which Kübler-Ross stage of grief?
    A. Denial
    B. Bargaining
    C. Anger
    D. Acceptance

77. Common symptoms of an exacerbation of multiple sclerosis can include which of the following?
    A. Hyperesthesia, fatigue, and hyporeflexia
    B. Paresthesias, urinary incontinence, and constipation
    C. Diplopia, ataxia, and emotional lability
    D. Ataxia, dementia, and temporal neuralgia

78. What is the postulated etiology of multiple sclerosis?
    A. Heredity
    B. Autoimmune disorder
    C. Chemical exposure
    D. Heavy metal poisoning

79. Lab studies for multiple sclerosis identification include
    A. Cerebrospinal fluid evaluation, sedimentation rate, and fluorescent treponomal antibody absorption
    B. Cerebrospinal fluid evaluation, syphilis, and a drug screen
    C. Cerebrospinal fluid evaluation, CBC, and HIV
    D. Cerebrospinal fluid evaluation, lipids, and sedimentation rate

80. What are the two major types of multiple sclerosis?
    A. Progressive and relapsing-resolving
    B. Relapsing-remitting and static
    C. Progressive and relapsing-relapsing
    D. Relapsing-remitting and progressive

81. What are the four types of Guillain-Barré syndrome?
    A. Ascending, progressive, relapsing-remitting, pure motor
    B. Ascending, descending, Miller-Fischer variant, pure motor
    C. Ascending, descending, relapsing, pure sensory
    D. Ascending, relapsing-remitting, pure motor, pure sensory

82. Myasthenia gravis is diagnosed using which of the following tests?
    A. Weber test
    B. Rinne test
    C. Tensilon test
    D. Clonus test

83. What is myasthenia gravis?
    A. A neuromuscular disorder where myelin is destroyed at varying rates
    B. A neuromuscular disorder at the neuromuscular junction
    C. A neuromuscular disorder seen after viral infections
    D. A fatal neuromuscular disorder of upper motor neurons and lower motor neurons causing muscle wasting

84. What are some common symptoms of myasthenia gravis?
    A. Ptosis, proximal muscle weakness, and spasticity
    B. Dysphonia, sialorrhea, and atrophy
    C. Fatigue, proximal muscle weakness, and respiratory weakness
    D. Generalized weakness, hyperreflexia, and dyspnea

85. Laura is a 50 year old woman admitted to the ED for acute coronary syndrome. She also has myasthenia gravis and has pyridostigmine in her purse so she does not miss a dose. The staff does not know she has this medication. Suddenly, Laura's monitor alarms and indicates a severe bradycardia. You suspect an overdose of pyridostigmine. If that is true, Laura's problem is
    A. Cholinergic crisis
    B. Acetylcholine crisis
    C. Myasthenia gravis crisis
    D. The bradycardia is related to the acute coronary syndrome, not myasthenia gravis

86. Which of the following statements about Bell's palsy is true?
    A. The patient will have to take long-term steroid treatments
    B. The patient will have to wear sunglasses when outside
    C. The patient will develop a secondary petechial rash
    D. The patient will no longer require the use of thermal packs to the face

87. An example of a mnemonic used to assess a patient's level of consciousness is
    A. TIPPS
    B. PQRST
    C. RRST
    D. AVPU

88. Giada is a 62 year old woman who has had several months of declining fine motor skills. Her family brought her to the ED because of a sudden onset of dementia and incontinence. Following a CT scan she was diagnosed with normal pressure hydrocephalus. What is the most common cause of normal pressure hydrocephalus?
    A. Cerebrovascular accident
    B. Deep vein thrombosis
    C. An idiopathic cause
    D. Recreational drug use

89. Your patient has suffered a stroke. He has been evaluated using the NIH stroke scale and received a score of 26. This score indicates that this patient has suffered
    A. A minor stroke
    B. A severe stroke
    C. A moderate stroke
    D. A moderate/severe stroke

90. One of the primary purposes of using the NIH scale is whether or not the degree of disability will merit
    A. Extended rehabilitation
    B. A DNR order
    C. Additional speech therapy
    D. Use of tPA

91. Which of the following is not considered a testable aspect of brain function when using the NIH stroke scale?
    A. Language
    B. Ethnicity
    C. Sensation
    D. Vision

92. Assessment of a patient indicated an abnormal response when the patient was tested for pronator drift. This response indicates that the patient probably has
    A. A forearm fracture
    B. Myasthenia gravis
    C. Upper motor neuron disease
    D. A skull fracture

93. Your patient is being evaluated for meningitis. The patient is placed supine, with hips and knees flexed. When the physician attempts to extend the leg past 135 degrees, the patient complains of pain. This response is known as
    A. Cullen's sign
    B. Moses' sign
    C. Trevell's sign
    D. Kernig's sign

94. When you attempt to passively flex your patient's neck and touch his chin to his chest, he complains of a stiff neck and pain. This response indicates
    A. Meningeal irritation
    B. A basilar skull fracture
    C. Labyrinthitis
    D. A peritonsilar abscess

95. Suspected cases of meningitis should be placed in which of the following type of isolation?
    A. Universal precautions are all that is needed
    B. Contact precautions
    C. Reverse isolation
    D. Droplet precautions

SECTION 7: NEUROLOGY ANSWERS

1. **Correct answer: B**
   The Glasgow Coma Scale measures eye opening, motor response, and verbal response. It rates each with a total scale from 3 to 15, with 15 being a fully responsive patient. A score of 6–7 is comatose level. The longer that the patient remains in the lower score ranges, the worse the projected outcome.

2. **Correct answer: B**
   A 6–7 is comatose level on the Glasgow Coma Scale. A score of 15 is a patient who is fully awake. A score of 3 means there is no eye, motor, or verbal response from the patient.

3. **Correct answer: A**
   Shingles on the trunk are characterized by lesions that follow a dermatome. Dermatomes are the path innervated by the spinal nerves. Shingles may be found anywhere on the body, including inside the mouth.

4. **Correct answer: B**
   Labs are often not required for shingles, but if the patient presents with sine shingles (symptoms without rash) the varicella-zoster viral culture may be necessary. Unless a secondary infection is suspected, blood cultures and a CBC would not be done. A varicella titer only shows immunity to varicella, not an acute illness.

5. **Correct answer: A**
   Contraindications for a lumbar puncture (LP) are signs of increased intracranial pressure, infection in the area where the LP would be performed, and anticoagulant therapy. If an LP is done when there is increased intracranial pressure, the sudden change in pressure in the cerebrospinal space can cause herniation of the brainstem and death.

6. **Correct answer: D**
   The cerebrospinal fluid in a patient with Guillain-Barré syndrome generally shows elevated protein but a normal cell count. A patient with meningitis or a subarachnoid hemorrhage would present with a decreased glucose level in the CSF. A high red blood cell count is indicative of an intracranial hemorrhage such as a ruptured aneurysm.

7. **Correct answer: C**
   With meningitis, the specific gravity is elevated, the CSF cloudy due to the infection, and the white blood cell count elevated. The glucose would be decreased in this case. Xanthochromia is a yellow, orange, or brown color of the CSF due to the breakdown of RBCs from a previous hemorrhage and is not seen with meningitis.

8. **Correct answer: B**
   The patient with a high cervical transection of the spinal cord can present with the following: sensation of the occiput, face, and ears; there is no diaphragmatic movement; no voluntary movement below the injury; and there is loss of bowel and bladder function. Patients with this level of injury often die due to pneumonia.

9. **Correct answer: A**

   This patient has autonomic dysreflexia also known as autonomic hyperreflexia. This is a life-threatening exaggerated sympathetic response to minor stimuli. The stimuli may be a drafty room, a full bladder, or a bowel obstruction. Treating the cause will fix the problem. The symptoms include hypertension, severe headache, tachycardia or bradycardia, profuse sweating or flushing.

10. **Correct answer: C**

    At C5-6 there is enough diaphragmatic movement to allow for adequate respiratory function. Injuries above C5-6 require some level of mechanical ventilation.

11. **Correct answer: D**

    The fifth thoracic spinal nerve innervates at the nipple line. The dermatome innervates not only the skin but the organs, muscles, and tendons along the same path. It is important to know the dermatomes when dealing with spinal injuries because they help locate the level of the injury.

12. **Correct answer: B**

    Eighty-five percent of cerebral aneurysms are located at the anterior bifurcations of the Circle of Willis and 15% at the posterior bifurcations.

13. **Correct answer: D**

    An explosive headache, often "worst headache of my life," is a common statement from patients suffering from rupturing cerebral aneurysms. It frequently is the last thing patients say before losing consciousness.

14. **Correct answer: B**

    Glasgow Coma Scale assessment is imperative and is helpful in monitoring for vascular spasm, a potentially life-threatening problem for a patient with a cerebral aneurysm. Vascular spasm occurs secondary to meningeal irritation from the blood in the subarachnoid space.

15. **Correct answer: B**

    Mean arterial pressure minus intracranial pressures equals cerebral perfusion pressure. Cerebral perfusion pressure is a calculated measurement of the pressure gradient that allows blood to flow to the brain. The CPP may also be calculated using the CVP instead of the ICP because it is a measure of vascular resistance.

16. **Correct answer: A**

    As cerebral perfusion pressure is a calculated measurement of the pressure gradient that allows blood to flow to the brain, the goal is a CPP of 50–80 mmHg.

17. **Correct answer: C**

    Nystagmus, rhythmic tremor or shaking of the eyes, indicates pressure or damage to cranial nerve VIII (acoustic) in the vestibular portion. Shaking is usually stronger on one side and may occur in any of the cardinal eye directions.

18. **Correct answer: D**

    The knee jerk, also known as the patellar reflex, is an example of a functional lower motor neuron. These reflexes are also known as deep tendon reflexes. The nerve impulse makes an arc from the tendon to the sensory portion of the spinal cord to the motor root and back to the patella, causing extension of the lower leg.

19. **Correct answer: A**
    Spinal shock is defined as an areflexia at or below the spinal cord injury. Spinal shock can occur hours to weeks after an injury to the spinal cord. The patient develops flaccidity, loss of sensation, and loss of bowel and bladder function. Hyperreflexia and spasticity after spinal cord injury occurs after spinal shock resolves.

20. **Correct answer: B**
    Neurogenic shock is a much more severe form of shock that may occur with spinal cord injuries at or above T6. The autonomic dysfunction causes increased vagal tone that results in severe bradycardia, decreased cardiac output, peripheral dilatation, and decreased SVR.

21. **Correct answer: C**
    AVMs are a complex tangle of misshapen blood vessels susceptible to hemorrhage. AVMs lack the normal blood flow from arterial to venous flow and do not go through a capillary bed. This high-pressure flow makes them more likely to bleed. They are not common, they occur slightly more often in men, and AVMs are the most common cause of stroke in children under 12 years of age.

22. **Correct answer: A**
    An altered mental state is the primary symptom of encephalopathy. The definition of encephalopathy is an umbrella term for a collection of symptoms of other illnesses. This can include liver or renal failure, infection, brain tumors, increasing hydrocephalus, and environmental hazard exposure.

23. **Correct answer: C**
    Because there are so many potential causes, encephalopathy must be treated at its cause first. Examples of treatment include antibiotics, hemodialysis, and electrolyte replacement.

24. **Correct answer: B**
    Blood tests for a patient with encephalopathy can include CMP, CBC, and sedimentation rate, tests for specific illness or toxin, lumbar puncture to rule out neurologic infection. Other tests include electroencephalogram (EEG) and imaging studies of specific structures—hepatic or renal imaging.

25. **Correct answer: A**
    A sympathetic response to a stimulus results in heightened awareness, increased blood pressure, bronchial dilation, and increased glucogenosis. Other responses include dilated pupils for increased visual acuity, increased heart rate, increased myocardial contractility, increased blood pressure, increased respiratory rate, decreased gastric motility, decreased gastric secretion, decreased urine output, decreased insulin production, and decreased renal blood flow.

26. **Correct answer: A**
    Symptoms of spinal shock include areflexia, autonomic dysfunction, loss of sensation, and eliminatory dysfunction. Spinal shock occurs hours to weeks after a cord injury, causing autonomic loss, and the severity of a spinal cord injury cannot be fully assessed until the shock has resolved.

27. **Correct answer: B**

    The most accurate method of measuring intracranial pressure is intraventriculostomy. Because the catheter is inserted directly into one of the lateral ventricles, it is the most direct and accurate method of measuring intracranial pressure. The drain is inserted on the right side of the head. The ventriculostomy allows for not only drainage of excess CSF but also sampling of CSF to monitor for infection.

28. **Correct answer: B**

    Four to 15 mmHg is the normal range for intracranial pressure.

29. **Correct answer: C**

    The transducer for any type of intracranial pressure monitoring system should be placed in the foramen of Monro. The foramen of Monro is the junction between the lateral ventricles and the third ventricle. It is located just above the ear.

30. **Correct answer: A**

    The effect of Cushing syndrome in a patient with increased intracranial pressure is increased systolic blood pressure, widening pulse pressure, and bradycardia. Cushing syndrome is also known as the triad of symptoms. These are late indicators of a serious deterioration of neurologic status. This patient is at very high risk for herniation and death.

31. **Correct answer: C**

    Cerebrospinal fluid absorbed at an increased rate decreases intracranial pressure. CO_2 retention, PaO_2 less than 50 mmHg, and increased metabolic activity contribute to increased intracranial pressure.

32. **Correct answer: C**

    A sudden increase in urine output from 30 to 1000 ml/hour of pale, clear urine indicates diabetes insipidus. Diabetes insipidus (DI) is a serious decrease in antidiuretic hormone (ADH). The most common causes of neurogenic DI are closed head injury and posterior pituitary tumor removal. ADH is produced by the posterior pituitary gland. Closed head injury and cerebral edema lead to pressure on the pituitary gland, thus decreasing ADH. Other common causes of DI are lung cancer (small or oat cell carcinoma), leukemia, and lymphoma.

33. **Correct answer: B**

    Treatment of diabetes insipidus includes intravenous replacement with D_5W/ ½ NS with 20 mEq of potassium is titrated to replace hourly urine output. Other therapies include DDAVP (desmopressin) nasal spray or a pitressin infusion. Strict I&O and daily weights, monitoring electrolytes, and serum and urine osmolalities are also done.

34. **Correct answer: C**

    The spinothalamic tract is tested by pinprick or monofilament testing. The spinothalamic tract carries impulses from the spine to the thalamus; thus, it is a sensory motor tract. The lateral spinothalamic senses pain and temperature, whereas the anterior tract senses light touch and pressure.

35. **Correct answer: C**

    Autonomic hyperreflexia, also known as autonomic dysreflexia, is caused by numerous stimuli such as bowel or bladder dysfunction, cool breezes, a clogged urinary catheter, and constipation.

Neurology | 165

36. **Correct answer: B**
Autonomic hyperreflexia is a potentially life-threatening response to a minor stimulus seen after spinal cord injury at T6 or higher. It occurs after the initial spinal shock has resolved. Symptoms can include severe hypertension, dysrhythmias, severe headache, and photophobia.

37. **Correct answer: D**
Brown Sequard causes ipsilateral (same side) motor paralysis and contralateral (opposite side) loss of pain and temperature sensation. This syndrome occurs because of the way the pyramidal tracts cross in the spinal column.

38. **Correct answer: B**
Neisseria meningitidis is the causative agent for meningococcal meningitis. *Streptococcus pneumonia* causes pneumococcal meningitis. *Haemophilius influenza* causes *Haemophilius meningitis*. *Staphylococcus aureus* is not likely to cause meningitis but can cause infection in the brain with ventriculostomy drains or bolts.

39. **Correct answer: B**
Petechiae are the hallmark symptom of meningococcal meningitis. Headache, malaise, and vomiting can be seen with any form of meningitis.

40. **Correct answer: C**
A positive Babinski or plantar reflex is a sign of an upper motor neuron lesion. It can be seen with spinal cord compression, head injury, and stroke. It is a pathologic sign.

41. **Correct answer: B**
The proper technique is stroking the lateral sole of the foot from the heel up to and across the ball of the foot. It should be done in one motion with a relatively sharp instrument like the end of a reflex hammer.

42. **Correct answer: B**
With a normal Doll's eyes or oculocephalic reflex, the eyes appear to move to the opposite direction from the head turn. For example, if the head is turned quickly to the patient's left, the eyes normally appear to move to the far right side. If the reflex is absent, the eyes appear fixed and do not move. This is a poor neurologic sign. It represents pontine and midbrain damage. It may be used in determining brain death.

43. **Correct answer: C**
Decerebrate posturing displays as both arms fully extended and internally rotated, legs fully extended with toes pointed. Decerebrate posturing demonstrates pressure on the midbrain and pons. It is a very poor neurologic sign, especially if it continues for more than 4 hours.

44. **Correct answer: B**
Ipsilateral, or same side, pupil dilation is the symptom seen with uncal herniation across the tentorium. The tentorium is a fold of dura mater that supports the temporal and occipital lobes. This herniation puts pressure directly on CN III, causing pupil dilation.

45. **Correct answer: B**
Cerebrospinal fluid is formed by the choroid plexus of the third ventricle. The arachnoid villi, projections from the subarachnoid space, reabsorb the cerebrospinal fluid.

46. **Correct answer: C**
    400ml – 800ml of cerebrospinal fluid is produced daily by the choroid plexus in the third ventricle. There is approximately 125–150ml circulating in the ventricular system and spinal column at one time.

47. **Correct answer: C**
    The cerebrospinal fluid should be clear and colorless with a protein count of 16–45 mg/dl, WBCs 0–5 cells/mm^2, and the glucose level should be approximately 80% of the serum glucose level.

48. **Correct answer: B**
    The six cardinal eye movements test CN III (oculomotor), CN IV (trochlear), and CN VI (abducens). CN III is assessed by having the patient follow the examiner's finger or light up and out, up and in, down and out, and inward toward the nose. CN IV is assessed by having the patient follow the examiner's finger down and in toward the tip of the nose. CN VI is assessed by following the examiner's finger out toward the ear.

49. **Correct answer: C**
    Personality changes and poor short-term memory are expected symptoms in a patient with left frontal lobe injury. The frontal lobe is responsible for personality, memory, motor function, Broca's area, and critical thinking skill.

50. **Correct answer: D**
    RIND is a reversible ischemic neurologic deficit. It is similar to a TIA, but symptoms last more than 24 hours and the patient recovers completely.

51. **Correct answer: A**
    TIAs typically last a very short time, sometimes less than an hour but no longer than 24 hours, and there are no neurologic deficits. With a RIND the symptoms last more than 24 hours but the patient still has a complete recovery. Both are possible precursors of a major stroke within a year.

52. **Correct answer: B**
    Alcohol use, smoking, and obesity are all modifiable risk factors in preventing stroke.

53. **Correct answer: C**
    Uncontrolled hypertension is the most common cause of stroke in the United States. More than 360,000 strokes per year are due to hypertension. Stroke can be the first symptom of hypertension for many patients. Diabetes mellitus can lead to cardiovascular disease and hypertension, but it is less common than hypertension alone.

54. **Correct answer: B**
    The two major types of stroke are ischemic and hemorrhagic. Hemorrhagic strokes are usually caused by hypertension and may include aneurysm rupture. Ischemic strokes are usually caused by an occlusion of an atherosclerotic cerebral artery secondary to an embolus or occlusion.

55. **Correct answer: C**
    Diabetes mellitus causes accelerated atherosclerosis in the large arteries of the cerebral circulation, thereby narrowing the lumen and increasing the risk for stroke.

56. **Correct answer: B**
    Uncontrolled hypertension is most likely to cause a lacunar stroke. A lacunar infarction is due to thrombosis of the small arteries that penetrate the cerebrum. It causes facial, arm, and leg deficits.

57. **Correct answer: B**
    A left-side cerebrovascular accident causes right-side deficits because of crossing of the cerebrospinal tracts in the brain and spinal cord. You would expect the patient to have speech deficits, loss of right visual field, and right facial droop.

58. **Correct answer: C**
    The dominant side of the brain, the left cerebral hemisphere, is the most likely site for a cerebrovascular accident. Because more than 90% of the population is right-side dominant, the left hemisphere is most likely to suffer a stroke.

59. **Correct answer: B**
    Prevention of aspiration should be the priority of the ED nurse. Prevention of decubitus ulcers, contractures, and depression are also a part of caring for a patient with a cerebrovascular accident, but the ABCs (airway, breathing, circulation) are always the first priority.

60. **Correct answer: B**
    Broca's area at the lower edge of the frontal lobe is responsible for verbal expression. A deficit in this area is called expressive aphasia. The patient can comprehend what is said but lacks the ability to form the words due to loss of motor skills.

61. **Correct answer: C**
    A left temporal cerebrovascular accident will likely cause receptive aphasia. This patient has had a stroke affecting Wernicke's area in the temporal lobe, which affects verbal reception. This causes an inability to interpret speech and can also affect comprehension of written words.

62. **Correct answer: B**
    The negative inspiratory force measures the ability of the patient to take a deep breath to minus 28 mmHg. Once the effort is less than 28 mmHg the patient should be evaluated for intubation to prevent respiratory arrest.

63. **Correct answer: B**
    Protein in the CSF is always increased with Guillain-Barré due to the destruction of the myelin sheath. Because Guillain-Barré is an autoimmune disorder, WBCs, abnormal glucose levels, and bacteria would not be present in the CSF.

64. **Correct answer: A**
    Guillain-Barré patients experience motor weakness, impaired respiratory function, and acute pain. The pain is due to accentuated sympathetic response secondary to loss of parasympathetic counterbalance.

65. **Correct answer: C**
    Autonomic dysfunction in Guillain-Barré is caused by lack of balance in the autonomic nervous system. The sympathetic nervous system is unopposed, causing heightened sensitivity and overresponse to minor stimuli, causing pain.

66. **Correct answer: B**
    Respiratory status and neurologic signs are the most important nursing management issues, especially during the early onset of the demylenating process.

67. **Correct answer: B**
    Risk for impaired respiratory function is the most important nursing diagnosis. Other nursing diagnoses include acute pain, risk for impaired verbal communication, and potential for neuromuscular weakness related to demyelination.

68. **Correct answer: A**
    Clipping of the aneurysm and endovascular coiling are the two common methods of managing aneurysms in the Circle of Willis. tPA is a thrombolytic and would not be given to this patient. Controlling the blood pressure involves maintaining a good cerebral perfusion pressure to reduce the risk of vasospasm. Amicar inhibits plasminogen activator, allowing fibrin production.

69. **Correct answer: B**
    Death from status epilepticus is usually caused by a hypermetabolic state within the brain. Status epilepticus results in decreased oxygen and glucose levels in the brain, leading to the release of glutamate. The increased glutamate causes the influx of calcium into the neurons, destabilizing them electronically, which leads to cell injury and death.

70. **Correct answer: B**
    The best action is to turn Beth to her right side and protect her airway. Because the seizure has already started, it would be impossible to safely insert an oral airway. Never try to restrain a patient having a seizure. Hitting the Code Blue button is certainly an option, but it doesn't help the patient immediately. Precipitating events, aura, onset, duration, nursing actions, and postictal state should be included in the nursing notes.

71. **Correct answer: C**
    This patient should be given a psychological evaluation. If he had a genuine grand mal seizure, the postictal state is expected to last several hours and the patient would not be able to request food.

72. **Correct answer: D**
    CBC, CMP, sedimentation rate, CRP, RPR, and a toxicology screen are the tests that need to be performed to help establish the cause of John Doe's seizures. Seizures can be caused by illness, infection, overdose on drugs or alcohol, tertiary syphilis, dehydration, electrolyte imbalance, and cardiac arrhythmia.

73. **Correct answer: C**
    Panic attacks, transient ischemic attacks, cardiac arrhythmias, and syncope are some causes of seizures.

74. **Correct answer: B**
    Aggrenox is a persantine-based medication given in twice daily dosing for stroke or TIA patients.

75. **Correct answer: B**
    Multiple sclerosis is a demyelinating disorder of the white matter of the brain and spinal cord. It can be intermittent, progressive, or relapsing. It follows an acute or a progressive course. It is the major cause of disability in young adults aged 16–40. It affects females more than males.

76. **Correct answer: C**
Fran is angry at her diagnosis and afraid she will suffer the same fate as her mother. The five stages of grief identified by Kübler-Ross in 1969 are denial, anger, bargaining, depression, and acceptance. The patient can move through the stages in any order and can revisit a stage at any time. The nurse should try to encourage the patient to express her feelings. The physician should also be notified, and the patient should receive counseling. Antidepressants may be considered.

77. **Correct answer: C**
Multiple sclerosis produces a wide variety of symptoms depending on the white matter being affected by the exacerbation. These symptoms include both motor and sensory problems. Symptoms include ataxia, positive Babinski reflex, vision disturbances (for example, diplopia), clumsiness, emotional lability, fatigue, paresthesias, paralysis, hyperactive deep tendon reflexes, loss of proprioception, loss of vibratory sense, impotence in men, and urinary problems in women.

78. **Correct answer: B**
Although the exact etiology of multiple sclerosis is unknown, it is thought to be an autoimmune disorder triggered by environmental exposure or viral illness. There are clusters in Northern European families, and there is a higher incidence in people who work with manganese.

79. **Correct answer: A**
Cerebrospinal fluid results will show a negative syphilis (RPR), abnormal colloid gold curve, increased IgG, myelin debris, and slightly increased protein. Other tests include fluorescent treponomal antibody absorption (FTA-ABS), sedimentation rate, HTLV-1 serology, and check for vascular disorders. Neurologic testing includes evoked responses that are highly predictive for MS. MRI shows plaques as white spots in the brain.

80. **Correct answer: D**
Relapsing-remitting and progressive are the most common forms of multiple sclerosis. The frequency of relapsing-remitting episodes is related to stress and illness. Progressive may follow a continuous but slow route or it may advance quickly to the patient's death. Relapsing-remitting may worsen to progressive MS.

81. **Correct answer: B**
Ascending, descending, Miller-Fischer variant, and pure motor are the four types of Guillain-Barré syndrome. Ascending is the classic form of weakness and numbness that starts in the legs and moves up the trunk to involve the cranial nerves in some patients. The weakness is symmetric. Descending affects the cranial nerves first and the weakness progresses caudally. Respiratory failure is a major problem for these patients. Miller-Fischer variant is a very rare form that has a triad of symptoms that includes ophthalmoplegia, areflexia, and pronounced ataxia. The pure motor form of Guillain-Barré is identical to ascending but there is limited sensory involvement and therefore no pain.

82. **Correct answer: C**
The tensilon test is often used to test for myasthenia gravis because of the ease of administration. The medication has a quick onset and half-life. Ten milligrams are given intravenously. If there is improvement in a weak muscle it is considered a positive tensilon test. The Weber and Rinne tests are for hearing. Clonus is a reflex used to test spasticity.

83. **Correct answer: B**

    Myasthenia gravis is a pure motor disorder that occurs when an autoimmune response at the neuromuscular junction destroys acetylcholine receptors on the muscle membrane.

84. **Correct answer: C**

    Most myasthenia gravis symptoms deal with the weakness caused by the lack of acetylcholine receptors at the neuromuscular junction. These symptoms include ptosis, diplopia, facial weakness, dysphagia, dysarthria, fatigue, neck weakness, proximal limb weakness, respiratory weakness, and generalized weakness.

85. **Correct answer: A**

    Cholinergic crisis is a life-threatening problem with any overdose—accident or otherwise. It causes bradycardia, severe weakness, cardiac arrest, and occasionally respiratory arrest.

86. **Correct answer: B**

    The patient with Bell's palsy will need to wear sunglasses when outside and use artificial tears because the blink reflex is absent. Steroids are often used short term for this condition. Thermal packs, especially cold, may exacerbate the condition.

87. **Correct answer: D**

    An example of a mnemonic used to assess a patient's level of consciousness is AVPU.
    A: alert
    V: responds to voice
    P: responds to painful stimuli
    U: unresponsive

88. **Correct answer: C**

    The most common cause of normal pressure hydrocephalus is idiopathic (unknown). For most patients the cause is idiopathic. The mnemonic for normal pressure hydrocephalus (NPH) is "wet, wobbly, and wacky" due to the symptoms of incontinence, instability, and dementia. This condition can be successfully treated with a ventriculoperitoneal (VP) shunt.

89. **Correct answer: B**

    The patient received a score of 26 after an evaluation for a stroke. This value indicates a severe stroke. The NIH scale rankings are
    0 = no stroke
    1–4 = minor stroke
    5–15 = moderate stroke
    15–20 = moderate/severe stroke
    21–42 = severe stroke

90. **Correct answer: D**

    One of the primary purposes of using the NIH scale is whether or not the degree of disability will merit use of tPA. The NIHSS also provides objective comparisons of efficacy between treatment and rehabilitation modalities.

91. **Correct answer: B**
    Ethnicity is not considered a testable aspect of brain function when using the NIH stroke scale. Components of the NIHSS include testing for language, sensation, vision, consciousness, movement, and speech.

92. **Correct answer: C**
    An abnormal response when testing for pronator drift indicates that the patient may have an upper motor neuron disease or weakness in the shoulder girdle. To elicit this response, have the patient stand for 20–30 seconds with both arms outstretched forward, palms up, and eyes closed.

    Tell the patient to hold that position while you tap the hands vigorously downward. The patient will not be able to maintain extension and supination and will drift into pronation.

93. **Correct answer: D**
    When the patient is placed supine, with hips and knees flexed and the physician attempts to extend the leg past 135 degrees, the patient complains of pain. This response is known as Kernig's sign and indicates meningeal irritation.

94. **Correct answer: A**
    When you attempt to passively flex your patient's neck and touch his chin to his chest, he complains of a stiff neck (nuchal rigidity) and pain. This response indicates meningeal irritation.

95. **Correct answer: D**
    Droplet precautions are indicated for suspected bacterial meningitis for the first 48 hours of antimicrobial therapy. This type of isolation is used for those types of infections spread when the patient talks, coughs, or sneezes. Reverse isolation is used to protect the immunocompromised patient. Contact isolation is for those patients with conditions such as MRSA or VRE.

SECTION 7: NEUROLOGY REFERENCES

Akopian, G., Gaspard, D. J., & Alexander, M. (2007). Outcomes of blunt head trauma without intracranial pressure monitoring. *American Surgeon, 73*(5), 447–450.

Bader, M. K., & Littlejohns, L. R. (2004). *AANN core curriculum for neuroscience nursing* (4th ed.). St. Louis, MO: Saunders.

Brabrand, M., Hosbond, S., & Folkestad, L. (2011). Capillary refill time: A study of interobserver reliability among nurses and nurse assistants. *European Journal of Emergency Medicine, 18*(1), 46–49.

Burns, S. M. (Ed.). (2007). *American Association of Critical-Care Nurses (AACN): AACN protocols for practice: healing environments* (2nd ed.). Sudbury, MA: Jones and Bartlett.

Center for Disease Control and Prevention. (2008). Spinal cord injuries: Acute injury care. Retrieved March 23, 2008, from http://www.cdc.gov/ncipc/dir/AcuteInjuryCare.htm

de Kruijk, J. R., Leffers, P., Meerhoff, S., Rutten, J., & Twijnstra, A. (2002). Effectiveness of bed rest after mild traumatic brain injury: A randomised trial of no versus six days of bed rest. *Journal of Neurology, Neurosurgery and Psychiatry, 73*(2), 167.

Emergency Nurses Association, & Newberry, L. (2007). *Sheehy's emergency nursing: Principles and practice* (6th ed.). St. Louis, MO: Mosby/Elsevier.

Gasparis Vonfrolio, L., & Noone, J. (1997). *Emergency nursing examination review* (3rd ed.). Staten Island, NY: Power Publications.

Hardin, S. R., & Kaplow, R. (Eds.) (2004). *Synergy for clinical excellence: The AACN synergy model for patient care*. Sudbury, MA: Jones & Bartlett.

Hardin, S. R., & Kaplow, R. (2010). *Cardiac surgery essentials for critical care nursing*. Sudbury, MA: Jones & Bartlett.

Hickey, J. V. (2002). *The clinical practice of neurological and neurosurgical nursing* (5th ed.). Philadelphia: Lippincott Williams & Wilkins.

Holleran, R. S. (2005). *Emergency transport nursing* (4th ed.). St. Louis, MO: Mosby.

Jacobs, B. B., & Hoyt, K. S. (2007). *Trauma nursing core course provider manual* (6th ed.). Bedford, IL: Emergency Nurses Association.

Jones & Bartlett Learning (2011). *2011 nurse's drug handbook* (10th ed.). Sudbury, MA: Jones & Bartlett Learning.

Lippincott. (2010). *Professional guide to signs and symptoms* (6th ed.). Philadelphia: Lippincott.

McMillan, T. M., McKenzie, P., Swann, I. J., Weir, C. J., & McAviney, A. (2009). Head injury attenders in the emergency department: the impact of advice and factors associated with early symptom outcome. *Brain Injury, 23*(6), 509–515.

Medina, J., & Puntillo, K. (2006). *AACN protocols for practice: Palliative care and end-of-life issues in critical care*. Sudbury, MA: Jones and Bartlett

Proehl, J. A. (2008). *Emergency nursing procedures* (4th ed.). St. Louis, MO: Saunders.

Rynn, B., Pynn, T. P., & Sandor, G. K. S. (2006). Snowmobile accidents and facial fractures. *Oral Health, 96*(6), 33.

Smeltzer, S., & Bare, B. G. (2003). *Brunner and Suddarth's textbook of medical-surgical nursing* (10th ed.). Philadelphia: Lippincott Williams & Wilkins.

Urdem, L. D., Stacy, K. M., & Lough, M. E. (2005). *Thelan's critical care nursing* (5th ed.). St. Louis, MO: Mosby.

Waninger, K. N., & Swartz, E. E. (2011). Cervical spine injury management in the helmeted athlete. *Current Sports Medicine Reports, 10*(1), 45–49.

Watson, S., & Gorski, K. A. (2011). *Invasive cardiology* (3rd ed.). Sudbury, MA: Jones & Bartlett Learning.

SECTION 8:

Obstetrics and Gynecology

Nothing strikes fear into the heart of an ED nurse like a patient who is 9 months and 10 minutes pregnant. ED nurses can deal with everything from multiple traumas to the most esoteric of medical conditions. However, the possibility of delivering a baby terrifies even the most experienced of nurses. I know of many ED nurses who have Labor and Delivery and the NICU on speed dial.

A few issues associated with obstetrics and gynecology are covered on the CEN exam. This section goes beyond the exam and covers information to help guide the ED nurse through assessment of the mother and baby to stabilization of the newborn.

Many emergency departments are now requiring the staff to take the American Academy of Pediatrics/American Heart Association Neonatal Resuscitation course. NRP is an excellent course, and I highly recommend it to help develop competency and allay anxiety if a birth occurs in the ED.

Another excellent course is S.T.A.B.L.E. The letters stand for sugar, temperature, airway, blood pressure, and lab work. This course is wonderful for those nurses who must prepare a baby for transport to another department or facility.

1. What is the treatment of choice for trichomonal vaginitis?
   A. Metronidazole 2000 mg orally for one dose
   B. Rocephin 250 mg intramuscularly, single dose
   C. Doxycycline 100 mg twice daily for 10 days
   D. Penicillin 500 mg every 8 hours for 10 days

2. A 21 year old woman is in the ED complaining of a vaginal discharge that is yellow-green in color and has a foul odor. Which diagnostic test do you anticipate the physician will order to help diagnose this condition?
   A. A urinalysis
   B. A vaginal wet mount
   C. No diagnostic tests are necessary
   D. A blood draw for an RPR study

3. Francine had delivered a 29-week gestation neonate 7 days ago who was admitted to the NICU. Also at that time, Francine was admitted to the ICU for hypovolemic shock, post uterine rupture, and a hysterectomy. She was discharged home yesterday. Today, Francine presents to the ED with a mild case of bronchitis. Francine states she still wants to breastfeed and has begun pumping. What effect will the week (or more) delay have on her total breastmilk supply?
   A. Francine will produce exactly the same total amount of breastmilk regardless of her complications
   B. Francine will likely produce less milk than the expected total if she had not had complications
   C. Francine will likely produce more milk than the expected total if she had not had complications
   D. Francine will probably not be able to breastfeed at all because the milk supply is dwindling

4. Minerva is 7 months pregnant and admitted to your unit for severe HELLP syndrome. She is also at risk for which of the following conditions?
   A. Intra-abdominal hypertension (IAH) and abdominal compartment syndrome (ACS)
   B. Decreased intracranial pressure (ICP)
   C. Hypocarbia
   D. Increased platelets

5. Joyce was prescribed steroids by her obstetrician. Antenatal corticosteroids affect fetal lung maturation and help prevent respiratory distress syndrome. Steroids work by
   A. Decreasing the size of the alveoli
   B. Accelerating the rate of glycogen depletion
   C. Reducing the number of lamellar bodies inside the cells
   D. Thickening the intra-alveolar septa

6. The respiratory therapist has just given Dolly an aerosol treatment and postural drainage. Dolly is 8 months pregnant. The postural drainage was inappropriate. Which of the following additional conditions is a contraindication for this type of treatment?
   A. Pleural effusions
   B. Head injury
   C. Asthma
   D. Stridor

7. Your patient has been diagnosed with maternal hyperglycemia. Maternal hyperglycemia ultimately causes
   A. Increased hepatic glucose uptake
   B. Microsomia
   C. Pierre-Robin sequence
   D. Decelerated lipogenesis

8. Maternal thyroid disease can have a substantial influence on fetal and neonatal thyroid function because
   A. Radiation stimulates thyroid function
   B. Thioamides can stimulate thyroid growth
   C. Immunoglobulin G (IgG) autoantibodies can cross the placenta
   D. Thyroid function is enhanced

9. The Kleihauer-Betke test identifies
   A. Sickle cell trait in utero
   B. Common blood group antigens
   C. Bone marrow lymphocyte precursors
   D. Fetal hemoglobin in maternal blood

10. Jane plans to breastfeed her newborn, just delivered in your emergency department. A mother's breastmilk contains the immunoglobulin known as
    A. IgG
    B. IgA
    C. IgM
    D. IgE

11. Which of the following statements about human breastmilk is true?
    A. Human breastmilk contains insoluble proteins
    B. Human breastmilk is always the best choice for an infant
    C. Human breastmilk is high in cytokines
    D. Human breastmilk provides absolute protection against bronchopulmonary dysplasia

12. Rhesus (Rh) hemolytic disease of the newborn is a severe, often fatal disease caused by
    A. An Rh-negative mother alloimmunized during the first Rh incompatible pregnancy
    B. An Rh-positive mother with an Rh-negative fetus
    C. An allergy to rhesus serum
    D. IgG Rh antibodies are unable to cross the placenta

13. If a mother received an incompatible transfusion of Rh-positive platelets following a placental rupture, it would be appropriate to administer
    A. Neostigmine
    B. FFP
    C. RhoGAM
    D. CuroSurf

14. A patient can be presensitized and is more likely to undergo organ rejection if she has a history of
    A. Multiple pregnancies
    B. Small or reduced lumens in the bile ducts
    C. Destruction of small airways
    D. Cytomegalovirus (CMV) infections

15. Abortion can best be defined as
    A. Intentional termination of a pregnancy after 24 weeks gestation
    B. Termination of a pregnancy prior to 20 weeks gestation
    C. Termination of a pregnancy after 23 weeks gestation
    D. Intentional termination of a pregnancy prior to 20 weeks gestation

16. Your patient has a diagnosis of placenta previa. As an ED nurse, you know this means
    A. Your patient was previously pregnant and has retained placental material
    B. Your patient is pregnant and the placenta has partially separated from the uterine wall
    C. Your patient is pregnant and the placenta is partially implanted into the endometrium
    D. Your patient is pregnant and the placenta is partially implanted over the inferior uterus and/or the cervix

17. Calculation of fetal gestational age is based on
    A. 210 days from conception
    B. 40 premenstrual weeks
    C. 10 lunar months counted from the first day of the last menstrual period
    D. A 29-day cycle

18. Beatrice is being seen in the emergency department for hyperemesis. She reports she is in her second trimester of pregnancy. You know the second trimester includes which of the following ranges for weeks of gestation?
    A. 6–24 weeks
    B. 13–27 weeks
    C. 15–30 weeks
    D. 20–29 weeks

19. Cara has just been told she is pregnant. What is the recommended caloric intake for most pregnant women?
    A. 1800 kcal/d
    B. 2000 kcal/d
    C. 2200 kcal/d
    D. 2400 kcal/d

20. Recommended daily minimum folic acid intake is _____ to _____
    A. 0.3 mg, to stimulate alveoli development
    B. 0.4 mg, to prevent neural tube defects
    C. 2.5 mg, to stimulate alveoli development
    D. 4 mg, to prevent neural tube defects

21. Danica asks what causes her morning sickness. You explain that morning sickness is affected by
    A. Increased human chorionic gonadotropin (hCG) levels
    B. Decreased progesterone levels
    C. Decreased estrogen levels
    D. Increased glucose levels

22. Josie is 5 months pregnant and presents to the emergency department with constant abdominal pain at the right costal margin, nausea, and low-grade fever. You note muscle rigidity and rebound tenderness. You suspect Josie may have
    A. Appendicitis
    B. Preterm labor
    C. Abruption
    D. Braxton-Hicks contractions

23. Lucy has a diagnosis of HELLP syndrome. What do the letters HELLP stand for?
    A. Headaches, emesis, lethargy, liver enzymes elevated, petechiae
    B. Headaches, elevated liver enzymes, lethargy, petechiae
    C. Hemolysis, emesis, lethargy, liver enzymes elevated, platelet deficiency
    D. Hemolysis, elevated liver enzymes, low platelets

24. Which of the following complications has not been associated with HELLP syndrome?
    A. DIC
    B. Abruption
    C. Placenta previa
    D. Acute renal failure

25. Which of the following statements regarding HELLP syndrome is true?
    A. HELLP syndrome can occur in the postpartum patient
    B. HELLP syndrome has a clearly defined etiology
    C. Classic symptoms of preeclampsia, hypertension, and proteinurea are always associated with HELLP syndrome
    D. Low platelet count in HELLP syndrome is caused by decreased production

26. Which of the following disease processes can mimic HELLP syndrome?
    A. Hepatitis and preterm labor
    B. ITP and preeclampsia
    C. Preterm labor and ITP
    D. Preeclampsia and abruption

27. Anna is a 28 year old gravida 8, para 1 and has been pregnant 33 weeks. She presents to the emergency department with headache, blurred vision, increased fatigue, +3 pitting edema, nausea, vomiting, and right abdominal pain. Which of the following lab results indicates a need for immediate intervention?
    A. Bilirubin 1 mg/dl
    B. Serum aspartate aminotransferase 120 units/L
    C. Lactate dehydrogenase 480 units/L
    D. Platelet count 200 mm$_3$

28. Heather is suspected of having HELLP syndrome. What initial action should be taken by the emergency department nurse before transfer to the Labor and Delivery department?
    A. Insert an IV
    B. Ensure a BMP is drawn
    C. Place a Foley catheter
    D. Verify history and physical—gravida, para, and gestation

29. Corticosteroids were ordered for a 30-week gestation, gravida 5, para 2, 32 year old in labor. Why was this patient prescribed corticosteroids as part of her therapy?
    A. To decrease inflammation in the feet and ankles
    B. To decrease destruction of platelets
    C. To increase fetal lung maturity
    D. To prevent seizures

30. Mikko is being transferred to a higher level medical center for treatment for HELLP syndrome. Her blood pressure is 150/88, heart rate 120, respiratory rate 28, and temperature 99.2°F. The physician orders a magnesium sulfate infusion. The magnesium is given to
    A. Treat hypertension
    B. Prevent seizures
    C. Decrease respiratory distress
    D. Decrease contractions

31. Lasix is ordered for a mother with HELLP syndrome. Her BP is 198/120, HR 110, and RR 20. Your first action should be to
    A. Administer the Lasix as ordered
    B. Ask to change the order to mannitol
    C. Refuse to administer the Lasix
    D. Ask for fluid restriction and orders for strict I and O.

32. Your facility does not have maternal child services. Should a laboring mother come to the emergency department, which of the following pieces of equipment or treatments is not usually needed in the first 15 minutes of a neonatal resuscitation?
    A. Epinephrine, naloxone, normal saline
    B. Self-inflating or flow-inflating bag
    C. Warming device and blankets
    D. Bulb syringe

33. Maria is a 25 year old presenting to the emergency department with mild respiratory distress, cough, night sweats, and fatigue. She reports she is 23 weeks pregnant. You receive orders to discharge her home for flu management (rest, fluids, and antivirals). Before the patient's discharge, what additional action should be performed?
    A. Discharge as ordered, nothing else is needed
    B. Ask the physician for a cough suppressant
    C. Ask the physician for an antibiotic for secondary infection
    D. Request that labor and delivery provide a nurse to assess fetal health

34. Jensen is a 19 year old presenting to the emergency department with unilateral pelvic pain, palpable pelvic mass, and abnormal vaginal bleeding. You should anticipate orders to
    A. Request an hCG test
    B. Administer glycerin suppository
    C. Suggest the patient walk the hall
    D. Request a CT scan

35. Althea is a 20 year old presenting to the emergency department in active labor. You are told that she is a gravida 2, para 3. This means
    A. Althea has been pregnant twice and delivered three viable children
    B. Althea has pregnant three times and delivered two viable children
    C. Althea has been pregnant three times and has had three miscarriages
    D. Althea has been pregnant twice and has had three miscarriages

36. Nancy is 30 years old. She presents with abdominal pain and vaginal bleeding. The physician writes that she is a nullipara, gravida 5. This means
    A. The physician wrote her history wrong and will need to correct it
    B. The patient has never been pregnant
    C. The patient has been pregnant five times but has never delivered a viable fetus
    D. The patient has been pregnant five times but has had five abortions

37. Sophia is a 32 year old presenting to the emergency department with vaginal bleeding, cramping, and abdominal pain. She is 20 weeks pregnant. During the vaginal exam, the physician reports that Sophia's cervical os is dilated to 5 cm. Sophia is experiencing a(n)
    A. Threatened abortion
    B. Inevitable abortion
    C. Incomplete abortion
    D. Missed abortion

38. Charlotte was brought into the emergency room by family members for heavy vaginal bleeding and severe cramping. Her hCG test is positive, the vaginal exam shows an open cervical os, and an enlarged uterus is noted. She is AB negative, serology negative, Hepatitis B negative, and GBS positive. She reports passing larger blood clots than normal in the last few days. Which of the following orders is contraindicated at this time?
    A. Place an IV for fluid resuscitation with lactated Ringer's
    B. Administer $Rh_o(D)$ immune globulin
    C. Consult obstetrical surgeon
    D. Infuse oxytocin 200 units per 1000 ml of lactated Ringer's

39. What is the most common cause of spontaneous abortion in the first trimester?
    A. Trauma
    B. Maternal anatomic abnormalities
    C. Infection
    D. Embryonic chromosomal defects

40. Complete abortions left untreated may result in a(n)
    A. Incomplete abortion
    B. Missed abortion
    C. Septic abortion
    D. Threatened abortion

41. Which of the following organisms is not considered normal vaginal flora?
    A. *Escherichia coli*
    B. Alpha-hemolytic *streptococci*
    C. Beta-hemolytic *streptococci*
    D. *Candida albicans*

42. Ava presents with severe abdominal distention, constant pelvic pain, fever, chills, and uterine tenderness. She reports that she had a dilation and curettage 3 days ago. She also reports passing green and black tissue clots. You should immediately
    A. Contact a surgical consult and prepare the patient for surgery
    B. Observe Ava for anaphylactic shock
    C. Administer spectinomycin hydrochloride
    D. Administer ganciclovir

43. Which of the following discharge instructions for a postabortion patient is true?
    A. Vaginal bleeding should stop within 4 to 5 days
    B. Slight cramping that lasts for 1 to 2 weeks is normal
    C. Avoid intercourse, douching, and tampons for at least 2 weeks
    D. Monitor blood pressure for 5 days

44. PIH stands for
    A. Pregnancy-induced hypoglycemia
    B. Pregnancy-induced headaches
    C. Pregnancy-induced hyperemesis
    D. Pregnancy-induced hypertension

45. Which of the following symptoms is consistent with a diagnosis of preeclampsia?
    A. Systolic blood pressure of 130 mmHg; oliguria
    B. Edema of the face, hands, and sacrum; vomiting
    C. Decreased deep tendon reflexes; albuminuria
    D. Weight gain of > 2 lbs per week; visual changes

46. Addison has been diagnosed with preeclampsia. While waiting for a bed in labor and delivery, the physician orders hydralazine. Which of the following dosages is correct?
    A. 40 mg IV
    B. 10 mg PO daily in divided doses
    C. 100 mg IM
    D. Hydralazine is contraindicated for pregnant women

47. What is the primary difference between preeclampsia and eclampsia?
    A. The systolic blood pressure of the preeclamptic patient is < 180 mmHg and > 180 mmHg for the eclamptic patient
    B. Albuminuria is noted only with preeclampsia
    C. Seizures are noted only with eclampsia
    D. HELLP syndrome is noted only with preeclampsia

48. Olivia was admitted to the emergency department for seizures. She had a seizure immediately upon arrival in the patient treatment area. The seizure has lasted for 7 minutes. Olivia is 30 weeks pregnant. Her BP is 210/130, RR is 40, and she has +4 pitting edema. After you administer magnesium sulfate, Olivia stops seizing. What position should you place her in while waiting for transfer to high-risk obstetrical unit?
    A. Supine
    B. Prone
    C. Right
    D. Left

49. Why is placenta previa a concern during late pregnancy?
    A. The placenta pulls away from the uterus with fetal growth
    B. As the fetus grows, the os thins and leads to bleeding
    C. High placenta implantation pulls away with contractions
    D. As the fetus grows the placenta thins and leads to preterm labor

50. Which signs and symptoms are consistent with placenta previa presentation?
    A. Sudden painless bleeding of bright red blood, hypotension, tachycardia, delayed capillary refill
    B. Sharp abdominal pain without bleeding, tachycardia and tachypnea
    C. Uterine rigidity, frank red blood, hypotension, tachycardia, back pain
    D. Foul vaginal discharge, constant pelvic pain, fever, chills

51. Amelia is 47 years old and pregnant at 35 weeks gestation. She was brought in to the ED after a motor vehicle accident. She was driving when the vehicle she was driving was T-boned on the passenger side. Amelia has multiple lacerations to face, chest, and abdomen. Her pants are saturated with blood and you note an open femur fracture to her right leg. She is at high risk for which of the following life-threatening conditions?
    A. Compartment syndrome
    B. Preterm labor
    C. Abruption
    D. Infection

52. Which of the following actions is a nursing priority when caring for a mother experiencing abruption?
    A. Two large-bore IVs with ½ normal saline infusions
    B. Consider administration of O+ blood
    C. Set up for intermittent fetal monitoring
    D. Mark fundal height and assess frequently

53. Which of the following signs is not an indication of impending delivery?
    A. Bloody show
    B. Bulging membranes
    C. Desire of the mother to void
    D. Crowning

54. Lily just delivered a term male infant with clear amniotic fluid in the emergency department. What is your immediate priority?
    A. Call nursery or NICU to come get the baby
    B. Remove wet blankets after drying
    C. Tracheal suctioning to clear airway
    D. Use hot water bottles or gloves to warm baby

55. Bartholin's cyst is a
    A. Unilateral cyst on the labia majora
    B. Unilateral cyst on the fallopian tubes
    C. Cyst caused by sexually transmitted diseases
    D. Cyst located near the clitoris

56. Zaida has been diagnosed with Skene's duct cyst. She is at high risk for
    A. Urinary retention
    B. Systemic infection
    C. An inguinal hernia
    D. Vaginitis

57. Per the 2011 NRP Guidelines, what major change to term newborn resuscitation is true?
    A. If positive pressure ventilation is required, 100% FiO_2 should be used
    B. All newborns requiring respiratory support should be monitored using pulse oximetry
    C. Use pulse oximetry to maintain saturation at 80–90% after 10 minutes of life
    D. Blow-by or free-flow oxygen should be at 8 Lpm to provide 100% FiO_2

58. Marcy just delivered a term infant in the emergency department. The umbilical cord was wrapped twice around the infant's neck. After you dried, stimulated, and suctioned the infant's airway with a bulb syringe, you determine the heart rate as 40 bpm. Your next action should be to
    A. Suction the airway using wall suction
    B. Begin chest compressions at a 15:2 ratio
    C. Use your fingertips to vigorously stimulate the infant
    D. Provide positive pressure ventilation at 40–60 bmp for 30 seconds and then reassess the heart rate

59. You are providing positive pressure ventilation (PPV) to an apneic newborn. You note increasing difficulty with obtaining chest rise. After repositioning the mask and head, your next action should be to
    A. Use wall suction to clear the mouth
    B. Place an orogastric tube
    C. Place a nasogastric tube to low intermittent wall suction
    D. Increase positive inspiratory pressure to > 40 mmHg

60. May is in active labor. Friends report she was "using this morning." She delivers a preterm female infant in the emergency department. The infant is apneic, floppy, cyanotic, and has a heart rate of 70. Which of the following actions is contraindicated in the care of this infant?
    A. Provide positive pressure ventilation for 30 seconds and then reassess HR, respiratory, and color
    B. Administer Narcan (naloxone) at 0.1 mg/kg
    C. Use pulse oximetry to titrate FiO_2 to keep oxygen saturation between 85% and 95%
    D. Wrap the infant in a polyethylene bag and place under heat source

61. Ella is a 20 year old seen in the emergency department 5 days ago for streptococcal pharyngitis. She returned with complaint of profuse, white, curdlike vaginal discharge. A vaginal exam shows vulvular inflammation and redness with red dermatitis and weeping areas on the inner thighs. Ella also reports painful urination with itching and burning. You suspect Ella is suffering from
    A. A trichomoniasis infection
    B. A gonorrheal infection
    C. Genital herpes
    D. A candidiasis infection

62. Gracie is a 35 year old seen in the emergency department for low back pain, severe muscle spasms, malaise, and dysmenorrhea. Her temperature is 102°F, HR 120, and RR 19. Assessment reveals an enlarged uterus with purulent, foul-smelling vaginal discharge. Which of the following diagnoses is likely given Gracie's symptoms?
    A. Atrophic vaginitis
    B. Chancroid
    C. Endometritis
    D. Gonorrhea

63. Layla is a 29 year old admitted to the emergency department after the metro train she was riding in derailed. She appears to be approximately 30 weeks pregnant. Witnesses reported that she was thrown into the back of the seat in front of her and she had initially complained of severe abdominal pain. She is now unresponsive and hypotensive. You are unable to detect fetal heart tones. You suspect uterine rupture. What findings support your suspicions?
    A. Copious vaginal bleeding
    B. Footling breech presentation in the vaginal canal
    C. Fetal legs in the abdominal cavity demonstrated by ultrasound
    D. A clot identified behind the placenta demonstrated by ultrasound

64. Abigail is a 40 year old patient who was struck in the head by a stray bullet during the July 4th holiday. She was brought into the emergency department with chest compressions in progress. Paramedics reported that CPR was started 2 minutes ago for ventricular fibrillation. Abigail is 35 weeks pregnant. After 2 more minutes of CPR in the ED, she becomes asystolic. The physician decides a postmortem cesarean delivery is indicated. Which of the following statements regarding postmortem cesarean delivery is true?
    A. Fetal outcome is best if postmortem cesarean delivery occurs within 10 minutes of maternal death
    B. Perimortem delivery may only be performed in surgery
    C. A neonatal resuscitation team should be on call should the infant survive delivery
    D. A classical abdominal incision is the best method for delivery

65. Glucose metabolism in a normal term newborn is
    A. 2–3 mg/kg/min
    B. 3–5 mg/kg/min
    C. 4–6 mg/kg/min
    D. 5–8 mg/kg/min

66. Which of the following infants is at risk for hyperglycemia?
    A. An infant of an insulin-dependent diabetic mellitus mother
    B. Term infant on prednisone for respiratory distress
    C. An intubated infant with meconium aspiration syndrome
    D. A premature infant

67. How soon after birth should you obtain an infant's blood glucose?
    A. Within 10 minutes
    B. Within 30 minutes
    C. Within 45 minutes
    D. Within 60 minutes

68. Actions should be taken to maintain an infant's blood glucose level at
    A. 40–100 mg/dl
    B. 50–120 mg/dl
    C. 60–160 mg/dl
    D. 80–150 mg/dl

69. Hypotonia, jitteriness, poor suck, apnea, and seizures indicate a hypoglycemic state in the
    A. Lungs
    B. Muscles
    C. Heart
    D. Brain

70. Initial IV fluids should be calculated at _____ for an infant newly born.
    A. 40 ml/kg/d
    B. 50 ml/kg/d
    C. 60 ml/kg/d
    D. 80 ml/kg/d

71. The mother of a newborn gave birth in a car on the way to the hospital. Your facility does not have a maternal-child department. The infant appears to be dehydrated. Appropriate solution and fluid orders for this 3.5-kg patient are
    A. $D_{10}W$ at 8.8 ml/h
    B. $D_{10}W$ at 11.7 ml/h
    C. $D_{12.5}W$ at 14.6 ml/h
    D. $D_{15}W$ at 8.8 ml/h

72. Micah is a newborn with a blood glucose level of 35 mg/dl after two $D_{10}W$ boluses have been given. What is the next action to be performed?
    A. Nothing, recheck in an hour
    B. Give a third bolus but use $D_{25}W$
    C. Hang $D_{12.5}W$ at 60 ml/kg/d
    D. Increase maintenance IV fluid of $D_{10}W$ to 120 ml/kg/d

73. How often should bedside glucose checks on a newborn be repeated?
    A. Only with labs and IV start
    B. Every 10 minutes
    C. Every 30 minutes
    D. Every hour

74. Which of the following statements regarding temperature of a newborn infant is accurate?
    A. Normal temperature is 36–37.5°C
    B. Moderate hypothermia is a core temperature 30–36°C
    C. Temperatures should be taken every 15–30 minutes until stable
    D. A radiant warmer on air mode is effective in controlling temperature

75. Which of the following initial reactions occurs with an infant suffering from cold stress?
    A. Hyptonia, peripheral vasoconstriction
    B. Increased metabolism of brown fat, decreased O_2 consumptions
    C. Increased glucose consumption, hypertonia
    D. Increased O_2 consumption, hypotonia

76. Effects of cold stress in infants is caused by a release of
    A. Norepinephrine
    B. Epinephrine
    C. Dopamine
    D. Glycogen

77. Which of the following warming methods is contraindicated for the care of a newborn?
    A. Heat stethoscope in hands before auscultation
    B. Use warmed, humidified oxygen
    C. Servo set radiant warmer
    D. Heat lamp set 6 inches away from the infant

78. Caleb was just born in the emergency department. He demonstrates cyanosis, tachypnea, and depressed mentation, and his PCO_2 is 30. The likely cause for his symptoms is
    A. Respiratory distress syndrome
    B. Congenital heart disease
    C. Aspiration
    D. Pneumothorax

79. Which acronym can be used to remember what information should be prepared prior to transport of a newborn infant aged 0–28 days from the emergency department to higher level of care within or outside the facility?
    A. STABLE
    B. TRANSPORT
    C. INFANT
    D. SEND

80. Which of the following does not affect the results of transillumination to determine pneumothorax in an infant?
    A. Skin pigmentation
    B. Edema
    C. Presence of an ETT
    D. Pulmonary interstitial emphysema

81. You are assisting with an emergency vaginal delivery. When the head is delivered, you note that the cord is wrapped tightly around the throat. What action should be performed at this time?
    A. Hold a hand to the head to prevent the infant from delivering until you can move the mother to labor and delivery
    B. Stretch the cord over the head
    C. Continue to deliver the infant and untangle the cord once the body is delivered
    D. Clamp the cord in two places and use sterile scissors to cut between the two clamps

82. Bailey is a 46 year old seen in the emergency room for cyclical abdominal cramping that is increasing in frequency and severity. When you assist her to undress you note a bulging bag with what appears to be a foot moving in it. As she lays down on the gurney, the rest of the bag delivers onto the bed. You should
    A. Rupture the amniotic sac and peel it away from the face and begin resuscitation
    B. Leave the sac intact and call Labor and Delivery
    C. Leave the sac intact and call the Neonatal Care Unit
    D. Wait for the physician to determine viability before starting resuscitation

83. Placental delivery should
    A. Occur typically within minutes of birth
    B. Be delayed until IV fluids can be initiated
    C. Be assisted by gently pulling on the cord
    D. Be assisted by pressing forcefully on the fundus to assist with expulsion

84. Which of the following statements is false?
    A. Once a mother delivers the placenta, massage the fundus
    B. Once the placenta is delivered, maternal bleeding should diminish immediately
    C. Examine the placenta for missing sections
    D. Dispose of placenta in biohazard bag

85. Which of the following actions is not helpful with controlling post-delivery bleeding?
    A. Administer oxytocin at 20 units per 1000 ml lactated Ringer's at 250 to 500 ml/hr
    B. Massage the fundus to keep it firm
    C. Assist the mother in breastfeeding
    D. Encourage the mother to drink ginseng tea to increase comfort after delivery

86. Fetal bradycardia is classified as a heart rate less than
    A. 60
    B. 80
    C. 100
    D. 120

87. Why is fetal breech positioning dangerous?
    A. Fetal breech positioning results in irreparable muscular skeletal damage
    B. Fetal breech positioning causes an increased risk of shoulder dystocia
    C. Fetal breech positioning causes an increased risk of uterine rupture
    D. Fetal breech positioning causes an increased risk of strangulation

88. Riley is 36 years old and pregnant at 39 weeks. She is in active labor and reports that her water broke an hour ago. Since then she has not felt the baby move. On inspection, you see the head engaged in the vagina with the umbilical cord pinched between the head and the wall of the vagina. Your first action should be to
    A. Transport the mother to the obstetrical unit
    B. Administer oxygen
    C. Use a gloved hand to support the head off the cord and leave the hand in place
    D. Push the cord back into the vagina

89. Postpartum hemorrhage can be described as
    A. Vaginal bleeding that continues for 3 weeks
    B. Blood loss that is less than 300 ml
    C. Hemorrhage that begins within 48 hours
    D. Blood loss post abortion

90. When planning care for a woman with vaginal bleeding, what is the most important parameter that should be taken into consideration?
    A. When was the last menstrual period
    B. Has an ultrasound been performed
    C. Is the cervical os open or closed
    D. Is the mother hemodynamically stable

91. A ruptured ovarian cyst often presents with similar symptoms to which of the following conditions?
    A. Appendicitis, ectopic pregnancy, and PIE
    B. PIE, diverticulitis, and appendicitis
    C. Appendicitis, PDI, and ectopic pregnancy
    D. Ectopic pregnancy, appendicitis, and PID

92. Allison has been diagnosed with a ruptured ovarian cyst. Her blood pressure is 85/60 and heart rate 160. While attempting to place a peripheral IV, she becomes unresponsive. What is your priority of care for this patient?
    A. Intubate
    B. Administer antibiotics
    C. Prepare to transfer the patient to surgery
    D. Obtain a central line

93. EMTALA regulations require emergency treatment to be given for all of the following persons except
    A. A pregnant woman in labor in her car outside the emergency room
    B. A gunshot victim found in the alley next to the hospital
    C. A visitor who suffers a heart attack in the deli next door to the emergency department
    D. A woman who exhibits stroke symptoms while attending a class in the education department

94. Which of the following situations is a violation of EMTALA?
    A. An apneic patient is intubated prior to transport to another facility for open heart surgery
    B. A woman has delivered a baby, but not the placenta, prior to transport to obstetrical unit
    C. Dopamine and dobutamine have been started to maintain blood pressure prior to transport to an intensive care unit
    D. A gunshot victim with a nicked artery requires manual pressure while being transported to surgery

95. Which of the following is true regarding gestational trophoblastic disease?
    A. There are three types of gestational trophoblastic diseases
    B. Gestational trophoblastic tumors are always cancerous
    C. Gestational trophoblastic tumors do not metastasize
    D. Ultrasound reveals a snowstorm pattern without observable fetus

96. Lizzy is a 20 year old homeless woman who presents to the emergency room with severe, bright red, vaginal bleeding. She reports that she has been pregnant for the last 11 months. Her β-hCG is elevated, but there are no fetal heart tones and the ultrasound reveals a snowstorm pattern. What should you do next?
    A. Prepare her for immediate surgery
    B. Assess blood pressure, temperature, and respiratory rate, and obtain urine for analysis
    C. Call for psychological assessment
    D. Transfer the patient directly to Labor and Delivery

97. Leila is a mentally challenged 20 year old admitted to the emergency department with a temperature of 103°F, headache, and sore throat. Her widowed father reports she has complained of worsening muscle pain over the last week. While assisting her into a gown you note general edema, a rash to the body, and blanching erythema. You suspect Leila may be suffering from
    A. Vaginitis
    B. Ruptured ectopic pregnancy
    C. Toxic shock syndrome
    D. Gestational trophoblastic tumor

98. Which organism is likely to cause toxic shock syndrome?
    A. *Staphylococcus aureus*
    B. *Escherichia coli*
    C. *Candida albicans*
    D. *Pseudomonas aeruginosa*

99. Which of the following is an appropriate treatment of toxic shock syndrome?
    A. Stabilize vascular pressure using colloids
    B. Provide O_2 support to maintain $PaO_2 > 80$ mmHg
    C. Transfer patient to an isolation room
    D. Remove identifiable sources of infection

100. Maylynn is seen in the emergency department for vaginal itching, odor, and heavy yellow-green vaginal discharge. You suspect she has vulvovaginitis caused by
    A. *Candida albicans*
    B. *Trichomonas vaginalis*
    C. Bacterial vaginosa
    D. *Escherichia coli*

101. The patient in bed one states she has endometriosis. What symptoms are consistent with that diagnosis?
    A. Dysmenorrhea, foul odor, and pelvic pain
    B. Dysuria, infertility, and no pain with intercourse
    C. Hematuria and vaginal bleeding between periods
    D. Dyspareunia and dysmenorrhea

102. Stella is admitted to the emergency room via ambulance after being found in a side ditch. Her clothing is torn and she has bruising noted to her face, chest, inner thighs, and buttocks. Her left eye is swollen shut and she is missing teeth. She has vaginal and rectal bleeding. Although she denies sexual assault, you should
    A. Contact police
    B. Provide medical care only
    C. Allow the patient to void if desired
    D. Begin washing and cleaning wounds

103. All the following professionals are considered a part of SART except
    A. Police officers
    B. Forensic examiners
    C. Laboratory personnel
    D. Patient advocates

104. The SART process should follow which of the following orders?
    A. Notify police, forensic evidence is collected, patient advocate is notified, counselors provided
    B. Notify police, SANE initiates assessment, evidence is transferred to attorney, patient is transferred to psych unit for evaluation and counseling
    C. Police are notified, patient advocate arrives to assist patient through process of hospitalization, disclosure is completed between hospital staff and police agency
    D. Police are notified, patient advocate and SANE are notified, initial disclosure with police and hospital staff, forensic evidence is collected

105. A woman has just been brought in by friends after she was sexually assaulted at a club. After initiating the SART process, you should
    A. Place the woman in a private room by herself until she can be examined
    B. Withhold notifying police until a history and physical can be taken
    C. Offer information on sexual assault attorneys
    D. Have a social services representative stay with the victim

106. Which of the following is not an important part of the history assessment of a victim of a sexual assault?
    A. Sexual history
    B. Childhood vaccinations
    C. Postassault activities
    D. Last menstrual period

107. Which of the following statements is true about the collection of evidence?
    A. Clothing should be removed via unbuttoning or unzipping if possible; if clothing must be cut, avoid cutting through bullet holes, knife cuts, tears, or button holes
    B. Collected evidence should be labeled with patient name, hospital name, collection site (ED), date and time of collection, description of specimen, and collector's initials
    C. All items released to police should be documented on the police report only
    D. Any biohazard materials related to the victim's care should be disposed of through hospital policy

108. Which of the following statements is false regarding consent when caring for a sexual assault victim?
    A. Additional medical care consents must be obtained before treating a sexual assault victim
    B. A consent for or against must be signed before an official forensic examination
    C. The consent for forensic examination implies consent to transfer evidence to police
    D. General medical consent implies permission to obtain photographs of injuries for documentation

109. Which of the following statements is true regarding physical collection of evidence during care of a sexually assaulted patient?
    A. Gloves should be changed when handling any new piece of evidence or with each new specimen collection
    B. The examiner may leave the room as often as needed to obtain supplies needed in assessment and care
    C. During vaginal assessment with a speculum, use water-based gel to prevent additional vaginal injury
    D. Only the examiner should remove patient clothing to preserve evidence

110. Which of the following is appropriate prophylactic treatment for STDs after a sexual assault?
    A. 350 mg ceftriaxone IM ×1
    B. 2 G azithromycin PO ×1
    C. 2 mg metronidazole PO ×1
    D. 100 mg doxycycline PO BID ×7 days

111. The physician orders a glucose bolus for a hypoglycemic newborn. The order should read
    A. $D_{10}W$ at 2 ml/kg IV push
    B. $D_{15}W$ at 4 ml/kg IV push
    C. $D_{25}W$ at 2 ml/kg IV push
    D. $D_{50}W$ at 0.5 ml/kg IV push

SECTION 8: OBSTETRICS AND GYNECOLOGY ANSWERS

1. **Correct answer: A**
   The treatment of choice for trichomonal vaginitis is metronidazole 2000 mg orally as a single dose. Rocephin and doxycycline are given in combination for pelvic inflammatory disease (PID).
   Penicillin is not appropriate for this patient.

2. **Correct answer: B**
   This patient most likely has trichomonal vaginitis, a sexually transmitted illness. A wet mount of the discharge is necessary so the organism can be viewed microscopically. The color and odor of the discharge give a clue to the diagnosis. Urinalysis might show few leukocytes but no nitrates. An RPR is a test for syphilis. A complete sexually transmitted illness panel should be ordered for this patient.

3. **Correct answer: B**
   Francine will likely produce less milk than the expected total because of her complications of hypovolemic shock with delayed pumping.

4. **Correct answer: A**
   Due to the pregnancy and resulting HELLP syndrome, there is an increased risk for fluid to collect in the abdominal cavity and for development of tissue edema resulting in intra-abdominal hypertension (IAH) and abdominal compartment syndrome (ACS). Signs and symptoms of IAH and ACS include an increased ICP, hypercarbia and decreased platelet values, decreased cardiac output, poor or absent urinary output, and abdominal wall rigidity.

5. **Correct answer: B**
   Antenatal corticosteroids affect fetal lung maturation and help prevent respiratory distress syndrome. Steroids work by accelerating the rate of glycogen depletion and glycerophospholipid biosynthesis. This process results in thinning the intra-alveolar septa and increases the size of the alveoli.

6. **Correct answer: B**
   If the patient has a head injury, the intracranial pressure will be increased. It is also best to avoid postural drainage on a woman in the last 2–3 months of pregnancy. The baby will shift toward the lungs and may cause respiratory distress. It is also a good idea to wait an hour after a patient eats to avoid nausea, vomiting, and possible aspiration.

7. **Correct answer: A**
   Maternal hyperglycemia ultimately causes increased hepatic glucose uptake secondary to fetal hyperinsulinemia and hyperglycemia. Increased glycogen synthesis, accelerated lipogenesis, and macrosomia will also occur.

8. **Correct answer: C**
   Maternal thyroid disease can have a substantial influence on fetal and neonatal thyroid function because immunoglobulin G (IgG) autoantibodies can cross the placenta and inhibit thyroid function. Thioamides used to treat maternal hyperthyroidism can obstruct fetal thyroid hormone synthesis. Most of these effects are transient. Radioactive iodine administered to a pregnant woman can destroy the fetus's thyroid gland.

9. **Correct answer: D**
The Kleihauer-Betke test identifies fetal hemoglobin in maternal blood. The results of this test allow for calculations to determine the amount of fetal-maternal hemorrhage and the amount of immune globulin (RhoGAM) necessary to prevent sensitization. If a patient has a positive test, follow-up testing at a postpartum check-up should be done to rule out the possibility of a false positive result. For example, a false-positive result in the mother could be caused by sickle cell trait, which causes persistent elevation of fetal hemoglobin.

10. **Correct answer: B**
A mother's breastmilk contains the immunoglobulin known as immunoglobulin A (IgA).

   This immunoglobulin is also secreted in human colostrum. IgA does not cross the placental barrier and is the most common immunoglobulin in the gastrointestinal and respiratory tracts.

   During pregnancy and lactation, because of hormonal stimuli, IgA B lymphocytes colonize mammary glands and produce a specific secretory IgA that may bind to a pathogen and prevent infection. The antimicrobial effects of IgA antibodies are related to immune exclusion, interference, or an inhibited ability to adhere to the epithelial cell wall. This helps provide protection to the neonate. Agglutination, neutralization, and immune elimination by phagocytosis and cytotoxicity may enhance the antimicrobial effects as well. HIV-infected mothers do not evidence protection. IgA antibodies may enhance transmission of HIV infection.

11. **Correct answer: C**
Human breastmilk is high in cytokines. Cytokines are soluble proteins that help stimulate the chemotaxis of neutrophils and help in epithelial cell propagation. Of all the factors associated with immunity—immunological, hormonal, and enzymatic—cytokines are believed to play a significant role in the immune modulation and immune protection of breastmilk. Most cytokines that are known to be deficient in the neonate, particularly in preterm infants, have been found in significant amounts in breastmilk. There are certain circumstances where human breastmilk is not safe for infant consumption.

12. **Correct answer: A**
Rhesus (Rh) hemolytic disease of the newborn (HDN) is a severe, often fatal disease caused by incompatibility between an Rh-negative mother and her Rh-positive fetus. The mother becomes alloimmunized to the D antigen present on fetal red blood cells (RBCs) during the first Rh-incompatible pregnancy. The first pregnancy is rarely affected because the number of Rh antibodies produced by the mother is low and the antibodies are usually IgM. When the mother is exposed to D-positive fetal RBCs during a subsequent Rh-incompatible pregnancy, the mother develops a secondary immune response. A large number of IgG Rh antibodies are produced that cross the placenta and make fetal red cells susceptible to attack by antibodies. The mother may also be alloimmunized from fetal-maternal hemorrhage, bleeding that occurs during normal delivery, ectopic pregnancies, spontaneous or induced abortions, and abdominal trauma.

13. **Correct answer: C**

    If the mother received an incompatible transfusion of Rh-positive platelets after a placental rupture, it is appropriate to administer RhoGAM. This medication may be used for prevention of Rh immunization in any Rh-negative person after transfusion of Rh-positive blood or blood products such as platelets or red blood cells.

14. **Correct answer: A**

    A patient can be presensitized and is more likely to undergo organ rejection if she has a history of multiple pregnancies. Other possible causes of rejection to be considered are transfusions, previous organ transplants, and blood type incompatibilities. Small or reduced lumens in the bile ducts, destruction of small airways, and cytomegalovirus infections are the results of organ rejections, not causes.

15. **Correct answer: B**

    Abortion can best be defined as termination of a pregnancy prior to 20 weeks gestation.

    Although viability is around 23 weeks, dates may be inaccurate up to 3 weeks either way. Some people think that abortion is only the result of an intentional act, but that is not true. Spontaneous abortion or miscarriage should be suspected in any woman of childbearing age presenting with vaginal bleeding. Many spontaneous abortions occur before discovery of the pregnancy due to a poor uterine environment (i.e., lack of implantation, infection, and structural abnormalities), malnutrition, abuse, and immunological incompatibilities.

16. **Correct answer: D**

    A diagnosis of placenta previa indicates the patient is pregnant and the placenta is partially implanted over the inferior uterus and/or over the cervix. This is highly dangerous as the patient enters the second and third trimesters when the uterus stretches and thins under the low implanted placenta. If the uterus stretches or the cervix thins, the placenta may separate and lead to bleeding. Partial separation from the uterine wall is abrupt placenta. A placenta that partially implants into the endometrium, and possibly the myometrium, is called a placenta accreta.

17. **Correct answer: C**

    Calculation of fetal gestational age is based on 10 lunar months counted from the first day of the last menstrual period. Other calculations include 280 days and 40 postmenstrual weeks. Assumption on months based on a 28-day cycle.

18. **Correct answer: B**

    The second trimester includes the range of 13–27 weeks of fetal gestation. It is during this trimester that a fetus reaches viability at 23 weeks. Unless the exact date of conception is known, weeks of fetal gestation may be off by ±3 weeks. The first trimester encompasses 0–12 weeks and the third trimester from 28–40 weeks, or until delivery.

19. **Correct answer: C**

    The recommended caloric intake for the average pregnant woman is 2200 kcal/d. This is 300 kcal/d more than the normal nonpregnant recommendation of 1900 kcal/d. Pregnant teens should consume 400–500 kcal/d more than regular intake to compensate for their already increased metabolic requirements.

20. **Correct answer: B**
Recommended daily minimum folic acid intake is 0.4 mg to prevent neural tube defects. Defects include encephalocele, anencephaly, and spina bifidas such as meningocele, myelomeningoceles, and myeloceles.

21. **Correct answer: A**
Increased human chorionic gonadotropin (hCG) levels contribute to morning sickness. Increased progesterone and estrogen levels as well as decreased glucose levels contribute to morning sickness.

22. **Correct answer: A**
Although the patient is pregnant, the patient's presenting symptoms indicate appendicitis. Due to fetal positioning, the appendix is displaced to the right costal margin, shifting the location of the rebound tenderness and pain. Pain would not be constant if the patient was in labor. An abruption presents with sudden, colicky abdominal pain and frank vaginal bleeding.

23. **Correct answer: D**
HELLP syndrome stands for hemolysis, elevated liver enzymes, and low platelets. This life-threatening condition occurs in approximately 4–12% of women with severe preeclampsia.

24. **Correct answer: C**
Placenta previa has not been associated with HELLP syndrome. HELLP syndrome has been associated with DIC, uterine abruption, and acute renal failure as well as premature delivery, intrauterine asphyxia, and ruptured liver hematoma. Placenta previa is not co-maternal morbidity.

25. **Correct answer: A**
HELLP syndrome can occur in the postpartum patient. Specific causes of HELLP syndrome are unknown. Although common, hypertension and proteinurea are not always seen in the patient with HELLP syndrome. Decreased platelet count is related to increased platelet consumption and not due to platelet production.

26. **Correct answer: B**
Idiopathic thrombocytopenic purpura (ITP), preeclampsia, hepatitis, and gallbladder diseases can present with symptoms similar to HELLP syndrome.

27. **Correct answer: B**
A serum aspartate aminotransferase level of 120 units/L indicates immediate intervention is required. This patient is developing HELLP syndrome. Findings that indicate possible HELLP syndrome include a serum aspartate aminotransferase > 70 units/L, bilirubin > 1.2 mg/dl, lactate dehydrogenase > 600 units/L, and platelets < 150 mm^3. Women who are multiparous (more than one pregnancy), older than 25 years, and who suffered previous miscarriages are at higher risk of HELLP syndrome. If the patient has a history of HELLP syndrome, then the patient is at even higher risk of developing HELLP syndrome.

28. **Correct answer: D**

    If the hospital has a labor and delivery unit, then the emergency department nurse should obtain as thorough a history and physical as possible prior to transfer. This provides the labor nurse with a clearer picture of risk and urgency. If the hospital does not have a maternal unit, then the emergency nurse should obtain a history and physical, insert an IV for fluid resuscitation and medication administration, and obtain a CBC with liver enzymes.

29. **Correct answer: C**

    Corticosteroids ordered for a 30-week gestation, gravida 5, para 2, 32 year old in labor are used to increase fetal lung maturity in case of premature delivery. Additional benefits include decreased inflammation in the mother's liver if she is at risk for HELLP syndrome.

30. **Correct answer: B**

    Magnesium sulfate should be started as a 4 to 6g-bolus with a maintenance dose via an IV infusion of 2 g per hour to prevent seizures. The magnesium sulfate should be administered regardless of the presence or absence of hypertension. If hypertension is also present, then an additional goal is to keep the SBP 90–100. Antihypertensives may also be administered to decrease the systolic blood pressure.

31. **Correct answer: C**

    A Lasix order received for a woman with HELLP syndrome should be refused. Lasix or any diuretic order should be questioned as they decrease circulating blood flow to the placenta and can inhibit nutrients available to the fetus and lead to fetal compromise. Fluid restriction should also be used with caution because of placental compromise. Magnesium sulfate and antihypertensives should be used to control blood pressure and prevent seizures.

32. **Correct answer: A**

    According to the new 2010 Neonatal Resuscitation Program guidelines, naloxone is not recommended to be administered during the first 15 minutes of neonatal life. Naloxone is used as an antagonist to opioid administration given to the mother within 4 hours of delivery. The primary goal, even if opioid use by the mother is known, is to provide resuscitation for the infant. The goal is to support the infant's heart rate and ventilation.

33. **Correct answer: D**

    Any woman presenting to the emergency room with respiratory and/or circulatory compromise and pregnant with a viable fetus should have a fetal assessment completed before discharge. Prolonged respiratory distress and/or circulatory compromise could lead to fetal asphyxia and fetal death. Early assessment and intervention may save the baby's life. The nurse should also question discharge of this patient due to her presentation consistent with a diagnosis of tuberculosis. The patient may require further assessment.

34. **Correct answer: A**

    If a woman of childbearing age presents to the emergency department with abdominal pain and vaginal bleeding, she should have an hCG test done. An hCG tests for pregnancy. Unilateral pelvic pain, palpable pelvic mass, and abnormal vaginal bleeding is indicative of an ectopic pregnancy. Underage females may be hesitant to report sexual activity if parents are present. Ectopic pregnancy occurs in approximately 2% of women. If ectopic pregnancy results in a rupture, additional symptoms include Kehr's sign (shoulder pain), tachycardia, hypotension, decreased level of consciousness, and cold, clammy skin. Failure to identify and intervene in the presence of ectopic pregnancy may lead to maternal death.

35. **Correct answer: A**
A woman who is gravida 2, para 3 has been pregnant twice and delivered three viable children. Gravida refers to the number of times the woman has been pregnant. Para refers only to the number of viable children delivered and does not indicate that those children survived infancy. It is important to also ask about number of abortions (spontaneous and voluntary), to more accurately determine maternal history.

36. **Correct answer: C**
A woman noted to be a nullipara means that she has never delivered a viable fetus regardless of number of pregnancies. Null refers to zero and para refers to viable deliveries.

37. **Correct answer: B**
A female of childbearing age who presents with vaginal bleeding, severe abdominal pain with cramping, and cervical os dilated > 3 cm is experiencing an inevitable abortion. Treatment includes bed rest, pain control, RhoGAM administration, and uterine evacuation. The type of uterine evacuation depends on the gestational age of the fetus and patient–physician discussion. Social services should be notified to provide emotional support and community resources for grief counseling if desired.

38. **Correct answer: D**
Infusion of oxytocin 200 units per 1000 ml of lactated Ringer's is contraindicated as the dosage is too high. The appropriate order would be for oxytocin 20 units per 1000 ml of lactated Ringer's. This patient has experienced an incomplete abortion and will need urgent surgical intervention to completely evacuate the remaining tissue and avoid complications.

39. **Correct answer: D**
Embryonic chromosomal defects are the most common cause of spontaneous abortion in the first trimester. Late spontaneous abortions are commonly caused by maternal anatomic abnormalities, infection, and maternal endocrine disorders.

40. **Correct answer: C**
Complete abortions left untreated may result in a septic abortion in the presence of infection. Septic abortion may occur after incomplete abortions or after an unsuccessful uterine evacuation. Normal vaginal flora that becomes opportunistic can lead to profound infection and sepsis.

41. **Correct answer: D**
Candida albicans is not a normal vaginal flora. *Escherichia coli,* alpha-hemolytic *streptococci,* and beta-hemolytic *streptococci* are all normal vaginal flora. Each of these organisms is opportunistic and can lead to septicemia in mother and infant before and during delivery.

42. **Correct answer: A**

    Contact a surgical consult and prepare the patient for surgery; this patient is experiencing septic abortion after a dilation and curettage. Severe abdominal distention, constant pelvic pain, fever, chills, and uterine tenderness indicate not only infection, but likelihood of infection of *Clostridium perfringens*. *Clostridium perfringens* is an anaerobic organism that produces gas gangrene, tissue necrosis, and uterine tissue sloughing. If the infection is severe enough, a hysterectomy is indicated. The emergency nurse will need to monitor for toxic shock and administer antibiotics as ordered. Spectinomycin hydrochloride is an antibiotic for gonorrhea and ganciclovir is an antiviral. Neither treatment is indicated for this patient.

43. **Correct answer: C**

    Postabortion discharge instructions should include avoiding intercourse, douching, and tampons for at least 2 weeks. This is to decrease exposure to infection. Other instructions include that vaginal bleeding should last for 1 to 2 weeks and mild cramping will occur during the first few days. To monitor for infection, her temperature should be taken both in the morning and evening, and to report any temperature > 100°F to her obstetrician.

44. **Correct answer: D**

    PIH stands for pregnancy-induced hypertension. Preeclampsia is a mild form of PIH. Eclampsia is a severe form of PIH and is life threatening.

45. **Correct answer: D**

    Weight gain of > 2 lbs per week and visual changes are indicative of preeclampsia. Additional symptoms include systolic blood pressure > 140 mmHg; diastolic blood pressure > 90 mmHg; albuminuria (+2 urine dipstick); oliguria; edema of the face, hands, and sacrum; headaches; upper right quadrant pain; and increased deep tendon reflexes with clonus.

46. **Correct answer: A**

    The correct dosage of hydralazine for a pregnant woman is 5 to 40 mg IV repeated prn, or 40 mg PO daily to a maximum of 400 mg daily.

47. **Correct answer: C**

    The primary difference between preeclampsia and eclampsia is that seizures are noted only with eclampsia. The presence of seizures indicates a life-threatening process for both mother and fetus. Fetal bradycardia, particularly during a seizure, can lead to asphyxia and fetal neurologic deficits. Albuminuria is noted with both preeclampsia and eclampsia. HELLP syndrome can be seen with both disease processes. The systolic blood pressure in preeclampsia is less than 140 mmHg, and in eclampsia the systolic blood pressure is > 140 mmHg.

48. **Correct answer: D**

    A woman experiencing seizures and eclampsia should be positioned on the left side to improve blood flow to the fetus. This position also increases renal blood flow and urine output and decreases edema. Supine positioning places the fetus under the diaphragm and inhibits full lung expansion. Supine positioning inhibits blood flow from the legs, kidneys, and intestines and causes pressure on the lower back and spine. Prone position places pressure on the uterus and increases fetal distress. Right side positioning is less beneficial than left side.

Obstetrics and Gynecology | 199

49. **Correct answer: B**
Placenta previa is a concern during late pregnancy because as the fetus grows and the cervical os thins, the placenta placement near or over the cervical os pulls away and leads to bleeding. During labor, the os also opens leading to more profound bleeding and increased maternal risk for hemorrhage. Complete placenta previa occurs when the placenta implants centered over the cervical os. Partial placenta previa has < 50% of the placenta over the cervical os. With a marginal placenta previa, only the margin is over the cervical os.

50. **Correct answer: A**
Sudden painless bleeding of bright red blood, hypotension, tachycardia, and delayed capillary refill are consistent with a placenta previa presentation. Uterine rigidity, frank red blood, hypotension, tachycardia, and back pain are consistent with abruption. Foul vaginal discharge, constant pelvic pain, fever, and chills are consistent with septic abortion. Sharp abdominal pain without bleeding, tachycardia, and tachypnea can be seen with labor.

51. **Correct answer: C**
This patient is at highest risk for abruption after the motor vehicle accident. The saturation of blood to her pants should be evaluated immediately to determine the source of the bleeding. Abruptions do not always present with bleeding after abdominal trauma, but should be considered whenever a pregnant woman suffers abdominal trauma. Preterm labor may result after an accident, but is not usually life threatening to the mother. Infection is a concern, but not immediately life threatening.

52. **Correct answer: D**
Nursing priorities when caring for a mother experiencing abruption include marking and frequently assessing fundal height for changes indicating the severity of occult bleeding. Two large-bore IVs should be placed for infusions of normal saline, lactated Ringer's, or O negative cross-matched blood. Continuous fetal monitoring should be initiated while surgical evaluation is performed. If the fetus is viable and maternal shock is severe, then immediate delivery is required to prevent loss of both mother and fetus.

53. **Correct answer: C**
The desire to void is not a sign of impending delivery. The desire is to bear down, presence of bloody show, bulging membranes, crowning, frequent contractions, and ruptured amniotic fluid are all indications of delivery.

54. **Correct answer: B**
Your immediate priority is to dry the infant and remove all wet linens from direct contact with the baby's skin. You do this first, to stimulate the baby to breathe and to limit the negative effects of cold stress on the infant. Avoid the use of hot water bottles or gloves to warm the infant. Direct contact may cause serious burns to exposed skin. The best method to warm the infant is to use warmed blankets, heat lamp, a radiant warmer, or place the baby on the mother's bare chest. Suctioning should include the use of a bulb syringe in the mouth and then nares, or use wall suction at 80 to 100 mmHg to the mouth. Avoid using a delee or large suction tubing in the nares.

It may cause irritation and swelling, further impeding airflow and increasing likelihood of respiratory distress. Tracheal suctioning prior to drying is only indicated if there was meconium and the infant was delivered apneic, bradycardic (HR < 100), and/or floppy. Although you will need to and want to call the NICU team or nursery to accept care of this infant, it is not the priority over providing resuscitation care to the infant.

55. Correct answer: A

Bartholin's cyst is a unilateral inflammation of the Bartholin duct located on the labia majora at the vestibule. Typically, the cyst is asymptomatic unless the duct occlusion is related to infection or results in painful intercourse or the ability to sit. Sexually transmitted diseases may worsen or increase risk of infection but do not cause Bartholin's cysts.

56. Correct answer: A

Skene's duct cysts can lead to urethral obstruction and urinary retention. The Skene's duct is located near the urethral meatus in the vestibule. With severe urinary retention the patient is also at risk for urinary tract infections, not vaginitis. Cysts may be due to blocked ducts or infection related to sexually transmitted diseases. Cysts of the canal of Nucka, located in the labia majora and pons, mimic inguinal hernias.

57. Correct answer: B

Per the 2011 NRP Guidelines, all term newborns requiring respiratory support should be monitored using pulse oximetry. This change is meant to decrease the effects of excessive oxygen use after delivery. Unused, free oxygen in the blood stream binds with water to form pockets of H_2O_2 and can damage tissue within the newborn, impairing or delaying normal transition to extrauterine life. If positive pressure ventilation (PPV) or bagging is required, place the infant on pulse oximetry and begin resuscitation using 21% and titrate to maintain desired oxygenation levels based on new guidelines of 85–95% within 10 minutes of life. When weaning off PPV to blow-by or free-flow oxygen, the flow rate should be decreased to around 5 Lpm. Excessive flow rate may lead to vagal stimulation and a decrease in heart rate. Blow-by or free-flow oxygen cannot provide 100% oxygen due to mixing of atmospheric air.

58. Correct answer: D

Any initial newborn heart rate less than 100/min requires positive pressure ventilation (PPV) at a rate of 40–60 breaths per minute for 30 seconds with FiO_2 titrated to keep oxygen saturations via pulse oximetry greater than 85%. If after 30 seconds of effective PPV with visible chest rise, the heart rate is < 60 bpm, then chest compressions at a 3:1 ratio should be initiated for 30–60 seconds. The heart rate should be continuously monitored while compressions are in progress. Suctioning should only be considered if the bulb syringe did not clear the airway of secretions and you cannot ventilate with chest rise.

59. Correct answer: B

If you are experiencing increasing difficulty obtaining chest rise when providing positive pressure ventilation (PPV) to an infant, reposition the mask and head, then insert an orogastric tube to aspirate stomach contents, and then place the OG open to air to vent the stomach. The vent will decrease pressures in the stomach and diaphragm to allow for increased lung expansion. Oral suctioning is indicated if secretions are noted, but the orogastric tube is the better choice. Low intermittent wall suction is indicated for gastric obstruction, diaphragmatic hernia, and ileus, not this scenario. PPV with positive inspiratory pressure (PIP) of 40 mmHg is excessive and likely to cause pneumothorax and sudden decompensation.

60. **Correct answer: B**
Narcan (naloxone) use is contraindicated to treat unknown drug exposure prior to delivery. If Narcan is used on an infant of a mother using methadone, the infant may begin to seize, impairing respiratory effort, and the seizures may lead to neurologic injury and death. Instead, provide positive pressure ventilation and titrate oxygen using pulse oximetry. For preterm infants under 28 weeks gestation or under 1000 grams, use a polyethylene bag with a heat source such as a heat lamp or radiant warmer to stabilize temperature. If using a polyethylene bag, do not dry the infant first. The moisture helps to prevent fluid and electrolytes loss through thin, permeable skin.

61. **Correct answer: D**
Candidiasis infections present with profuse, white curdlike vaginal discharge that may be yeasty or sweet smelling. Vulvular inflammation, redness, and dermatitis to inner thighs are also symptoms of this infection. Complaints often include itching, burning, and painful urination. The history includes sudden onset, recent or current antibiotic use, or coincides with menses. Frequent candidiasis infections should be assessed for causes such as frequent douching, sexual activity, hygiene habits, and work environment of both patient and sexual partners.

62. **Correct answer: C**
Gracie is most likely suffering from endometritis. As bacteria infect the endometrial lining of the uterus, patients may present with low back pain, severe muscle spasms, malaise, and dysmenorrhea. Assessment reveals an enlarged uterus with serosanguineous or purulent, foul-smelling vaginal discharge and fever. Gonorrhea may present with fever in severe cases but not with an enlarged uterus. Chancroid presents with headaches and mucopurulent, foul-smelling discharge with vulvular lesions. Atrophic vaginitis presents with scant, watery, white discharge without abdominal pain.

63. **Correct answer: C**
Uterine rupture should be suspected of any pregnant female with history of abdominal trauma resulting in sudden deceleration or extreme abdominal compression. Patients present with severe abdominal pain and decreased or absent fetal heart tones and movement. Fetal parts or the entire fetus may be located in the abdominal cavity outside of the uterus, with minimal to no vaginal bleeding. Due to internal bleeding from the ruptured uterus and placental injury, the mother will become hypovolemic and hypotensive. Shock may develop, leading to both fetal and maternal death. Upon diagnosis, the mother should be treated immediately with volume replacement and prepared for surgery. Emergency cesarean delivery is indicated to save the fetus with probable hysterectomy to preserve maternal life.

64. **Correct answer: D**
A classical abdominal incision is the best method for postmortem cesarean delivery of a viable fetus. Delivery should occur within 5 minutes of maternal death to increase positive fetal neurologic outcome. Perimortem delivery may occur in the emergency department if indicated to save fetal life. The neonatal resuscitation team should be physically present, not on call, if postmortem cesarean delivery is indicated.

65. **Correct answer: C**
    Glucose metabolism in a normal term newborn is 4–6 mg/kg/min. Maintenance IV fluids must contain glucose to compensate for this level of metabolism and maintain adequate blood glucose. As an illness becomes progressively worse, the glucose requirements and the consumption of glucose by the infant are greater.

66. **Correct answer: B**
    An infant receiving prednisone or other steroids is at risk for hyperglycemia. An infant of an insulin-dependent diabetic mother, intubated with respiratory distress, and prematurity all predispose an infant to hypoglycemia. Blood glucose should be assessed as soon as possible to initiate treatment if needed. Disease processes that increase glucose consumption or cause fetal hyperinsulinemia require close monitoring after delivery up to 28 days of life.

67. **Correct answer: B**
    An infant's blood glucose should be assessed within 30 minutes of birth. Illness, respiratory distress, and shock increase glucose consumption and can lead to hypoglycemia quickly. The condition is worsened if the infant is not consuming sufficient calories.

68. **Correct answer: B**
    Actions should be taken to maintain an infant's blood glucose at 50 to 120 mg/dl. If unable to consume sufficient calories to maintain adequate glucose levels, insert an IV and provide dextrose boluses and maintenance fluids with dextrose. If the glucose is too high, decrease IV flow rate or amount of glucose concentration.

69. **Correct answer: D**
    Hypotonia, jitteriness, poor suck, apnea, and seizures indicate hypoglycemic state in the brain. The brain is extremely sensitive to fluctuations in oxygen and glucose. Most signs and symptoms of hypoglycemia initiate in the brain.

70. **Correct answer: D**
    Initial IV fluids should be calculated at 80 ml/kg/d for an infant newly born.

71. **Correct answer: B**
    The newborn weighing 3.5 kg should begin maintenance fluids of $D_{10}W$ at 11.7 ml/h. This would equal 80 ml/kg/d. Calculate rate by multiplying 80 by 3.5 kg divided by 24 hours in a day. Glucose solutions greater than 12.5% must be infused via central line to avoid injury to vessels. $D_{10}W$ at 80 ml/kg/d provides 5.5 mg/kg/min. $D_{10}W$ at 8.8 ml/h only provides 4.2 mg/kg/min, which is insufficient glucose or fluid volume for a dehydrated infant. $D_{12.5}W$ at 14.6 ml/h is 100 ml/kg/h. This is too high a glucose concentration. $D_{15}W$ at 8.8 ml/h is 60 ml/kg/h. This is too much glucose and too little volume.

72. **Correct answer: D**
    If two boluses of $D_{10}W$ fail to increase blood glucose, then the next step is to increase the rate of maintenance glucose infusion, and then increase the concentration of glucose. Waiting an hour to recheck glucose could result in worsening hypoglycemia. $D_{25}W$ should never be used; the concentration is too high and would damage vessels. $D_{12.5}W$ at 60 ml/kg/d provides the same glucose as maintenance IV fluids of $D_{10}W$ at 80 ml/kg/d and would not improve glucose levels. The only option is to increase the rate up to 120 ml/kg/d before increasing concentration to $D_{12.5}W$.

73. **Correct answer: C**
    Bedside glucose checks on a newborn should be repeated every 30 minutes.

74. **Correct answer: C**
    The temperature of the infant should be taken every 15–30 minutes until stable. Normal infant temperature should be 36.5 to 37.5°C. Moderate hypothermia is defined as a core temperature of 32–35.9°C. Radiant warmer on servo/skin mode is more effective in maintaining temperature.

75. **Correct answer: C**
    Hypertonia, increased glucose and O_2 consumption, increased brown fat metabolism, and vasoconstriction are all physiological reactions to cold stress.

76. **Correct answer: A**
    In response to cold stress, the body releases norepinephrine. The norepinephrine triggers an increase in metabolic rate, increased O_2 and glucose utilization, hypoxia, pulmonary constriction, and hypoxemia. If the cold stress continues, the infant is at risk for death as the body converts to anaerobic metabolism in the lack of oxygen.

77. **Correct answer: D**
    Using a heat lamp at 6 inches away from the patient is too close and risks burning the infant's skin. The size and wattage of the bulb also determine how close the heat lamp should be without causing injury to skin. Please avoid using chemical heat gels or gloves filled with hot water against the skin. These methods may cause up to third-degree burns. Servo radiant warmer setting, using warmed, humidified oxygen, and warming stethoscopes all are appropriate to warm an infant or decrease risk of heat loss.

78. **Correct answer: B**
    Tachypnea with a decreased PCO_2 is linked to congenital heart disease and other nonpulmonary disease processes. Pulmonary causes of tachypnea, such as respiratory distress syndrome, aspiration, and pneumothorax, lead to increased PCO_2.

79. **Correct answer: A**
    The STABLE acronym can be used to remember what information should be prepared prior to transport of an infant aged 0–28 days from the emergency department to higher level of care within or outside the facility. STABLE stands for sugar, temperature, airway, blood pressure, lab work, and emotional support for family and patient. The speed at which the ED staff can stabilize an infant for transport improves patient outcomes by decreasing injury to tissues and lessening risk of complications. The transporting team is better able to quickly transport the infant for a higher level of care.

80. **Correct answer: C**
    The presence of an ETT does not affect the results of transillumination to determine pneumothorax in an infant. Skin pigmentation can result in a false negative. Edema and pulmonary interstitial emphysema can result in a false positive.

81. **Correct answer: D**
    If an infant's head has been delivered with the cord wrapped tightly around the neck (nuchal cord), then clamp the cord in two places and use sterile scissors to cut between the two clamps. If the body is delivered without releasing the pressure of the cord around the neck, the pressures might strangle the infant or irregularly tear the cord and cause bleeding in the infant and mother. Stretching the cord over the head

without relieving the pull on the cord could also result in tearing of the cord. Once the head is delivered, especially with a nuchal cord, the infant does not receive oxygen from the mother or is unable to take a breath. The anoxic episode may lead to profound neurologic compromise.

82. Correct answer: A

    If an amniotic sac delivers with the infant inside, then rupture the sac and peel it away from the face and provide resuscitation by drying and suctioning the infant and initiate ventilation. Remember to suction the mouth first and then the nares. If the infant is estimated to be greater than 23 weeks gestation and weighs greater than 400 grams, then continue resuscitation until neonatal staff can arrive. Remember to keep the infant warm and dry and continue to provide ventilation that produces visible chest rise.

83. Correct answer: A

    Placental delivery should occur typically within minutes of birth up to 30 minutes after infant delivery. Placental delivery should not be delayed by waiting for IV fluids. IV fluids should be started as soon as able. The placenta should not be rushed or forcefully pulled out as this may result in retained placenta leading to infection and internal bleeding. Gentle fundal massage can aid in placental delivery but should not cause acute pain. Pulling on the cord may lead to tearing and increase maternal bleeding.

84. Correct answer: D

    A delivered placenta should be bagged and sent with the mother to the obstetrical unit for assessment by the obstetrician as well as examined by the ED physician for missing sections. Missing sections indicate retained placenta and potential bleeding and infection complications. With delivery of the placenta, vaginal bleeding should diminish immediately. The mother should be monitored closely for degree of bleeding. Massaging the fundus triggers cramping that assists in slowing bleeding.

85. Correct answer: D

    Mothers should be discouraged to drink or consume ginkgo or ginseng preparations after delivery. Both substances have been identified as platelet antiaggregators and may lead to additional bleeding. Oxytocin, fundal massages, and breastfeeding all release hormones and chemicals that result in uterine contractions and decreased bleeding.

86. Correct answer: C

    Fetal bradycardia is classified as a fetal heart rate less than 100 bpm. Immediate interventions to increase fetal heart rate include providing oxygen, repositioning, IV fluids, and transfer to an obstetrical unit.

87. Correct answer: D

    Breech positioning during vaginal delivery is dangerous as risk of strangulation is increased. If the cord is wrapped around the neck during delivery or if the infant is pulled on while the neck is at the cervix without a contraction, the risk of strangulation also exists. Assisting delivery by pulling on the infant should only be done with contractions. The infant is also at risk for prolapsed cord if portions of the cord exit the vagina before the infant. This inhibits blood flow and oxygen to the infant during delivery and increases the risk for neonatal resuscitation. Breech positioning is called a frank breech if both feet are near the head, a full breech with feet near the abdomen, and a singling footling breech if only one foot presents through the vagina.

88. **Correct answer: C**

    If you note that the umbilical cord precedes any portion of the infant in the vaginal canal, then use a sterile gloved hand to support the head or presenting part off the cord and leave your hand in place. This allows blood and oxygen to pass through the cord to the infant. You will need to leave your hand in place during transfer to the obstetrical unit or surgical suite for an emergency cesarean. Oxygen should be administered to the mother. Do not push the cord back into the vagina as this may result in further compression or kinking of the cord. If able, reposition the mother on her hands and knees with her buttocks in the air to decrease pressure on the vaginal canal and allow for gravity to release pressure on the cord.

89. **Correct answer: D**

    Postpartum hemorrhage can be described as blood loss after abortion or delivery for up to 6 weeks. Consistent frank blood loss exceeds 500 ml with the mother exhibiting signs of hypovolemic shock. Hemorrhage noted within 24 hours is clarified as primary postpartum hemorrhage.

90. **Correct answer: D**

    The most important thing to consider for a woman who is vaginally bleeding is to first determine if she is hemodynamically stable. If she is not stable, treat shock aggressively. Determining the last menstrual period is used to rule out likelihood of pregnancy and pregnancy-related bleeding complications. Ultrasound is used to rule out placenta previa, abruption, gestational age, and pregnancy. Cervical os status assists in determining impending delivery and abortion.

91. **Correct answer: D**

    Ectopic pregnancy, appendicitis, PID, diverticulitis, and ovarian torsion present with similar symptoms to those of ruptured ovarian cysts. Symptoms include sudden, sharp, unilateral lower back pain and peritoneal irritation. Patients may also complain of nausea and vomiting, low-grade fever, and hemoperitoneum.

92. **Correct answer: C**

    The immediate priority is to prepare the hemodynamically unstable patient for surgery. If the patient is spontaneously breathing, provide oxygen support as necessary. Intubation requires precious time and is not a priority if positive pressure ventilation/bagging produces a visible chest rise. Antibiotics should be administered as long as it does not delay surgical intervention. A central line placement requires too much time and delays surgical intervention.

93. **Correct answer: C**

    EMTALA regulations do not mandate the hospital provide emergency care to be given on property not belonging to the hospital. If an individual experiences a medical emergency anywhere on hospital grounds or within 250 yards, then the hospital is obligated to assess, stabilize, and treat as necessary. Exceptions to the rules include if the emergency occurs on property covered by another Medicare or other licensed facility such as an adjoining medical office building, surgicenter, or urgent care.

94. **Correct answer: B**

Transportation of a woman who has delivered a baby, but not the placenta, is a violation of EMTALA. Complications may occur if the placenta is expelled during transport; therefore, it is required that the mother be held in the emergency department until the placenta is delivered. Intubation, medication administration, and treatments that initiate stabilization must be completed prior to transport. Interventions are not expected to necessarily fix the problem but allow for safe transport without greater complications.

95. **Correct answer: D**

A woman with gestational trophoblastic disease will have an ultrasound that reveals a snowstorm pattern without an observable fetus. Initial presentation is similar to pregnancy as the woman will have elevated β-hCG levels and an enlarged uterus larger than appropriate for gestation, yet fetal heart tones and the fetus are not seen on ultrasound. There are two types of gestational trophoblastic tumors. Hydatidiform moles develop at conception to form a cystic tumor that is typically benign and does not metastasize. Choriocarinomas may develop from hydatidiforms or uterine tissues and are cancerous and will metastasize.

96. **Correct answer: B**

This patient is presenting with severe vaginal bleeding. Regardless of history, obtain vital signs immediately to determine hemodynamic stability and whether the patient is preeclamptic. Obtain a urine specimen if possible. Although initial presentation may indicate that she is pregnant, the length of "pregnancy," elevated β-hCG, and lack of identifiable fetus suggest a gestational trophoblastic tumor. Next, you should prepare for surgical intervention such as dilatation and curettage or dilatation and evacuation. There may be an underlying psychological history, but it is not a priority at this time. If signs of preeclampsia are noted, monitor closely for seizures.

97. **Correct answer: C**

Leila may be suffering from toxic shock syndrome. Toxic shock syndrome (TSS) presents with a temperature > 102°F, headache, sore throat, and myalgias. Dermatological assessment reveals general edema, a rash to the body, and blanching erythema. The patient may also present with nausea, vomiting, and hypotension. The patient has an existing developmental compromise and may not have sufficient cognition regarding gynecologic hygiene. Toxic shock syndrome has been linked in the past to tampon use. If Leila has been using tampons inappropriately and has not followed directions, she is at risk for TSS. Other correlations have been found with diaphragms and contraceptive sponge use. TSS may be noted after tubal ligation, hysterectomy, and carbon dioxide lasering of genital condyloma.

98. **Correct answer: A**

Staphylococcus aureus is the organism to most likely to cause toxic shock syndrome.

99. **Correct answer: D**

Removing identifiable sources of infection is an important step in effectively treating toxic shock syndrome. Potential sources of TSS include tampons, diaphragms, contraceptive sponges, and intimacy toys. Blood pressure should be stabilized with isotonic crystalloids, vasopressors, and inootropes. PaO_2 should be maintained over 60 mmHg with appropriate oxygen support devices. The patient does not need to be transferred to an isolation room, unless contact isolation cannot be maintained in her current location. In addition, antibiotics should be initiated as soon as available and the patient transferred to an intensive care unit.

100. **Correct answer: B**
Trichomonas vaginalis can cause a vulvovaginitis presenting with vaginal itching, odor, and heavy yellow-green vaginal discharge.

101. **Correct answer: D**
Dyspareunia (painful intercourse) and dysmenorrhea are common presenting symptoms of endometriosis. Additional symptoms include pelvic pain, dysuria, hematuria, and history of infertility. Analgesics and hormonal therapy may be prescribed to lessen symptoms.

102. **Correct answer: A**
As mandatory reporters, we have an obligation to report an alleged crime to police. Before providing any nonemergent care, thoroughly document injuries with pictures whenever possible. Stella's injuries are consistent with sexual assault and should be investigated. Stigma of rape and fear if the assailant is known may hinder the victim from reporting the assault and filing charges. You cannot force a victim to file a complaint or to submit to forensic examination. Until the patient refuses forensic examination, continue collecting evidence according to policy.

103. **Correct answer: C**
Laboratory personnel are not considered to be members of the SART (Sexual Assault Response Team). However, their training includes specific techniques and policies for special handling of forensic evidence that could be later used in court.

104. **Correct answer: D**
The SART process for reporting and collection when sexual assault is known or suspected begins with police notification, a patient advocate and sexual assault nurse examiner (SANE) are notified, initial disclosure occurs between staff and police, and forensic evidence is collected. The patient's advocate and SANE may assist patient through the hospital system to receive appropriate counseling, medical treatment, and follow-up care. Once evidence is collected, it is turned over to the appropriate authorities for judicial proceedings.

105. **Correct answer: D**
If the hospital does not have a designated patient advocate or counselor, then contact social services to have a worker sit with the victim. It is crucial not to leave the woman alone at this time. Not only may she inadvertently destroy forensic evidence, but she may be at risk for suicide or may walk away from treatment for fear or shame. A counselor as well as patient support, friends, and family should be included in providing support to the victim. Notify police as soon as sexual assault is suspected or determined to fully initiate appropriate SART processes. Should the case go to court, the district or city attorney represents the victim. The counselor, advocate, or social worker can explain appropriate procedures and provide community resources and compensation programs to the victim. Medical personnel should continually explain the purpose of all medical procedures and provide support as needed.

106. **Correct answer: B**

Childhood vaccinations are not an important part of history assessment. The nurse should obtain a complete sexual history including last menstrual period, contraception used, sexual activities within the last 72 hours, reproductive history, and sexually transmitted diseases. General and mental health histories should also be obtained. Make sure to document data regarding the assault including abuser's actions, weapons or items used in the assault, location, abuser's description, and postassault activities. Any postassault activities, including showering, voiding, eating, drinking, and changing of clothing, can damage forensic evidence collection.

107. **Correct answer: A**

Clothing collected as forensic evidence should be removed via unbuttoning or unzipping if possible; if clothing must be cut, avoid cutting through bullet holes, knife cuts, tears, or button holes. Cutting though any existing hole, tear, or break in fabric can damage evidence and impede future investigation. All collected evidence should be labeled with patient name, hospital name, collection site (ED), date and time of collection, description of specimen, and collector's full name. All items released to police should be documented on the medical chart as well as in the police report. Any biohazard materials related to the victim's care should be turned over to police for documentation; this includes weapons, bullet or knife fragments, fibers, blood samples, and clothing.

108. **Correct answer: B**

It is not true that a consent for or against must be signed before an official forensic examination. Additional consents include a general consent for medical assessment and specific consents for disposition of physical and diagnostic evidence to police. Consents should be specific regarding types of evidence collected and disposition, such as DNA sampling, fibers, clothing, weapons, photographs, and all written documentation.

109. **Correct answer: A**

When collecting physical evidence during care of a sexually assaulted patient, gloves should be changed when handling any new piece of evidence or with each new specimen collection to prevent cross-contamination. Before beginning the examination, ensure that all necessary equipment is available in the room because the examiner may not leave the room once the examination begins. If an examiner leaves the room, the chain of custody will be broken, impairing future litigation. The patient should be allowed to remove clothing as able. Use a clean sheet on the floor to recover any soil or debris dropped from clothing during removal. Photos should be taken before removal of clothing and serially when performing the assessment. During the vaginal assessment with a speculum, tap water, not gels or lubricants, should be used. Gels and lubricants may alter sperm and dilute specimen collection.

110. **Correct answer: D**

Although each of the medications is appropriate prophylactic treatment for STDs after a sexual assault, only 100 mg doxycycline PO BID ×7 days is the appropriate dosage. The correct dosage for the other drugs is as follows: 125 mg ceftriaxone IM ×1, 1 g azithromycin PO ×1, and 2 g metronidazole PO ×1.

111. **Correct answer: A**

Glucose boluses for infants under 28 days old should read $D_{10}W$ at 2 ml/kg IV push. Avoid concentrations greater than 12.5% peripherally and 20% centrally that will cause severe injury to vessels.

SECTION 8: OBSTETRICS AND GYNECOLOGY REFERENCES

Adam, A. C., Rubio-Texeira, M., & Polaina, J. (2004). Lactose: The milk sugar from a biotechnological perspective. *Critical Reviews in Food Science and Nutrition, 44*(7/8), 553–557.

American Heart Association. (2010). Guidelines 2010 for cardiopulmonary resuscitation and emergency cardiovascular care. Retrieved October 18, 2010, from www.americanheart.org

American Heart Association. (2010). Guidelines 2010 for cardiopulmonary resuscitation and emergency cardiovascular care. Retrieved from www.americanheart.org

Anonymous. (2009, March). HELLP syndrome. American Pregnancy Association. Retrieved online at www.americanpregnancy.com

Bachman, T., Marks, N., & Rimensberger, P. (2008). Factors affecting adoption of new neonatal and pediatric respiratory technologies. *Intensive Care Medicine, 34*(1), 174–178.

Balasubramanian, S., & Ganesh, R. (2008). Vitamin D deficiency in exclusively breast-fed infants. *Indian Journal of Medical Research, 127*(3), 250–255.

Barnett, R., & Kendrick, B. (2010). HELLP syndrome—A case study. *New Zealand Journal of Medical Laboratory Science, 64*(1), 14–17.

Bashore, T. M., Granger, C. B., Hranitzky, P., & Patel, M. R. (2010). Heart disease. In S. J. McPhee & M. A. Papadakis (Eds.), *Lange 2010 current medical diagnosis and treatment* (49th ed., pp. 358–366). New York: McGraw-Hill Medical.

Bellad, M. B., Dhumale, H., and Shravage, J. C. (2009). Preterm labor: A review. *Journal of South Asian Federation of Obstetrics & Gynecology, 1*(3), 1–4.

Bialk, J. L. (2004). Ethical guidelines for assisting patients with end-of-life decision making. *Medsurg Nursing, 13*(2), 87–90.

Buxton, I. L., Singer, C. A., & Tichenor, J. N. (2010). Expression of stretch-activated two-pore potassium channels in human myometrium in pregnancy and labor. *Plos One, 25*(5), e12372.

Calonge, N., Teutsch, S., & Botkin, J. (2008). Expanding newborn screening: Process, policy, and priorities. *Hastings Center Report, 38*(3), 32–39.

Cardwell, C. R., Carson, D. J., Yarnell, J., Shields, M. D., & Patterson, C. C. (2008). Atopy, home environment and the risk of childhood-onset type 1 diabetes: A population-based case control study. *Pediatric Diabetes, 9*(3 pt 1), 191–196.

Casanova, B. C., Sammel, M. D., Chittams, J., Timbers, K., Kulp, J. L., & Barnhart, K. T. (2009). Prediction of outcome in women with symptomatic first-trimester pregnancy: Focus on intrauterine rather than ectopic gestation. *Journal of Women's Health, 18*(2), 195–200.

Cunningham, F. G., Leveno, K. L., & Bloom, S. L. (2005). Obstetrical hemorrhage. In F. G. Cunningham, K. L. Leveno, S. L. Bloom, et al. (Eds.), *Williams obstetrics* (22nd ed., pp. 619–670). New York: McGraw-Hill.

Danes, A. F., Cuenca, L. G., Rodriguez Bueno, S., Mendarte Barrenechea, L., & Ronsano, J. B. (2008). Efficacy and tolerability of human fibrinogen concentrate administration to patients with acquired fibrinogen deficiency and active or in high-risk severe bleeding. *Vox Sanguinis, 94*(3), 221–226.

Desai, N. R, Gupta, S., Said, R., Desai, P., & Dai, Q. (2010). Choriocarcinoma in a 73-year-old woman: A case report and review of the literature. *Journal of Medical Case Reports, 4*(4), 379.

Deutchman, M., Tubay, A. T., & Turok, D. (2009). First trimester bleeding. *American Family Physician, 79*(11), 985–994.

Dhulkotia, J. S., Alazzam, M., & Galimberti, A. (2009). Tisseel for management of traumatic postpartum haemorrhage. *Archives of Gynecology and Obstetrics, 279*(3), 437–439.

DiGiulio, D. B., Gervasi, M. T., Romero, R., Vaisbuch, E., Mazaki-Tovi, S., Kusanovic, J. P., . . . Relman, D. A. (2010). Microbial invasion of the amniotic cavity in pregnancies with small-for-gestational-age fetuses. *Journal of Perinatal Medicine, 38*(5), 495.

Doheny, K. (2010). Diet drinks linked with preterm labour risk. *Midwives, 13*(4), 7.

Dolapcioglu, K., Gungoren, A., Hakverdi, S., Hakverdi, A. U., & Egilmez, E. (2009). Twin pregnancy with a complete hydatidiform mole and co-existent live fetus: Two case reports and review of the literature. *Archives of Gynecology and Obstetrics, 279*(3), 431–436.

Domen, R. E., & Hoeltge, G. A. (2003). Allergic transfusion reactions: An evaluation of 273 consecutive reactions. *Archives of Pathology & Laboratory Medicine, 127*(3), 316–320.

Emergency Nurses Association, & Newberry, L. (2003). *Sheehy's emergency nursing: Principles and practice* (5th ed.). St. Louis, MO: Mosby/Elsevier.

Emergency Nurses Association, Newberry, L., & Criddle, L. M. (2007). *Sheehy's manual of emergency care* (6th ed.). St. Louis, MO: Mosby.

Eskild, A., & Vatten, L. J. (2009). Abnormal bleeding associated with preeclampsia: A population study of 315,085 pregnancies. *Acta Obstetricia et Gynecologica Scandinavica, 88*(2), 154–158.

Fejzo, M. S., Poursharif, B., Korst, L. M., Munch, S., MacGibbon, K. W., Romero, R., & Goodwin, T. M. (2009). Symptoms and pregnancy outcomes associated with extreme weight loss among women with hyperemesis gravidarum. *Journal of Women's Health, 18*(12), 1981–1987.

Figueiredo, B., & Costa, R. (2009). Mother's stress, mood and emotional involvement with the infant: 3 months before and 3 months after childbirth. *Archives of Women's Mental Health, 12*(3), 143–153.

Finch, R. (2009). Antimicrobials: Past, present and uncertain future. *Clinical Medicine, 9*(3), 257–258.

Folashade, O., Simmons, B. J., & Hacker, Y. (2003). Management of Bartholin's duct cysts and gland abscess. *American Family Physician, 68*(1), 135–140.

Fosmire, M. S. (2009). *EMTALA FAQ*. Retrieved January 15, 2011, from www.emtala.com

Gambol, P. (2007). Maternal phenylketonuria syndrome and case-management implications. *Journal of Pediatric Nursing, 22*(2), 129–138.

Gasparis Vonfrolio, L., & Noone, J. (1997). *Emergency nursing examination review* (3rd ed.). Staten Island, NY: Power Publications.

Ghanizadeh, A., Ghanizadeh, M. J., Moini, R., & Ekramzadeh, S. (2009). Association of vaginal bleeding and electroconvulsive therapy use in pregnancy. *Journal of Obstetrics and Gynaecology Research, 35*(3), 569–571.

Gien, J., Seedorf, G., Balasubramaniam, V., Markham, N., & Abman, S. H. (2007). Intrauterine pulmonary hypertension impairs angiogenesis in vitro: Role of vascular endothelial growth factor–nitric oxide signaling. *American Journal of Respiratory and Critical Care Medicine, 176*(11), 1146–1153

Guyton, A. C., & Hall, J. E. (2005). *Textbook of medical physiology* (11th ed.). Philadelphia: Saunders.

Hardin, S. R., & Kaplow, R. (2010). *Cardiac surgery essentials for critical care nursing*. Sudbury, MA: Jones & Bartlett Learning.

Hasan, R., Funk, M. L., Herring, A. H., Olshan, A. F., Hartmann, K. E., & Baird, D. D. (2010). Accuracy of reporting bleeding during pregnancy. *Paediatric and Perinatal Epidemiology, 24*(1), 31–34.

Heng, Y. J., Waterhouse, M. K., Quinzio, D., Permezei, M., Rice, G. E., & Georgiou, H. M. (2010). Temporal expression of antioxidants in human cervicovaginal fluid associated with spontaneous labor. *Antioxidants & Redox Signaling, 13*(7), 951.

Hermansen, C., & Lorah, K. (2007). Respiratory distress in the newborn. *American Family Physician, 76*(7), 987–994.

Holleran, R. S. (2005). *Emergency transport nursing* (4th ed.). St. Louis, MO: Mosby.

Howell, E. A., Mora, P. A., Chassin, M. R., & Leventhal, H. (2010). Lack of preparation, physical health after childbirth, and early postpartum depressive symptoms. *Journal of Women's Health, 19*(4), 703–708.

Jacobs, B. B., & Hoyt, K. S. (2007). *Trauma nursing core course provider manual* (6th ed.). Bedford, IL: Emergency Nurses Association.

Jones & Bartlett Learning (2011). *2011 nurse's drug handbook* (10th ed.). (2011). Sudbury, MA: Jones & Bartlett Learning.

Kalelioglu, I., Uzum, A. K., Yildirim, A., Ozkan, T., Gungor, F., & Has, R. (2007). Transient gestational diabetes insipidus diagnosed in successive pregnancies: Review of pathophysiology, diagnosis, treatment, and management of delivery. *Pituitary, 10*(1), 87–93.

Karlsen, K. (2006). *The S.T.A.B.L.E. program* (5th ed.). Park City, UT: American Academy of Pediatrics.

Kattwinkel, J. (Ed.). (2006). *Neonatal resuscitation textbook* (5th ed.). American Academy of Pediatrics & American Heart Association. Park City, UT: American Academy of Pediatrics.

Kattwinkel, J., Perlman, J. M., & Aziz, K. (2010). Special report neonatal resuscitation: 2010 American Heart Association guidelines for cardiopulmonary resuscitation and emergency cardiovascular. *Pediatrics, 126*(5), 1319–1344.

Kealey, G. P. (2009). Carbon monoxide toxicity. *Journal of Burn Care and Research, 30*(1), 146–147.

Kirsch, J. D., & Scoutt, L. M. (2010). Imaging of ectopic pregnancy. *Applied Radiology, 39*(3), 10–12, 14–17, 21–22.

Koren, G., & Maltepe, C. (2004). Pre-emptive therapy for severe nausea and vomiting of pregnancy and hyperemesis gravidarum. *Journal of the Institute of Obstetrics and Gynaecology, 24*(5), 530–533.

Levi, M., & Cate, H. T. (1999). Disseminated intravascular coagulation. *New England Journal of Medicine, 341*(8), 586–592.

Lippincott. (2010). *Professional guide to signs and symptoms* (6th ed.). Philadelphia: Lippincott.

Lipson, J. G., Dibble, S. L., & Minarik, P. A. (Eds.). (1996). *Culture and nursing care: A pocket guide*. San Francisco: UCSF Nursing Press.

MacDorman, M. F., Declercq E., & Zhang J. (2010). Obstetrical intervention and the singleton preterm birth rate in the United States from 1991–2006. *American Journal of Public Health, 100*(11), 2241–2247.

Madan, I., Romero, R., Kusanovic, J. P., Mittal, P., Chaiworapongsa, T., Dong, Z., . . . Hassan, S. S. (2010). The frequency and clinical significance of intra-amniotic infection and/or inflammation in women with placenta previa and vaginal bleeding: An unexpected observation. *Journal of Perinatal Medicine, 38*(3), 275–279.

Maggiorini, M. (2010). Prevention and treatment of high-altitude pulmonary edema. *Progress in Cardiovascular Diseases, 52*(6), 500–506.

Mahdi, B. M. (2010). Estimation of CA-125 level in first trimester threatened abortion. *Internet Journal of Gynecology and Obstetrics, 12*(2).

Malee, M. P. (2007). Pituitary and adrenal disorders in pregnancy. In S. G. Gabbe, J. R. Niebyl, & J. L. Simpson (Eds.), *Obstetrics: Normal and problem pregnancies* (5th ed., pp. 1038–1043). Philadelphia: Elsevier Churchill Livingstone.

Martin, B. (2010). Family presence during resuscitation and invasive procedures: AACN practice alert. Retrieved from http://www.aacn.org

McCormack, R. A., Doherty, D. A., Magann, E. F., Hutchinson, M., & Newnham, J. P. (2008). Antepartum bleeding of unknown origin in the second half of pregnancy and pregnancy outcomes. *International Journal of Obstetrics and Gynaecology, 115*(11), 1451–1457.

Mikolajczyk, R. T., Louis, G. M., Cooney, M. A., Lynch, C. D., & Sundaram, R. (2010). Characteristics of prospectively measured vaginal bleeding among women trying to conceive. *Paediatric and Perinatal Epidemiology, 24*(1), 24–30.

Moraes, C. L., Reichenheim, M., & Nunes, A. P. (2009). Severe physical violence among intimate partners: A risk factor for vaginal bleeding during gestation in less privileged women? *Acta Obstetricia et Gynecologica Scandinavica, 88*(9), 1041–1048.

Myers, L. (2010). Postpartum plasma exchange in a woman with suspected thrombotic thrombocytopenic purpura (TTP) vs. hemolysis, elevated liver enzymes, and low platelet syndrome (HELLP): A case study. *Nephrology Nursing Journal, 37*(4), 399–402.

Nama, V., & Manyonda, I. (2009). Tubal ectopic pregnancy: diagnosis and management *Archives of Gynecology and Obstetrics, 279*(4), 443–453.

Nishimura, T., Suzue, J., & Kaji, H. (2009). Breastfeeding reduces the severity of respiratory syncytial virus infection among young infants: A multi-center prospective study. *Pediatrics International: Official Journal of the Japan Pediatric Society, 51*(6), 812–816.

Nwosu, Z. C., & Omabe, M. (2010). Maternal and fetal consequences of preeclampsia. *Internet Journal of Gynecology and Obstetrics, 13*(1).

Ohara Padden, M. (1999). HELLP syndromes: Recognition and perinatal management. *American Academy of Family Physicians, 60*(3), 829–842.

Patsouras, K., Panagopoulos, P., Sioulas, V., Salamalekis, G., & Kassanos, D. (2010). Uterine rupture at 17 weeks of a twin pregnancy complicated with placenta percreta. *Journal of Obstetrics & Gynaecology, 30*(1), 60–61.

Penaloza, D., Sime, F., & Ruiz, L. (2008). Pulmonary hemodynamics in children living at high altitudes. *High Altitude Medicine & Biology, 9*(3), 199–207.

Perry, S. E., Hockenberry, M. J., Lowdermilk, D. L., & Wilson, D. (Eds.). (2010). Musculoskeletal or articular dysfunction. In *Maternal child nursing care* (4th ed., pp. 1705–1708). Philadelphia: Mosby Elsevier.

Persson, R., Hitti, J., Verhelst, R., Vaneechoutte, M., Persson, R., Hirschi, R., . . . Eschenbach, D. (2009). The vaginal microflora in relation to gingivitis. *BMC Infectious Diseases, 9,* 6.

Prescribing reference. (2009, Summer). *NPPR: Nurse Practitioner's Prescribing Reference, 16*(2).

Proehl, J. A. (2008). *Emergency nursing procedures* (4th ed.). St. Louis, MO: Saunders.

Quinla, J. D., & Hill, D. A. (2003). Nausea and vomiting of pregnancy. *American Family Physician, 68*(1), 121–128.

Sarkar, S., Hagstrom, N. J., Ingardia, C. J., Lerer, T., & Herson, V. C. (2005). Prothrombotic risk factors in infants of diabetic mothers. *Journal of Perinatology, 25*(2), 134–138.

Sela, H. Y., & Einav, S. (2011). Injury in motor vehicle accidents during pregnancy: A pregnant issue. *Expert Review of Obstetrics & Gynecology, 6*(1), 69.

Soleymani Majd, H., Srikantha, M., Majumdar, S., B-Lynch, C., Choji, K., Canthaboo, M., & Ismail, L. (2009). Successful use of uterine artery embolisation to treat placenta increta in the first trimester. *Archives of Gynecology and Obstetrics, 279*(5), 713–715.

Spooner, L. M., & Liu, E. (2009). Tuberculosis, CNS. In F. J. Domino, R. A. Baldor, A. M. Erlich, & J. Golding (Eds.), *The 5-minute clinical consult 2010* (18th ed., pp. 1358–1359). Philadelphia: Lippincott Williams & Wilkins.

Steyn, N. P., Lambert, E. V., & Tabana, H. (2009). Conference on "Multidisciplinary approaches to nutritional problems." Symposium on "Diabetes and health." Nutrition interventions for the prevention of type 2 diabetes. *Proceedings of the Nutrition Society, 68*(1), 55–70.

Tan, P. C., Jacob, R., Quek, K. F., & Omar, S. Z. (2007). Pregnancy outcome in hyperemesis gravidarum and the effect of laboratory clinical indicators of hyperemesis severity. *Journal of Obstetrics and Gynaecology Research, 33*(4), 457–464.

Thapa, K., Shrestha, M., Sharma, S., & Pandey, S. (2010). Trend of complete hydatidiform mole. *Journal of the Nepal Medical Association, 49*(177), 10–13.

Turner, M. (2007). Hyperemesis gravidarum: Providing woman-centered care. *British Journal of Midwifery, 15*(9), 540–544.

U.S. Organ Procurement and Transplantation Network (OPTN). (2005). Scientific Registry of Transplant Recipients (SRTR): OPTN/SRTR annual report. Retrieved February 20, 2005, from http://www.optn.org

Urdern, L. D., Stacy, K. M., & Lough, M. E. (2005). *Thelan's critical care nursing* (5th ed.). St. Louis, MO: Mosby.

Utz-Billing, I., & Kentenich, H. (2008). Female genital mutilation: an injury, physical and mental harm. *Journal of Psychosomatic Obstetrics and Gynaecology, 29*(4), 225–229.

Verklan, M. T., & Walden, M. (2010). *Core curriculum for neonatal intensive care nursing.* St. Louis, MO: Saunders.

Voigt, M., Henrich, W., Zygmunt, M., Friese, K., Straube, S., & Briese, V. (2009). Is induced abortion a risk factor in subsequent pregnancy? *Journal of Perinatal Medicine, 37*(2), 144–149.

Wang, D., Hu, Y., He, Y., Xie, C., & Yin, R. (2009). Pure ovarian choriocarinoma mimicking ectopic pregnancy in true hermaphroditism. *Acta Obstetricia et Gynecologica Scandinavica, 88*(7), 850–852.

Wang, L. M., Wang, P. H., Chen, C. L., Au, H. K., Yen, Y. K., & Liu, W. M. (2009). Uterine preservation in a woman with spontaneous uterine rupture secondary to placenta percreta on the posterior wall: A case report. *Journal of Obstetrics and Gynaecology Research, 35*(2), 379–384.

Watson, S., & Gorski, K. A. (2011). *Invasive cardiology* (3rd ed.). Sudbury, MA: Jones & Bartlett Learning.

Wood, L., & Quenby, S. (2010). Exploring pregnancy following a pre-term birth or pregnancy loss. *British Journal of Midwifery, 18*(6), 350–356.

Yildizhan, R., Kolusari, A., Adali, F., Adali, E., Kurdoglu, M., Ozgokce, C., & Cim, N. (2009). Primary abdominal ectopic pregnancy: A case report. *Cases Journal, 1*(2), 8485.

Yuan, W., Duffner, A. M., Chen, L., Hunt, L. P., Sellers, S. M., & Bernal, A. L. (2010). Analysis of pre-term deliveries below 35 weeks' gestation in a tertiary referral hospital in the UK. A case-control survey. *BMC Research Notes, 3*, 119.

Zefer, N. B., Greer, V., & Woolard, R. H. (2009). The use of transvaginal ultrasound by emergency physicians in medical student education. *Donald School Journal of Ultrasound in Obstetrics & Gynecology, 3*(4), 59–64.

Zeqiri, F., Paçarada, M., Kongjeli, N., Zeqiri, V., & Kongjeli, G. (2010). Missed abortion and application of misoprostol. *Medicinski Arhiv, 64*(3), 151–153.

SECTION 9:

Shock States

1. Your patient with severe acute pancreatitis now has a blood pressure of 68/40. She has a heart rate of 138 and a respiratory rate of 32. You suspect hypovolemic shock. The hypovolemic shock is probably due to
   A. Blood loss from a ruptured gallbladder
   B. Third spacing related to capillary leaking
   C. Insufficient volume intake related to vomiting
   D. Excessive fluid loss due to diarrhea

2. When evaluating a CVP pressure monitoring tracing, the c wave represents
   A. Mechanical atrial diastole
   B. The decrease in RA volume during relaxation
   C. Emptying of the right atrium into the RV
   D. The increase in RA pressure from closure of the tricuspid valve

3. When evaluating the CVP pressure waves, the v wave represents
   A. Mechanical atrial diastole
   B. The increase in RA pressure from closure of the tricuspid valve
   C. Emptying of the right atrium into the RV
   D. The decrease in RA volume during relaxation

4. Mast cell degranulation with resultant histamine release and vasodilation is an appropriate definition of
   A. Septic shock
   B. Pleural effusion
   C. Anaphylaxis
   D. MODS

5. Systemic inflammatory response syndrome (SIRS) can best be defined as
   A. Sepsis with cardiovascular failure
   B. Sepsis with accompanying organ failure
   C. Tachycardia or tachypnea with a fever
   D. Systemic organ dysfunction

6. Jane had a pulmonary artery catheter placed and has a PAOP (PCWP) of 4. She is restless and mildly tachycardic. Absent any specific cardiac issue, you anticipate which of the following interventions?
    A. Administration of an inotrope
    B. Volume replacement
    C. Increase afterload with a vasoconstrictor
    D. Administration of nitroprusside to decrease preload

7. Your patient is a Jehovah's Witness and was admitted with chest and abdominal injuries. His Hgb and Hct is falling and his Hgb is now 6.5 and Hct 24. His chest tubes have drained 460 ml in the last half hour. The anticipated treatment is to
    A. Administer 500 cc of albumin
    B. Administer one unit of type-specific whole blood
    C. Administer 250 ml of fresh frozen plasma
    D. Administer continuous-circuit autotransfusion

8. Your patient is in cardiogenic shock. At this time she is awaiting placement on an intra-aortic balloon pump. In any patient with cardiogenic shock, an undesirable outcome would produce
    A. Increased cardiac output
    B. Increased systemic vascular resistance
    C. Decreased ventricular preload
    D. Decreased pulmonary artery pressures

9. Shaun took his sister's skateboard out for a ride. He was wearing a helmet and protective gear. Shaun rode too fast downhill and could not stop, striking a car. Shaun suffered a fractured left tibia, a left flail chest, a cervical sprain, a right Colle's fracture, and road rash on his face and neck. He is admitted with a blood pressure of 82/40, HR 126, RR 26 and shallow, T 98.4°F. His 12-lead EKG shows ST elevation in the anterior leads. Shaun's initial CXR shows a normal cardiac silhouette and no infiltrates. His Hgb is 9.3 and Hct 30. MB is 19%. He is restless and complains of pain in the neck, chest, and left leg. Shaun is probably suffering from
    A. Pulmonary edema
    B. Pulmonary hypertension
    C. Hypovolemic shock
    D. Cardiogenic shock

10. Your patient was transferred from a tertiary care facility and is in decompensated shock. You have dobutamine infusing via a peripheral IV line with TPN and intralipids. You have just received an order to give sodium bicarbonate intravenously and to give ampicillin intravenously as well. As an ED nurse you know the most appropriate actions to take would be to
    A. Stop the intralipids and infuse the sodium bicarbonate while waiting for pharmacy to send the ampicillin
    B. Start a peripheral heparin lock to infuse the sodium bicarbonate and follow with the ampicillin infusion
    C. Ask the physician to place a central line or PICC line for additional venous access ports
    D. Piggyback the ampicillin on the main IV line and start another peripheral line on the other arm

11. You are treating a patient with suspected sepsis. His blood pressure is 76/50, heart rate is 144, respiratory rate is 20, and O_2 saturation is 84% in room air. Prior to initiating an infusion of dopamine, which of the following actions is a priority for the nurse?
    A. Obtain consent for a central line
    B. Prepare to infuse dobutamine and dopamine together
    C. Verify the number of isotonic crystalloid boluses already given
    D. Ensure phentolamine mesylate is at bedside

12. Martina is an asthmatic who is rapidly decompensating. You are preparing to initiate vasoactive support. Which of the following is the most appropriate vasoactive drug of choice?
    A. Isuprel
    B. Dopamine
    C. Vasopressin
    D. Neosynephrine

13. Your patient is severely hypotensive. Norepinephrine bitartrate (Levophed) is infusing via his central line. Which of the following orders should you question?
    A. Monitor blood pressure every 30 minutes
    B. Administer with dopamine
    C. Dilute in D_5W
    D. Titrate off over a period of 6 to 24 hours

14. Luigi is being seen in the ED after falling from his roof. He sustained a right fractured tibia and fibula and a fractured right clavicle. Your initial assessment results are as follows:
    EKG: ST at 122 with isolated PVCs
    Art line BP 74/50 cuff BP 76/54 skin pale, cool, clammy
    RR 26, breath sounds clear, slightly diminished RLL O_2 2 L/min via NC
    Mentation: Responds to questions slowly, oriented to self and time
    Pulmonary artery catheter readings:
      PAP 22/10
      PAOP 6
      RAP 5
    Cardiac output 3.4   Cardiac index 1.7
    Which of the following conditions do you believe Luigi is developing?
    A. Cardiogenic shock
    B. Left ventricular failure
    C. Septic shock
    D. Hypovolemic shock

15. Adrian is a professional skier. When he returned home from the airport this afternoon he was short of breath, overly fatigued, and somewhat slow to answer questions. Adrian went to watch TV and then collapsed. Adrian arrived in your ED about 20 minutes ago. He required immediate intubation and is now being mechanically ventilated at TV 750, FiO_2 0.70, AMV 16. He remains unresponsive. A pulmonary artery catheter was placed. Adrian's assessment findings are as follows:
EKG: ST at 124
Art line BP 76/42 cuff BP 70/52 Doppler only to DP, no pressure obtained
Skin pale, cool, clammy   T 98.0°F
RR 16, breath sounds = bilateral crackles Marked pretibial and pedal edema
Mentation: Unresponsive to painful stimuli
Pulmonary artery catheter readings:
    PAP 48/28
    PAOP 24
    RAP 22
Cardiac output 3.0   Cardiac index 1.0
Adrian is probably developing
  A. Pulmonary hypertension
  B. A cardiac tamponade
  C. Cardiogenic shock
  D. Right heart failure

16. Darlene was traveling home with the choir on the church bus and ate a snack her seatmate provided. After about 5 minutes Darlene began to wheeze and her respirations were labored. A choir member administered epinephrine via an EpiPen and Darlene's symptoms abated. The next day Darlene saw her family physician. This physician did not explain the reason for the reaction to Darlene. Two days later Darlene was sharing some of her snack mix with her nephew and again began wheezing. She became severely tachypneic and she was transported to the ED. She required treatment with epinephrine and steroids and was intubated, and a pulmonary artery catheter placed. Darlene is 7 months pregnant. She is currently exhibiting the following signs and symptoms:
EKG: ST at 118 without ectopy
Cuff BP 94/68 skin cool, pale capillary refill 3 seconds
Ventilator settings; SIMV 12, TV 600, FiO_2 100%
RR 14, breath sounds: clear   T 99.4°F (rectal)
Mentation: Awake, restless
Pulmonary artery catheter readings:
    PAP 28/18
    PAOP 18
    RAP 7
    SVR 816
Cardiac output 3.3   Cardiac index 2.1
Darlene is probably developing
  A. Anaphylactic shock
  B. Cardiogenic shock
  C. Hypovolemic shock
  D. Obstructive shock

17. Harold was standing on a second-story balcony 2 days ago when it collapsed, impaling his right arm on the metal fence. The piece of fence was removed at the scene, and Harold refused treatment by paramedics. Harold planned to see his physician next week. Harold became progressively nauseous overnight and exhibits the following parameters and symptoms:
    EKG: ST at 112 without ectopy
    Arterial line BP 98/60   Cuff BP 92/54 skin warm, dry capillary refill 2 seconds
    RR 26, breath sounds: clear O_2 3 L/min via NC
    T 100.4°F
    Mentation: Alert, oriented ×4
    Because of his history and current symptoms, Harold had a pulmonary artery catheter placed and the initial readings are as follows:
       PAP 20/8
       PAOP 6
       RAP 4
       SVR 820
    Cardiac output 7.6   Cardiac index 4.0
    Harold is probably developing
    A. A pericardial tamponade
    B. Left heart failure
    C. Distributive shock
    D. Septic shock

18. Malignant hyperthermia is most likely to occur after the administration of
    A. Morphine
    B. Tetracycline
    C. Halothane
    D. Lidocaine

19. An early sign of malignant hyperthermia is
    A. Rhabdomyolysis
    B. Bleeding from venipuncture sites
    C. Increased temperature
    D. Elevated serum creatinine phosphokinase

20. A late sign of malignant hyperthermia is
    A. Jaw rigidity
    B. Rhabdomyolysis
    C. Tachycardia
    D. Metabolic acidosis

21. To determine if your patient has a genetic predisposition for malignant hyperthermia, which of the following drugs might be used for sensitivity testing?
    A. Halothane
    B. Caffeine
    C. Accolate
    D. Singulaire

22. Your patient has malignant hyperthermia. Which of the following arterial blood gas results is expected from a patient with this condition?
    A. pH 7.35, pCO_2 40, pO_2 80
    B. pH 7.28, pCO_2 49, pO_2 60
    C. pH 7.40, pCO_2 38, pO_2 90
    D. pH 7.42, pCO_2 41, pO_2 70

23. Your patient was in full arrest following a root canal. After a successful resuscitation, the patient has developed Ludwig's angina. This type of angina can be defined as
    A. A type of painful bradycardia in which the QT interval is lengthened
    B. An infectious process
    C. Dysrhythmia with severe pain secondary to inhalation of noxious gases
    D. Cardiac ischemic postcode syndrome

24. In patients with sepsis, endotoxins stimulate production of tumor necrosis factor (TNF). The TNF in turn stimulates
    A. Neutrophil activation and platelet aggregation
    B. Parathyroid
    C. Increased CO_2 retention
    D. Increased CPP

25. Patients who are stung by bees numerous times are in danger of developing
    A. Anemia
    B. Kidney failure
    C. Long QT interval
    D. Hydrocephalus

26. A possible side effect of cocaine use is
    A. Malignant hyperthermia
    B. Cherry red skin
    C. Paralytic ileus
    D. Constricted pupils

27. Which of the following drugs may promote anaphylaxis in a patient receiving treatment for status asthmaticus?
    A. Oxygen
    B. N-acetyl-cysteine
    C. Codeine
    D. Guaifenesin

28. Which of the following is a nursing consideration with administration of norepinephrine (Levophed)?
    A. Do not administer with alkaline solutions
    B. Do not administer for low coronary artery perfusion states
    C. It is not indicated for vasogenic shock
    D. Do not use for hypotensive states

29. Levophed may cause tissue necrosis. You should treat extravasations with
    A. An antihistamine
    B. Benadryl
    C. Phentolamine
    D. Hydralazine

30. If your patient was in the early stage of septic shock, you would expect which of the following hemodynamic parameters?
    A. SVR elevated, PAOP elevated, CO decreased
    B. CO decreased, RAP elevated, PAOP elevated
    C. RAP elevated, SVR decreased, PAOP increased
    D. CO increased, PAOP decreased, SVR decreased

31. You accompanied your patient to the radiology department for a renal arteriogram. After the dye was injected the patient complained of a "salty taste" in his mouth. You know
    A. This is the first sign of an anaphylactic reaction
    B. This will result in termination of the arteriogram
    C. This reaction is expected and should pass after about 5 minutes
    D. This is an emergency

32. Grace is 73 years old and is admitted to your unit with tachycardia (138), RR 28, BP 94/60, T 96.4°F. Her white count is 16,000. Grace states she was treated for a "kidney infection" 2 weeks ago while on vacation. She denies pain at this time. Grace probably has
    A. MODS
    B. Kidney stones
    C. SIRS
    D. Appendicitis

33. Your patient with pneumonia was just intubated and placed on mechanical ventilation. His urine output dropped significantly. This is probably due to
    A. Third spacing
    B. Sepsis
    C. Underresuscitation
    D. MODS

34. Allessio is 20 years old. He got in a street fight with gang members and was stabbed in the right anterior chest. Allessio lost about 1400–1600 ml of blood. Which of the following signs and symptoms are expected with this volume of blood loss?
    A. Decreased, pulse pressure normal, RR 20–30/min
    B. BP normal, RR increased, capillary refill normal
    C. RR increased, BP normal, pulse pressure normal
    D. BP decreased, RR increased, CO decreased

35. Pulmonary artery catheter infections may be best prevented by which of the following actions?
    A. Using an antibiotic-coated catheter
    B. Removing the catheter within 48–72 hours of insertion
    C. Using prophylactic antibiotics
    D. Avoiding continuous heparin infusions

36. The body's systemic inflammatory immune hormonal response to severe injury or illness arising from a variety of causes is known as
    A. MODS
    B. SSCM
    C. SIRS
    D. PACC

37. Which of the following substances is not considered a highly influential mediator of gram-negative septic shock?
    A. Myocardial depressant factor
    B. TNF
    C. Interleukin-1
    D. Endotoxin

38. If your patient is in a cardiogenic shock, which set of parameters would be accurate?

	HR	CI	SVR	PVR
A.	↑	↓	↑	Normal or ↑
B.	↓	↑	↑	↓
C.	↑	↓	↑	↓
D.	↑	↑	↑	↓

39. The classic initial presentation of septic shock is
    A. Tachypnea, vasoconstriction, and tachycardia
    B. Fever, tachycardia, and vasodilation
    C. Pale, cool skin, positive blood culture, and tachycardia
    D. Vasoconstriction, hypothermia, and cool skin

40. SIRS is the acute development of two or more of the following criteria, which are
    A. Hypothermia (< 36°C) and bradycardia (age related)
    B. Fever (> 38°C) and leukocytosis (WBC > 12,000/mm^3)
    C. Leukopenia (WBC > 10,000/mm^3) and tachypnea
    D. Weak central pulses and neutropenia

41. Your patient is suffering from cardiogenic shock and requires ECMO therapy. Which of the following statements about extracorporeal membrane oxygenation (ECMO) is true?
    A. ECMO is used for treatment of pulmonary hypoplasia
    B. ECMO replaces nitric oxide as the therapy of choice for PPHN
    C. ECMO should not be used in cases of intravascular hemorrhage
    D. ECMO is not a treatment for cardiogenic shock

42. The autonomic nervous system is not responsible for the control of which of the following body functions?
    A. Pupil constriction
    B. Cardiac muscle
    C. Smooth muscle
    D. Glands

43. A patient has lost 1500–2000 ml of blood, has a HR of > 120, a decreased blood and pulse pressure, and a RR of 30–40. In addition, the patient is very anxious and somewhat confused. What classification of hypovolemic shock due to hemorrhage is appropriate for this patient?
    A. Class IV
    B. Class II
    C. Class I
    D. Class III

44. Which of the following conditions is not a cause of obstructive shock?
    A. Spinal shock
    B. Tension pneumothorax
    C. Air embolus
    D. Cardiac tamponade

45. Which of the following conditions is not considered to be a cause of distributive shock?
    A. Pregnancy
    B. Anaphylaxis
    C. Neurogenic shock
    D. Spinal shock

46. In shock states the liver is stimulated by _____ to activate glycogenolysis.
    A. Renin
    B. Angiotensinogen
    C. Aldosterone
    D. Epinephrine

47. Your patient is 30 years old with an unknown blood type. She was given multiple units of O-positive packed cells following a car accident. A nursing consideration for future treatment should include
    A. Vital signs every hour
    B. A CT scan
    C. Rho(D) immune globulin
    D. A pelvic exam

SECTION 9: SHOCK STATES ANSWERS

1. **Correct answer: B**
   Patients with pancreatitis undergo massive fluid shifting to the third spacing related to capillary leaking due to the inflammatory response to pancreatic self-digestion. Mediators released during the inflammatory response lead to vasodilation and increased capillary permeability. Fluid may shift into the bowel, mucosal lining, and within the lungs leading to acute lung injury (ALI). The drop in blood pressure may lead to acute kidney injury (AKI) and renal failure. Immediate fluid replacement with crystalloids and colloids is required to maintain intravascular volume. A history of poor volume intake only worsens the hypovolemia but not the primary and most severe cause of the hypovolemic shock.

2. **Correct answer: D**
   During CVP pressure monitoring, the c wave represents the increase in RA pressure from closure of the tricuspid valve.

3. **Correct answer: A**
   When evaluating the CVP pressure waves, the v wave represents mechanical atrial diastole.

4. **Correct answer: C**
   Mast cell degranulation with resultant histamine release and vasodilation is an appropriate definition of anaphylaxis. Anaphylaxis is a form of distributive shock. The histamine release may cause normal peripheral vascular tone to become inappropriately relaxed. Vasodilation results in increased venous capacitance, causing a relative hypovolemia even if the patient has not actually lost any net fluid. The common physiologic disturbance in all forms of distributive shock is a decrease in preload.

5. **Correct answer: C**
   The International Consensus Conference in 2002 standardized the definition of systemic inflammatory response syndrome (SIRS). SIRS is defined as tachycardia or tachypnea with fever or high leukocyte count. Sepsis is defined as SIRS in the presence of suspected or proven infection, and severe sepsis is defined as sepsis with accompanying organ dysfunction. When cardiovascular failure occurs in the setting of severe sepsis, then it is classified as septic shock.

6. **Correct answer: B**
   The low wedge pressure of 4 indicates hypovolemia, and the patient will require volume replacement.

7. **Correct answer: D**
   The religious preference of the patient must be respected. The only acceptable form of transfusion in this case is via autotransfusion.

8. **Correct answer: B**
   In any patient with cardiogenic shock, an undesirable outcome would produce increased systemic vascular resistance. A primary goal in cardiogenic shock is to improve the pumping action of the heart (improve myocardial contractility), reduce the workload (decrease SVR) and oxygen demand, and improve cardiac output.

If possible, systemic vascular resistance should be decreased and the left ventricle augmented with an inotrope. Nitroprusside will reduce preload and afterload. The cardiac workload will be decreased as is the myocardial oxygen demand.

9. **Correct answer: D**
Shaun is in the first stage of cardiogenic shock secondary to systolic dysfunction. The injuries to the chest may have caused a pulmonary artery laceration or a cardiac contusion, which is more likely. His blood pressure is low, and the EKG shows ST segment elevation in the anterior leads. If the myocardium is contused, it will react the same way as if an MI had occurred. The pumping function of the myocardium is compromised and may need additional support with inotropes. Shaun will probably undergo volume replacement, angiography, and surgery.

10. **Correct answer: B**
Dobutamine is not compatible with either sodium bicarbonate or ampicillin, so the nurse cannot infuse the medications together. The appropriate choice is to start another peripheral line to administer sodium bicarbonate while waiting for the ampicillin to arrive from pharmacy. If the patient remains hemodynamically unstable and unable to obtain or maintain peripheral venous access, then it is appropriate to speak with the physician regarding more stable access such as a central line or a PICC line.

11. **Correct answer: C**
When starting dopamine, it is important to ensure that hypovolemia has been treated appropriately. In septic shock the patient may receive multiple fluid boluses until pulmonary edema is noted or the boluses fail to impact blood pressure. Central venous access is the preferred route, but the physician is responsible for obtaining consent. If central access is unavailable, peripheral access is acceptable. However, the site must be monitored closely for infiltration and additional IV access points must be available. Phentolamine mesylate should be available in case infiltration does occur, but it is not the first action to be performed.

12. **Correct answer: A**
Isuprel (isoproterenol) is the better choice for vasoactive support for the asthmatic patient in decompensated shock. Isuprel is a catecholamine that causes smooth muscle relaxation, bronchodilation, and pulmonary vasodilation to decrease PVR and increase heart rate and contractility. Dopamine causes increases peripheral vasoconstriction to increase blood pressure but does not affect pulmonary blood flow. Vasopressin results in systemic vasoconstriction and acts on the renal tubules to increase water reabsorption. Neosynephrine causes arteriolar vasoconstriction resulting in greater PVR and more VQ shunting. There is also the possibility of the patient becoming hypoxemic.

13. **Correct answer: A**
Norepinephrine bitartrate (Levophed) infusions require blood pressure monitoring at least every 5 minutes. Direct arterial monitoring is preferred for more accurate evaluation. The solution should be clear without particulates and mixed in D_5W, D_5W with normal saline, or normal saline and covered from direct light. Levophed may be infused with dopamine, but monitor peripheral circulation closely due to severe vasoconstriction and possible extravasation. Levophed should also be weaned off over at least 6 to 24 hours to prevent rebound hypotension.

14. **Correct answer: D**
    Luigi's blood pressure, PAS/PAD pressures, and RAP are low. The cardiac output and cardiac index are low, and the heart rate and respiratory rate are low. His mentation is diminished. The values indicate hypovolemic shock.

15. **Correct answer: C**
    Adrian is developing cardiogenic shock. When the left ventricle fails, fluid backs up into the pulmonary vasculature. Because the wedge pressure is high, it means the fluid is already backed up in the left heart. The PAP and RAP are high, and bilateral crackles indicate pulmonary congestion. Cardiac output and cardiac index are low, and BP is not being maintained.

16. **Correct answer: D**
    Darlene was admitted for anaphylactic shock. However, she now appears to be in obstructive shock. She is 7 months pregnant, and the baby is probably pressing on her aorta and vena cava. A simple change of position might fix the problem. In anaphylactic shock, the PAP would be low in the initial stages because of vasodilation. In obstructive shock the PAP and PAOP can be normal or high. Symptoms usually resolve once the problem is eliminated.

17. **Correct answer: D**
    Harold is in the hyperdynamic or warm stage of septic shock. The endotoxins are causing an increase in metabolism and act as vasodilators. The temperature is up because of the increased metabolism and infection. The RAP, PAP, SVR, and PAOP are decreased because of vasodilation. The cardiac output and cardiac index are high because they are compensating. Hypotension occurs because of vasodilation. Urine output should be quite high. Harold needs immediate treatment with large quantities of fluids, vasopressors, antibiotics, and antiendotoxins.

18. **Correct answer: C**
    Induction agents such as halothane, succinylcholine, or desflurane may initiate an episode of malignant hyperthermia. Stress and depolarizing muscle relaxants may also trigger MH. In malignant hyperthermia excess calcium builds up in microplasm. The patient then suffers from sustained skeletal muscular contractions. This leads to a hypermetabolic state.

19. **Correct answer: D**
    Early signs of malignant hyperthermia include elevated serum creatinine phosphokinase (CPK), jaw rigidity, tachycardia, respiratory and metabolic acidosis. Please note that MH can develop up to 24 hours postoperatively.

20. **Correct answer: B**
    Late signs of malignant hyperthermia include rhabdomyolysis, increased temperature, and bleeding from venipuncture sites.

21. **Correct answer: B**
    Caffeine is used diagnostically because it can contract muscles at higher doses without the danger of depolarizing cell membranes. In malignant hyperthermia, the use of anesthetic agents like halothane causes muscles to contract and the patient to become hyperthermic. The antidote for malignant hyperthermia is dantrolene.

22. **Correct answer: B**
    Malignant hyperthermia is a hypermetabolic state and results in metabolic and respiratory acidosis (pH 7.28, pCO$_2$ 49, pO$_2$ 60).

23. **Correct answer: B**
    Ludwig's angina is a submaxillary infection. It is a cellulitis of the neck and floor of the mouth that usually occurs with, or after, dental disease.

24. **Correct answer: A**
    In patients with sepsis, endotoxins stimulate production of tumor necrosis factor (TNF). The TNF in turn stimulates neutrophil activation and platelet aggregation. In addition, TNF stimulates increased capillary permeability and release of IL-1, IL-6, and IL-8.

25. **Correct answer: B**
    Patients who are stung by bees numerous times are in danger of developing kidney failure. Bee stings have proteins in the venom that act as enzymes. The enzymes lyse the cells, and the cellular debris accumulates very quickly and actually clogs the kidneys. The patient then dies from kidney failure. Any patient who has been stung multiple times needs to be monitored for at least 2 weeks after the incident.

26. **Correct answer: A**
    A possible side effect of cocaine use is malignant hyperthermia. The antidote is dantrolene. Malignant hyperthermia is usually seen in patients receiving anesthetics. This patient may also require ice packs and a hypothermia blanket. On occasion, bowel irrigations with cold water and cold NG tube irrigations have been necessary. The cherry red skin is a possible effect with carbon monoxide poisoning.

27. **Correct answer: B**
    Anaphylaxis may be caused or exacerbated by the use of N-acetyl-cysteine (Mucomyst). Mucomyst may actually cause bronchospasm, so it must be used with a bronchodilator. Usually, Mucomyst is contraindicated. Codeine is generally not used in status asthmaticus. Guaifenesin is Robitussin—a mild cough syrup.

28. **Correct answer: A**
    Alkaline solutions may cause the norepinephrine to precipitate. Also, do not use it if the solution is discolored. Norepinephrine is used for low coronary perfusion states, vasogenic shock, and hypotension.

29. **Correct answer: C**
    Regitine (phentolamine) is used to counteract tissue necrosis caused by Levophed. It should be administered subcutaneously around the area of extravasation.

30. **Correct answer: D**
    A patient in the early stages of septic shock may have a mild fever and will be in a hyperdynamic state. The endotoxins that are circulating have vasodilatory effects, so RAP, PAOP, and SVR are decreased. The increase in CO is compensatory.

31. **Correct answer: C**
    The salty taste is normal and the patient may be slightly nauseous, feel like he or she wants to cough, or feel flushed. This sensation will pass in about 5 minutes.

32. **Correct answer: C**

    SIRS is a systemic infection that can present in the elderly with hypothermia and even a WBC of < 4000 or > 12,000. MODS is usually the result of a direct injury to an organ. A kidney stone or appendicitis should present with pain and tenderness.

33. **Correct answer: C**

    Underresuscitation is probably due to miscalculation of possible insensible losses and third spacing.

34. **Correct answer: D**

    This patient is in hypovolemic shock. The normal blood volume in an adult is about 5000 ml. Blood loss in the amount of 1500 ml is equal to about one third of the total blood volume. You would expect the HR to increase to 120–150, BP to decrease with a narrowed pulse pressure, the RR to increase to 25–40, CO to decrease, and delayed capillary refill to occur. The skin would be cool and clammy, and there may be some neurologic issues like restlessness, anxiety, and confusion.

35. **Correct answer: B**

    Pulmonary artery catheter infections may be best prevented by removing the catheter within 48–72 hours of insertion. If the catheter remains in place more than 72 hours, there is significant risk of infection. One of the major complications of pulmonary artery catheters is infection. Studies have shown the initial source of the infection is from an initial colonization of skin bacteria that migrate down the catheter. Additional studies have shown that coating the catheter with antibiotics has not been particularly effective. The point of insertion (subclavian or jugular) also has been found to have no bearing on the risk of infection. Heparin may keep the catheter from clotting but does not have any bearing on potential infections. Prophylactic antibiotics do not prevent catheter infections and may lead to more antibiotic-resistant strains colonizing the catheter.

36. **Correct answer: C**

    SIRS is the body's systemic inflammatory immune hormonal response to severe injury or illness arising from a variety of causes. SIRS is not dependent on an infection. SIRS is, however, accompanied by an infectious process (sepsis).

37. **Correct answer: A**

    Myocardial depressant factor is not considered a highly influential mediatory of gram-negative septic shock.

38. **Correct answer: A**

    A patient in cardiogenic shock would present with these parameters.

    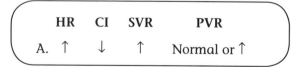

39. **Correct answer: B**

    The classic presentation of septic shock is fever, tachycardia, and vasodilation.

40. **Correct answer: B**

    SIRS is the acute development of two or more of the following criteria, which are fever (> 38°C) and leukocytosis (WBC > 12,000/mm^3).

41. **Correct answer: C**
    ECMO should not be used for intravascular hemorrhage because systemic heparinization is required.

42. **Correct answer: A**
    The autonomic nervous system is not responsible for the control of pupil constriction.

43. **Correct answer: D**
    This patient has lost 1500–2000 ml of blood, has a HR of > 120, a decreased blood and pulse pressure, and a RR of 30–40. In addition, the patient is very anxious and somewhat confused. This patient is considered to be in class III hypovolemic shock due to hemorrhage.

44. **Correct answer: A**
    Spinal shock is not a type of obstructive shock. Obstructive shock is the result of inadequate blood volume secondary to compression or obstruction of the aorta, pulmonary arteries, great veins, or the heart.

45. **Correct answer: A**
    Pregnancy is not considered a cause of distributive shock. However, in late stages of pregnancy, the baby can rest on the vena cava and cause an obstructive shock state. Relief usually comes from a change in the mother's position. Distributive shock results from a low blood volume or poor distribution of blood.

46. **Correct answer: D**
    The liver stores excess glucose as glycogen. In shock states the liver is stimulated by epinephrine to activate glycogenolysis. The glycogen is converted to glucose to help maintain cell metabolism. Epinephrine constricts the hepatic so blood is diverted to vital organs. However, if the liver is ischemic for too long, liver failure may result.

47. **Correct answer: C**
    This patient had an unknown blood type and was given O-positive packed cells. After the patient stabilizes it might be necessary to administer Rho(D) immune globulin because the patient is premenopausal.

SECTION 9: SHOCK REFERENCES

American Association of Critical-Care Nurses (AACN). (2009). Pulmonary artery pressure monitoring: AACN practice alert. Retrieved October 30, 2010, from http://www.aacn.org

American Heart Association. (2010). *Congenital cardiovascular defects: Statistics*. Retrieved September 12, 2010, from http://www.americanheart.org/presenter.jhtml?identifier=4576

Anonymous. (2008). Medication-related complications in the trauma patient. *Journal of Intensive Care Medicine, 23*(2), 91–108.

Anonymous. (2010). Compartment syndrome: Studies from Umea University describe new findings in compartment syndrome. *Obesity, Fitness & Wellness Week,* 1412.

Balogh, Z. J., van Wessem, K., Yoshino, O., & Moore, F. A. (2009). Postinjury abdominal compartment syndrome: Are we winning the battle? *World Journal of Surgery, 33*(6), 1134–1141.

Bauer, M. P., van Dissel, J. T., & Kuijper, E. J. (2009). *Clostridium difficile*: Controversies and approaches to management. *Current Opinion in Infectious Diseases, 22*(6), 517–524.

Berg, R. A., Hemphill, R., Abella, B. S., Aufderheide, T. P., Cave, D. M., Hazinski, M. F., . . . Swor, R. A. (2010). Part 5: Adult basic life support: 2010 American Heart Association Guidelines for Cardiopulmonary Resuscitation and Emergency Cardiovascular Care. *Circulation 122* (suppl 3): S685–S705.

Boland, M. R., & Heck, C. (2009). Acute exercise-induced bilateral thigh compartment syndrome. *Orthopedics, 32*(3), 218.

Cauwels, A. (2007). Nitric oxide in shock. *Kidney International, 72*(5), 557.

Chernecky, C., & Berger, B. (2004). *Laboratory tests and diagnostic procedures* (4th ed.). Philadelphia, PA: Saunders.

Darovic, G. O. (2002). *Hemodynamic monitoring: Invasive and noninvasive clinical application* (3rd ed.). Philadelphia, PA: Saunders.

den Uil, C. A., Lagrand, W. K., Valk, S. D., Spronk, P. E., & Simoons, M. L. (2009). Management of cardiogenic shock: Focus on tissue perfusion. *Current Problems in Cardiology, 34*(8), 330–349.

Emergency Nurses Association, & Newberry, L. (2003). *Sheehy's emergency nursing: Principles and practice* (5th ed.). St. Louis, MO: Mosby/Elsevier.

Emergency Nurses Association, Newberry, L. & Criddle, L. M. (2005). *Sheehy's manual of emergency care* (6th ed.). St. Louis, MO: Mosby.

Gandhi, S. K., Powers, J. C., Nomeir, A. M., Fowle, K., Kitzman, D. W., Rankin, K. M., & Little, W. C. (2001). The pathogenesis of acute pulmonary edema associated with hypertension. *New England Journal of Medicine, 344*(1), 17–22.

Gasparis Vonfrolio, L., & Noone, J. (1997). *Emergency nursing examination review* (3rd ed.). Staten Island, NY: Power Publications.

Hardin, S. R., & Kaplow, R. (Ed.). (2010). *Cardiac surgery essentials for critical care nursing*. Sudbury, MA: Jones & Bartlett Learning.

Holleran, R. S. (2005). *Emergency transport nursing* (4th ed.). St. Louis, MO: Mosby.

Huffmyer, J. L., Groves, D. S., Scalzo, D. C., DeSouza, D. G., Littlewood, K. E., Thiele, R. H., & Nemergut, E. C. (2011). The effect of the intrathoracic pressure regulator on hemodynamics and cardiac output. *Shock, 35*(2), 114–116.

Hungerer, S., Ebenhoch, M., & Buhren, V. (2010). 17 Degrees Celsius body temperature—Resuscitation successful? *High Altitude Medicine & Biology, 11*(4), 369.

Jacobs, B. B., & Hoyt, K. S. (2007). *Trauma nursing core course provider manual* (6th ed.). Bedford, IL: Emergency Nurses Association.

Jones & Bartlett Learning. (2011). *2011 nurse's drug handbook* (10th ed.). Sudbury, MA: Jones & Bartlett Learning.

Jeger, R. V., Radovanovic, D., Hunziker, P. R., Pfisterer, M. E., Stauffer, J. C., Erne, P., & Urban, P. (2008). Ten-year trends in the incidence and treatment of cardiogenic shock. *Annals of Internal Medicine, 149*(9), 618–626.

Kapoor, A., & Thiemermann, C. (2011). Targeting CCR2: A novel therapeutic strategy for septic shock? *American Journal of Respiratory and Critical Care Medicine, 183*(2), 150.

Lippincott. (2010). *Professional guide to signs and symptoms* (6th ed.). Philadelphia, PA: Lippincott.

Malik, A. A., Khan, W. S., Chaudhry, A., Ihsan, M., & Cullen, N. P. (2009). Acute compartment syndrome—A life and limb threatening surgical emergency. *Journal of Perioperative Practice, 19*(5), 137–142.

Martin, B. (2010). Family presence during resuscitation and invasive procedures: AACN practice alert. Retrieved from http://www.aacn.org

McMahon, C. G., Kenny, R. A., Bennett, K., Little, R., & Kirkman, E. (2011). Effect of acute traumatic brain injury on baroreflex function. *Shock, 35*(1), 53–58.

Megarbane, B., Voicu, S., Deye, N., & Baud, F. (2011). Defining refractory myocardial infarction-associated cardiogenic shock: An ongoing elusive challenge. *Critical Care Medicine, 39*(2), 422.

Menon, T., Nandhakumar, B., Jaganathan, V., Shanmugasundaram, S., Malathy, B., & Nisha, B. (2008). Bacterial endocarditis due to group C streptococcus. *Journal of Postgraduate Medicine, 54*(1), 64.

Morrison, L. J., Deakin, C. D., Morley, P. T., Callaway, C. W., Kerber, R. E., Kronick, S. L., ... Nolan, J. P.; on behalf of the Advanced Life Support Chapter Collaborators (2010). Part 8: Advanced life support: 2010 International Consensus on Cardiopulmonary Resuscitation and Emergency Cardiovascular Care Services With Treatment Recommendations. *Circulation 122* (suppl 2): S345-S421.

Patanwala, A. E., Amini, A., & Erstad, B. L. (2010). Use of hypertonic saline injection in trauma. *American Journal of Health-System Pharmacy, 67*(22), 1920–1928.

Patel, G. P., Grahe, J. S., Sperry, M., Singla, S., Elpern, E., Lateef, O., & Balk, R. A. (2010). Efficacy and safety of dopamine versus norepinephrine in the management of septic shock. *Shock, 33*(4), 375–380.

Peel, D. A. (2007). Endocarditis due to a nutritionally variant *Streptococcus*: A lesson in recognition and isolation. *British Journal of Biomedical Science, 64*(4), 175.

Prescribing reference. (2009, Summer). *NPPR: Nurse practitioner's prescribing reference, 16*(2).

Proehl, J. A. (2008). *Emergency nursing procedures* (4th ed.). St. Louis, MO: Saunders.

Spaniol, S. R., Knight, A. R., Zebley, J. L., Anderson, D., & Pierce, J. D. (2007). Fluid resuscitation therapy for hemorrhagic shock. *Journal of Trauma Nursing, 14*(3), 152.

University of California Davis. (2003). Safety of droperidol in the emergency department reviewed. *Biotech Week,* Jul 16, 2003, p. 327

Urdern, L. D., Stacy, K. M., & Lough, M. E. (2005). *Thelan's critical care nursing* (5th ed.). St. Louis, MO: Mosby.

Waibel, B. H., & Rotondo, M. F. (2010). Damage control in trauma and abdominal sepsis. *Critical Care Medicine, 38*(9), S421–S430.

Wan, Z., Ristagno, G., Sun, S., Li, Y., Weil, M. H., & Tang, W. (2009). Preserved cerebral microcirculation during cardiogenic shock. *Critical Care Medicine, 37*(8), 2333–2338.

Watson, S., & Gorski, K. A. (2011). *Invasive cardiology: A manual for cath lab personnel* (3rd ed.). Sudbury, MA: Jones & Bartlett Learning.

SECTION 10:

Genitourinary and Renal

1. The current definition of acute renal failure is
   A. Trauma to one or both kidneys
   B. Decrease in renal perfusion from shock or anaphylaxis
   C. A sudden or rapid decline in renal filtration function
   D. An obstruction to passage of urine

2. Intrinsic AKI is most commonly caused by
   A. Arteriolar vasoconstriction
   B. Acute ischemic or cytotoxic injury
   C. Amphotericin
   D. Hypercalcemia

3. Sudden anuria may be due to
   A. An embolic event
   B. Congestive heart failure
   C. Prostate enlargement
   D. Azotemia

4. Postrenal AKI may be caused by
   A. Malignant hypertension
   B. Transplant rejection
   C. Neurogenic bladder
   D. Preeclampsia

5. BUN may be elevated in patients
   A. Undergoing steroid treatments
   B. Taking streptomycin
   C. Taking chloramphenicol
   D. With a low protein intake

6. A renal transplant that results from humoral rejection or acute cellular rejection may be definitively diagnosed only via
   A. Ultrasound
   B. Nuclear scan
   C. Doppler scan
   D. Renal biopsy

7. In the polyuric phase of AKI, it is important for the nurse to carefully monitor
   A. Nitrogen balance
   B. Potassium and phosphorus
   C. Dopamine and mannitol levels
   D. Desmopressin levels

8. Anuria is defined as a urine output of
   A. < 30 ml/h
   B. 200 ml/d
   C. 300 ml/d
   D. < 100 ml/d

9. Oliguria is a urine output of 100–400 ml/d and is usually the result of
   A. Pyelonephritis
   B. Rhabdomyolysis
   C. Prerenal syndrome
   D. Acute glomerular nephritis

10. Mrs. G was sent to the ED directly from her physician's office. She had been complaining of fatigue and generalized pain. Her lab work indicated a rapidly rising BUN, and she is now undergoing further tests. While assessing Mrs. G, you note she has severe acne around the face and neck. You suspect that the rise in BUN may be due to
    A. Tetracycline
    B. HCTZ
    C. Bumetanide
    D. Mannitol

11. Mannitol and loop diuretics may be used in the treatment of AKI. Mannitol is nontoxic but must be used with caution because
    A. Mannitol may damage the eighth cranial nerve
    B. Mannitol may cause vestibular impairment
    C. Mannitol may produce a hyperosmolar state
    D. Mannitol may bind with proteins in the renal tubule

12. Nephrotoxicity may be caused by
    A. Furosemide
    B. Aspirin
    C. Thioguanine
    D. Acyclovir

13. NSAIDs may cause
    A. Prerenal AKI
    B. Intrinsic AKI
    C. Postrenal AKI
    D. Increased urine osmolality

14. Medications that can decrease BUN levels include
    A. Neomycin and rifampin
    B. Chloral hydrate and furosemide
    C. Bacitracin and gentamicin
    D. Chloramphenicol and streptomycin

15. Which of the following statements about creatinine is true?
    A. A normal range is 0.8 to 1.4 mg/dl
    B. Creatinine levels are higher in females
    C. Lower than normal levels may indicate pyelonephritis
    D. Low levels are a precursor to eclampsia

16. Allergic nephritis may be caused by
    A. Inadequate protein consumption
    B. Weight loss
    C. Cimetidine
    D. Water intoxication

17. The primary site for urea synthesis is in the
    A. Kidneys
    B. Liver
    C. Lungs
    D. Pancreas

18. Increased production of urea may be due to
    A. GI bleeding
    B. Low protein diet
    C. Congenital kidney disease
    D. Hypothermia

19. Your patient was involved in a head-on collision and had to be freed from under the steering column. Your patient has been diagnosed with a ruptured bladder. It is important to also assess for signs of
    A. Bowel perforation
    B. A ruptured spleen
    C. A shearing injury
    D. Rectal injury

20. You notice your patient's hand spasming when the automatic blood pressure cuff inflates. When you attempt a manual blood pressure measurement, the same thing happens when you inflate just past the systolic pressure and keep the pressure in place. This carpopedal spasm is indicative of
    A. Hypokalemia
    B. Hyperphosphatemia
    C. Hypocalcemia
    D. Hypernatremia

21. Your patient is becoming confused, is lethargic, and has muscle weakness. A review of her lab reports shows a calcium level of 11.7. A common way to treat this condition is to use
    A. D_5W and a Kayexalate enema
    B. Normal saline and a loop diuretic
    C. Glucose followed by insulin
    D. Nothing—this is a normal value

22. While assessing your patient you notice significant pretibial and pedal edema. When the patient is weighed you note he stated he has gained 1.5 kilograms of weight in 24 hours. This is equal to at least _____ml of excess fluid.
    A. 2000
    B. 1500
    C. 3000
    D. 500

23. Your patient has a calcium level of 7.8. You would expect which of the following EKG changes to be observed on the EKG tracing?
    A. Tall, peaked T-waves
    B. A prominent U wave
    C. A first-degree AV block
    D. A prolonged QT interval

24. One way to check for low calcium levels is to tap over a branch of the facial nerve. If the patient is hypocalcemic, the upper lip on the same side (ipsilateral) will twitch. This is known as
    A. Trousseau's sign
    B. Chvostek's sign
    C. Grey-Turner's sign
    D. Homan's sign

25. What is the primary acid-base disturbance exhibited by patients with AKI?
    A. Metabolic acidosis
    B. Respiratory acidosis
    C. Metabolic alkalosis
    D. Respiratory alkalosis

26. Jorgen, a 63 year old retired schoolteacher, is admitted to the ED for cocaine intoxication. He begins to complain of severe epigastric pain. Labs are as follows: WBC 17.5 with 76% neutrophils, hematocrit 41%, LDH 341, platelets 226, BUN 7, creatinine 1.0. Urine analysis shows trace of proteins, few RBCs, and + urine toxicology for cocaine. What is the likely cause of his pain?
    A. Peptic ulcer disease
    B. Renal infarction
    C. Gastroenteritis
    D. Infarcted mesenteric artery

27. Aldosterone is secreted when the extracellular sodium level is _____ and/or when extracellular potassium is _____.
    A. Low, low
    B. Low, high
    C. High, low
    D. High, high

28. June is a 24 year old graduate student admitted to the ED for an exacerbation of her cystic fibrosis. June is at a high risk for developing
    A. Hypernatremia
    B. Hypocalcemia
    C. Hyponatremia
    D. Hypercalcemia

29. Amelia came to the ED for severe abdominal pain. It was determined that she has peritonitis and had a J-tube placed while waiting for an ICU bed. Amelia is at risk for which of the following electrolyte deficits?
    A. Sodium
    B. Magnesium
    C. Manganese
    D. Phosphorus

30. Your patient is a 66 year old diabetic with congestive heart failure. After 4 days of no contact, her daughter found her in bed, unresponsive. She has a red, dry, swollen tongue, temperature of 102°F, and flushed dry skin. She is tachycardic, hypotensive, and has decreased reflexes. Her urine specific gravity is 1.050. You suspect this patient is suffering from
    A. Hypernatremia
    B. Hypocalcemia
    C. Hypermagnesemia
    D. Hypokalemia

31. _____ is the major extracellular cation, and _____ is the major intracellular cation.
    A. Calcium, magnesium
    B. Sodium, calcium
    C. Potassium, sodium
    D. Sodium, potassium

32. What percentage of the body's potassium may be found in the extracellular fluid?
    A. 2%
    B. 5%
    C. 10%
    D. 98%

33. Potassium is reabsorbed in the
    A. Proximal tubules
    B. Distal tubules
    C. Ascending colon
    D. Descending colon

34. Increased aldosterone secretions _____ potassium excretion.
    A. Decrease
    B. Increase
    C. Bind and prevent
    D. Do not affect

35. Your patient is exhibiting severe delirium tremens and is an alcoholic. What will happen to the potassium level in this patient?
    A. Potassium moves from the vascular circulation into the interstitium
    B. Potassium moves out of the cell into vascular circulation
    C. Potassium moves out of the cell into the interstitium
    D. Potassium from the vascular circulation moves into the cell

36. Hypokalemia may cause
    A. Respiratory alkalosis only
    B. Metabolic alkalosis only
    C. Both respiratory and metabolic alkalosis
    D. Metabolic acidosis only

37. Hypokalemia due to excessive urinary excretion is caused by all of the following except
    A. Oliguria
    B. Renal disease
    C. Lasix
    D. Increased adrenal cortical hormones

38. If your patient is hypokalemic, what changes would you expect to see on an EKG tracing?
    A. Peaked T waves
    B. U waves
    C. Shortened QT intervals
    D. Absent P waves

39. Michael suffered a crush injury when a beam dropped on him. You would expect to see which of the following results on his electrolyte panel?
    A. Hyperphosphatemia
    B. Hypomagnesemia
    C. Hypocalcemia
    D. Hyperkalemia

40. It is recommended that adults consume approximately _____ mg of potassium daily.
    A. 500
    B. 1000
    C. 2000
    D. 3500

41. All of the following foods are high in potassium except
    A. Avocados
    B. Raisins
    C. Potatoes
    D. Carrots

42. Harold originally came to the ED for exercise intolerance and shortness of breath. It was determined he had excess fluid retention secondary to mild CHF. Harold was placed on diuretics, and you have been educating him about dietary issues. You discussed cooking methods for vegetables with your patient and his wife. Which of the following cooking techniques leaches out the greatest amount of potassium from vegetables?
    A. Boiling
    B. Baking
    C. Steaming
    D. Microwaving

43. Your patient is receiving potassium in his IV fluid, and the physician has ordered a potassium rider. What is the maximum rate of infusion for potassium solutions in a peripheral IV line?
    A. 2 mEq/hour
    B. 4 mEq/hour
    C. 10 mEq/hour
    D. 15 mEq/hour

44. In Addison's disease, what condition occurs secondary to the altered aldosterone levels?
    A. Hyperkalemia related to the decrease in aldosterone secretion
    B. Hyperkalemia related to the increase in aldosterone secretion
    C. Hypokalemia related to the decrease in aldosterone secretion
    D. Hypokalemia related to the increase in aldosterone secretion

45. All of the following are treatments for hyperkalemia except
    A. Glucose and insulin
    B. Kaon
    C. Calcium gluconate
    D. Bicarbonate administration

46. Maria has congestive heart failure and was prescribed Lasix for water retention by her nurse practitioner. Maria's feet and legs continued to swell, so she took an extra Lasix this morning. She became dizzy and nauseous and then came to the ED. Now she has profound muscle weakness and flat T waves. You would expect Maria's potassium level this morning to be in the range of
    A. 1.8 mEq/L
    B. 3.8 mEq/L
    C. 4.2 mEq/L
    D. 6.1 mEq/L

47. Normal magnesium levels for an adult are in the range of
    A. 0.5–1.5 mg/dl
    B. 1.5–2 mg/dl
    C. 2–3 mg/dl
    D. 4–5 mg/dl

48. Magnesium is required for all of the following physiologic functions except
    A. To act as an antagonist to calcium
    B. For enzyme activation
    C. Synthesis of nucleic acid and proteins
    D. Sodium-potassium pump operation

49. Magnesium alters intracellular calcium by impacting which of the following hormones?
    A. Parathyroid
    B. Aldosterone
    C. Cortisol
    D. Glycosol

50. Magnesium is most prevalent in which of the following areas of the body?
    A. Extracellular fluid
    B. In the liver
    C. In the bone
    D. In the spleen

51. As part of his discharge teaching, you are helping Joe to determine what foods are rich in magnesium. He asks you what the recommended daily intake of magnesium is for an adult. Your answer is
    A. 50–100 mg per day
    B. 100–200 mg per day
    C. 200–350 mg per day
    D. 350–420 mg per day

52. Your patient was admitted and treated for torsades de pointes. You are teaching about adding foods to his diet that are rich in magnesium. Your patient asks which of the following foods is a poor source of magnesium.
    A. Honey
    B. Broccoli
    C. Almonds
    D. Chocolate

53. Kathy had gastric bypass surgery 2 weeks ago. Which of the following electrolytes is she at most risk for an imbalance?
    A. Potassium
    B. Magnesium
    C. Calcium
    D. Sodium

54. Edna eats a diet high in calcium because her family has a history of osteoporosis. She was admitted to the ED for a fractured pelvis and pulmonary embolism suffered when she fell down her stairs. She has been experiencing increasing weakness and muscle tremors. She has noted an increase of "skipping" beats. She stated she was very dizzy and disoriented just before she fell. Based on the symptoms, which of the following labs should you assess immediately?
    A. Calcium level
    B. Sodium level
    C. Hemoglobin and hematocrit
    D. Magnesium level

55. Chloe has major abdominal trauma after a motor vehicle accident. She is exhibiting signs and symptoms of hypomagnesemia related to excessive urinary loss. How long will this loss occur?
    A. 12 hours
    B. 24 hours
    C. 36 hours
    D. 48 hours

56. Your patient was admitted in ketoacidosis. Her magnesium level is 0.5 mEq/L. What symptoms would you expect to see demonstrated by this patient?
    A. Convulsions
    B. Lethargy
    C. Negative Babinski sign
    D. Decreased reflexes

57. Nancy was diagnosed with breast cancer 8 years ago. The cancer has now metastasized to the bone. She came to the ED because her current pain medication is ineffective and her physician cannot be reached by phone. You would expect to see which changes in her electrolyte levels?
    A. Decrease in magnesium and increase in calcium levels
    B. Decrease in both magnesium and calcium levels
    C. Increase in both magnesium and calcium levels
    D. Increase in magnesium and decrease in calcium levels

58. Your patient is in cardiac arrest. Magnesium replacement is ordered. What is the usual dose of magnesium for a patient in cardiac arrest?
    A. 0.5 grams
    B. 1–2 grams
    C. 3–4 grams
    D. 4–5 grams

59. Magnesium is ordered for your patient. During the infusion you note flaccidity, absent patellar reflexes, shallow respirations, and a flushed face. Your next nursing action should be
    A. Give the magnesium—the patient is just sleeping
    B. Hold the dose for 1 hour
    C. Give the dose over 3 hours
    D. Hold the dose, contact the physician, and obtain a magnesium level

60. The most common cause of hypermagnesemia is
    A. Gastrointestinal bypass
    B. Gastrointestinal fistulas
    C. Renal failure
    D. Overdose

61. The family of your patient with hypermagnesemia asks why his face is flushed. You answer,
    A. "He has a temperature"
    B. "His magnesium level is a little high and causes his face to look flushed"
    C. "He is embarrassed because the hospital gown does not provide enough coverage"
    D. "He just completed his physical therapy"

62. What percentage of calcium is stored in the bone?
    A. 99%
    B. 85%
    C. 80%
    D. 75%

63. Which of the following statements about calcium is true?
    A. Approximately 40% of calcium is ionized in the serum
    B. Calcium levels cannot be correlated with albumin levels
    C. Calcium bonded to protein cannot pass the capillary wall
    D. Calcium is not necessary for coagulation

64. Serum calcium is decreased by all of the following except
    A. Increases in vitamin D
    B. Renal tubular excretion
    C. Gastrointestinal excretion
    D. Bone demineralization

65. As calcium levels _____, the parathyroid gland _____ secretions.
    A. Increase, decreases
    B. Increase, increases
    C. Decrease, decreases
    D. Decrease, remains consistent

66. You are testing for hypocalcemia by trying to elicit Trousseau's sign. You elicit this response by
    A. Tapping the cheek
    B. Lifting the left leg up and looking for head movement toward the chest
    C. Inflating a BP cuff to greater than the systolic pressure for 3 minutes and waiting for a carpal spasm
    D. Taking a sharp object up from the heel to the toes and watching for the toes to spread

67. Ginger is scheduled to undergo continuous renal replacement therapy (CRRT) this week. Your patient teaching should include which of the following drugs that need to be stopped 2–3 days prior to therapy?
    A. Beta-blockers
    B. ACE inhibitors
    C. Heparin
    D. Calcium channel blockers

68. For a nonpumped continuous renal replacement therapy (CRRT) to function appropriately, the minimal mean arterial blood pressure must be
    A. 40 mmHg
    B. 30 mmHg
    C. 60 mmHg
    D. 80 mmHg

69. Joyce has renal failure and will be undergoing continuous renal replacement therapy (CRRT). She asks if she can have visitors during the procedure. You tell her
    A. "Of course. There are no restrictions"
    B. "No. They would be in the way of the equipment"
    C. "No. They will increase your risk of infection"
    D. "Probably, but if they are sensitive to the sight of blood, they may want to wait until after the procedure"

70. Which of the following continuous renal replacement therapies require only venous access and pumping function?
    A. CVVHDF, SCUF
    B. CVVH, CVVHD
    C. CAVH, CAVHD
    D. CVVH, CAVH

71. Bob is in renal failure after cardiac arrest. He has continued cardiovascular instability. The best method for removal of his extra fluid is by using
    A. Hemodialysis
    B. Peritoneal dialysis
    C. Continuous renal replacement therapy
    D. Plasmapheresis

72. William is undergoing hemodialysis in your ED for acute renal failure as a result of uncontrolled type 2 diabetes. His wife asks how you know the hemodialysis is effective. Adequacy of dialysis is measured by
    A. Urine creatinine clearance
    B. Sodium, chloride, and potassium levels
    C. Blood pressure
    D. Urea clearance

73. You are assessing your patient's existing shunt prior to emergency hemodialysis. You note there is no thrill or bruit at the shunt site. Your next nursing action is to
    A. Call the surgeon to do a new graft
    B. Use a Doppler to determine graft patency
    C. Administer a bolus of heparin
    D. Continue with the hemodialysis; there is nothing wrong

74. Hemodialysis is used to treat many metabolic abnormalities as well as renal failure. One possible use for hemodialysis is to administer
    A. Vitamin C and calcium carbonate for patients with osteoporosis
    B. Erythropoietin for excessive iron
    C. Phosphate binders for hyperphosphatemia
    D. Glucose for hyperglycemia

75. Communication between all staff is vital. When transferring your patient with a graft, which of the following information is a priority to communicate to all staff that may come in contact with this patient?
    A. Last dialysis date
    B. Location of the graft
    C. Type of dialysis machine used
    D. Total fluid removed with last dialysis

76. The usual amount of dialysate used in peritoneal dialysis is
    A. 0.5–1 L
    B. 1–2 L
    C. 2–3 L
    D. 3–4 L

77. Which of the following is the correct fluid exchange sequence in peritoneal dialysis?
    A. Dump, dwell, and drain
    B. Installation, dwell, and drain
    C. Drain, instillation, and dwell
    D. Instillation, drain, and dwell

78. Peritoneal dialysis functions by using which two principles?
    A. Diffusion and ultrafiltration
    B. Osmotic pressure and osmosis
    C. Ultrafiltration and oncotic pressure
    D. Diffusion and osmosis

79. You are preparing to teach your patient about peritoneal dialysis. It is important to tell the patient which one of the following findings is normal?
    A. During the instillation phase the insertion site may leak
    B. During the dwell phase you may feel abdominal fullness and shortness of breath
    C. During the dwell phase subcutaneous fluid may be seen in the groin
    D. During the drain phase you will feel dizzy and have palpitations

80. During the drain phase you note only 50% return in the collection bag. Your next action should be to
    A. Position the patient prone
    B. Check for kinks, bends, or cracks in the tubing
    C. Double check the amount instilled
    D. Assess for subcutaneous fluid

81. You are providing discharge teaching to the family of a patient who received peritoneal dialysis. The patient will undergo at least three more treatments at your rural ED. As part of the discharge teaching you give the patient a home glucometer. The daughter questions this action because her mother is not a diabetic. You should tell the daughter
    A. Peritoneal dialysis can cause diabetes
    B. Her mother was just diagnosed with diabetes
    C. The dialysate contains glucose and can lead to hyperglycemia
    D. Peritoneal dialysis may lead to pancreatitis

82. For which of the following disease processes is immunoadsorption used as a treatment?
    A. Paraneoplastic neurologic syndromes
    B. Multiple sclerosis
    C. Cutaneous T-cell lymphomas
    D. Heart transplant rejection

83. Apheresis is best defined as
    A. The removal of plasma and/or proteins from the blood
    B. The selective removal of cells, plasma, and substances from the blood
    C. The selective removal of cellular components from the blood
    D. The removal of an antigen in the blood

84. Exchange plasma volume used in apheresis is usually given in a ratio of
    A. 1.5:1
    B. 2:1
    C. 2.5:1
    D. 3:1

85. Your patient was undergoing lymphocytopheresis and plasma exchange for progressive multiple sclerosis with citrate as the anticoagulant. She was receiving treatment at a dialysis center when she began to feel tingling all over her body. The patient was transported across the street to your ED for possible additional treatment. Which of the following lab results are you initially most concerned with?
    A. ABG, ionized calcium, PT/PTT levels
    B. Potassium, magnesium, PT/PTT levels
    C. INR, potassium, sodium, chloride levels
    D. ACT, ionized calcium level, ABGs

86. Maxim has been diagnosed with hypertension. He states that to control his blood pressure he "will never eat another thing with salt." You should tell him
    A. "That is not easy. Most fresh vegetables and fruit have tons of sodium"
    B. "Great. Sodium only plays a minor part in water balance and cellular activity, so your body won't know the difference"
    C. "You cannot completely eliminate sodium from your diet. Your body has an intricate system of safety measures to protect the level of sodium in your body"
    D. "Good idea. That should work fine"

87. The recommended sodium daily intake for someone limiting sodium from their diet ranges between
    A. 100 and 900 mg
    B. 1000 and 2000 mg
    C. 3000 and 5000 mg
    D. 4000 and 6000 mg

88. Ben was put on a limited sodium diet and has been working with a nutritionist. He was admitted to your ED for chest pain and pulmonary edema. Ben reports that he had stopped all additional sodium intake, has been following his diet regimen closely, stopped eating out, and is drinking 8–10 eight-ounce glasses of tap water every day. He also states he is voiding sufficient amounts. His sodium level is 155 mEq/L. What is the likely cause of Ben's hypernatremia?
    A. Renal failure
    B. Hypotonic fluids
    C. Diabetes mellitus
    D. His water softener system

89. Which of the following fruits has the lowest sodium content per 3.5-ounce serving?
    A. Cantaloupe
    B. Grapes
    C. Peaches
    D. Blackberries

90. Lucas is trying to limit his salt intake. Which of the following meat products would you recommend for Lucas to eat?
    A. Chicken without the skin
    B. Canned beef hash
    C. Fresh pike
    D. Canned crab

91. Alec was having chest pain while lifting boxes into his attic. The symptoms abated immediately when he stopped lifting the weight. Alec's wife brought him to the ED anyway. Alec's EKG and tests were normal. Alec's wife says he does not eat a good diet and that may cause a heart attack. Alec loves cheese but wants to limit his sodium intake. Which of the following cheeses has the highest sodium per 3.5 ounces?
    A. Swiss cheese
    B. Mozzarella cheese
    C. Cheddar cheese
    D. Parmesan cheese

92. You are receiving report on John who was injured when he suffered a seizure while working on his roof. His sodium level on admission was 120 mEq/L. What symptoms of hyponatremia would you expect John to exhibit?
    A. Twitching
    B. Tachypnea
    C. Lethargy
    D. Flattened T waves

93. A common cause of hyponatremia is
    A. Saltwater drowning
    B. Overhydration
    C. Administration of hypertonic solutions
    D. Hyperoxia

94. A 19 year old man comes to the ED complaining of a terrible rash on his penis he has had for the past 3 days. The rash looks like blisters in a small cluster on the shaft of the penis. This patient's symptoms are suspicious for which sexually transmitted infection?
    A. Herpes zoster
    B. Syphilis
    C. *Molluscum contagiosum*
    D. Herpes simplex I or II

95. An elderly patient presents to the ED with a fever, chills, dysuria, frequency, and pain at the costovertebral angle. It is likely this patient is suffering from
    A. Pyelonephritis
    B. Urinary calculi
    C. A lower urinary tract infection
    D. Prerenal AKI

96. The primary causative organism for urinary tract infections is
    A. *Escherichia coli*
    B. *Staphylococcus aureus*
    C. Proteus species
    D. *Klebsiella*

97. Your female patient presents to the ED with fever, chills, pain on urination, moderate burning at the supra pubic area, and diarrhea. This patient is most likely suffering from
    A. Acute renal failure
    B. A kidney infection
    C. A lower urinary tract infection
    D. An upper urinary tract infection

98. Urinary calculi most often form in the
    A. Ureters
    B. Glomerulus
    C. Bladder
    D. Renal pelvis

99. An elderly male patient requires urinary catheterization. As you attempt to advance the catheter you meet resistance and cannot advance the catheter more than about 3 inches into the urethra. The probable cause of this blockage is
    A. A urinary calculus
    B. Benign prostatic hyperplasia
    C. A large catheter
    D. A small catheter that has curled on itself

100. Which of the following is the most common sexually transmitted infection (STI)?
    A. Syphilis
    B. Gonorrhea
    C. Chlamydia
    D. Genital herpes

101. What symptoms do you expect with genital herpes?
    A. Dysuria, myalgia, and burning pain
    B. Dyspareunia, pustules, and itching
    C. Single, crusted lesion that is painful
    D. Fever, groin pain, and lymphadenopathy

102. Which of the following drugs would be used for an initial outbreak of genital herpes?
    A. Penicillin VK 500 mg every 8 hours for 10 days
    B. Acyclovir 400 mg every 8 hours for 10 days
    C. Septra DS 160/800 mg every 12 hours for 10 days
    D. Doxycycline 100 mg every 12 hours for 10 days

103. Your patient has been diagnosed with pelvic inflammatory disease (PID). What antibiotics do you anticipate being prescribed for this patient?
    A. Ceftriaxone 250 mg IM as a single dose, plus doxycycline 100 mg PO every 12 hours for 14 days
    B. Metronidazole 2% vaginal cream QHS for 10 days
    C. Cephalexin 500 mg orally every 6 hours for 10 days and levofloxacin 500 mg PO daily for 7 days
    D. Ciprofloxacin 500 mg PO twice daily for 10 days

104. What is the hallmark symptom of primary syphilis?
    A. Painful vesicular lesions on genitalia
    B. Painless chancre or lesion on the genitalia
    C. Painless maculopapular lesions on the groin
    D. Painful papules on genitalia

105. What are the most common symptoms of candida vaginitis?
    A. Thick, odorless discharge, pruritis
    B. Pruritis and thin, watery, yellow-green vaginal discharge
    C. Fishy smelling milky adherent discharge
    D. Gray-green vaginal discharge with pelvic pain

106. What is the treatment of choice for candida vaginitis?
    A. Ampicillin 500 mg every 8 hours for 7 days
    B. Doxycycline 1000 mg BID for 7 days
    C. Metronidazole 500 mg BID for 7 days
    D. Fluconazole 150 mg PO as a single dose

107. A 36 year old woman was brought to the ED after being raped in a parking lot. What should your initial assessment include?
    A. Physical exam and treatment for any physical injuries
    B. Psychiatric evaluation of the patient's mental state
    C. Patient's birth control status
    D. Identification of the rapist

108. How should a rape victim's clothing be managed in the collection of evidence?
    A. After a preliminary examination is done, clothing is returned to the patient
    B. Clothing should be labeled and placed in a paper bag
    C. Place clothing in a plastic belongings bag with the patient's name
    D. Have her loved ones hold onto the clothing

109. Which of the following diagnosis is appropriate for a victim of rape?
    A. Depression
    B. Posttraumatic stress disorder
    C. Rape-trauma syndrome
    D. Impaired adjustment

110. Julio took 100 mg of Viagra 6 hours ago and has had an erection since. What is the treatment of choice for this condition?
    A. Observation only
    B. Atropine 0.4 mg IV every 2 hours
    C. Cavernosal injection of phenylephrine
    D. Ice packs to the scrotum

111. What symptoms would you expect to find in a patient with priapism?
    A. Painful erection, history of penile trauma, cardiovascular disease
    B. Antidepressants, cardiovascular disease, an erection lasting more than 4 hours
    C. Recreational drugs, painful erection, beta-blockers
    D. Erection lasting more than 4 hours, history of priapism, antidepressants

SECTION 10: GENITOURINARY AND RENAL ANSWERS

1. **Correct answer: C**
   The current definition of acute renal failure is a sudden or rapid decline in renal filtration function. Acute renal failure is now known as acute renal injury (AKI) and can be classified as prerenal, intrinsic, or postrenal. Because material covered on the CEN exam reflects practice up to about a year ago, the new terminology should be added. Some item writers may use this new terminology on the exam.

2. **Correct answer: B**
   Intrinsic AKI is most commonly caused by acute ischemic or cytotoxic injury. Other causes include cell detachment, dilatation of the lumen, and injury to the distal nephron. Arteriolar vasoconstriction, amphotericin, and hypercalcemia are causes of prerenal AKI.

3. **Correct answer: A**
   Anuria is usually due to postrenal AKI, such as from an embolic event. Mechanical obstruction of the urinary collection system is involved. The collection system is comprised of the renal pelvis, the ureters, the bladder, and the urethra.

4. **Correct answer: C**
   Postrenal AKI may be caused by a neurogenic bladder. Other causes include tumor, tricyclic antidepressants, fibrosis, BPH, prostate CA, urethral obstruction, stone disease, and ligation during surgery. Malignant hypertension, transplant rejection, DIC, and preeclampsia are causes of intrinsic failure/injury.

5. **Correct answer: A**
   The BUN may be elevated in patients undergoing steroid treatments. The BUN may also be elevated in cases of GI or mucosal bleeding or excessive protein intake.

6. **Correct answer: A**
   A renal transplant that results from humoral rejection or acute cellular rejection may be definitively diagnosed only via ultrasound. Ultrasound may be difficult to obtain or interpret due to ascites, obesity, or fluid in the retroperitoneal area. Doppler scans measure blood flow, and the flow is diminished due to prerenal and intrinsic AKI. Nuclear scans are of limited value because the excretion rates may be slowed by disease. The renal biopsy is the gold standard for diagnosing rejection.

7. **Correct answer: B**
   Potassium and phosphorus must be diligently monitored during the polyuric phase of AKI because of the potential for dysrhythmias.

8. **Correct answer: D**
   Anuria is defined as a urine output < 100 ml/d.

9. **Correct answer: C**
   Oliguria is a urine output of 100–400 ml/d and is usually the result of prerenal syndrome or hepatorenal syndrome. Pyelonephritis, rhabdomyolysis, and acute glomerular nephritis are causes of nonoliguria (> 400 ml/d of urine output.).

10. **Correct answer: A**
    Tetracycline decreases anabolism and thereby increases the BUN.

11. **Correct answer: C**
    Mannitol is nontoxic but must be used with caution because it may produce a hyperosmolar state. Damage to the eighth cranial nerve, vestibular impairment, and renal tubule binding of proteins are characteristics of loop diuretics. Loop diuretics include furosemide, bumetadine, and torsemide.

12. **Correct answer: D**
    Acyclovir is nephrotoxic and can crystallize in the kidney and cause AKI. It is important for the ED nurse to carefully monitor the infusion time and the amount of fluid used to dilute intravenous drugs. Additional drugs that can crystallize in the kidney are sulfonamides, idinivir, and triamterine.

13. **Correct answer: A**
    NSAIDs block prostaglandin production, which alters glomerular arteriolar perfusion and may cause prerenal AKI.

14. **Correct answer: D**
    Medications that can decrease BUN levels include chloramphenicol and streptomycin. Chloral hydrate, furosemide neomycin, rifampin, bacitracin, and gentamicin are medications that increase BUN levels.

15. **Correct answer: A**
    A normal range for creatinine is 0.8 to 1.4 mg/dl. Females have less muscle mass than males, so they have lower levels of creatinine. Higher levels than normal may indicate pyelonephritis or eclampsia.

16. **Correct answer: C**
    Allergic nephritis may be caused by cimetidine. Cimetidine interferes with creatinine excretion in the renal tubule. Renal function does not decrease, but the creatinine does rise. If diminished renal function exists, an allergic nephritis may develop.

17. **Correct answer: B**
    Over 99% of urea synthesis occurs in the liver. Dietary protein is converted into amino acids and peptides. About 90% of these molecules are absorbed and transferred to the liver. Any excess nitrogen is converted into urea.

18. **Correct answer: A**
    Increased production of urea may be due to GI bleeding. Approximately 500 ml of whole blood equals 100 grams of protein. The extra protein must be converted to urea.

19. **Correct answer: D**
    Patients trapped under a steering column often have rectal injures, pelvic fractures, and injured iliac vessels.

20. **Correct answer: C**
    The carpopedal spasm is indicative of hypocalcemia and is known as Trousseau's sign. You can also elicit this response by having the patient hyperventilate. When the patient becomes alkalotic, the serum calcium level decreases and a carpopedal spasm occurs.

21. **Correct answer: B**
    The patient has hypercalcemia, as evidenced by the calcium level of 11.7. A loop diuretic prevents reabsorption of calcium, and normal saline is used to increase the

patient's glomerular filtration rate. If you were to administer a thiazide diuretic, it would actually decrease calcium excretion. Use of glucose, insulin, and Kayexalate is not indicated because they are treatments for hyperkalemia.

22. **Correct answer: B**

    1 kilogram = 2.2 pounds = 1000 ml. Thus, 1.5 kilograms equals 1500 ml. Although you may believe this is too basic a piece of information for a CEN review, it is the little pieces of information like this that trip people up on the exam.

23. **Correct answer: D**

    This patient is hypocalcemic. Lack of calcium slows cardiac contractility (the prolonged QT) and the patient might develop torsades de pointes (polymorphic ventricular tachycardia). Torsades is also caused by hypokalemia.

24. **Correct answer: B**

    One way to check for low calcium is to tap over a branch of the facial nerve. If the patient is hypocalcemic, the upper lip on the same side (ipsilateral) will twitch. This is known as Chvostek's sign. Trousseau's sign utilizes a BP cuff to elicit a carpopedal spasm indicative of hypocalcemia. Grey-Turner's sign is ecchymosis around the umbilicus, indicating abdominal issues, and Homan's sign may indicate DVT.

25. **Correct answer: A**

    The primary acid-base disturbance exhibited by patients with AKI is metabolic acidosis. The AKI patient cannot excrete ammonium or acid ions in quantities that are necessary to aid in the excretion of hydrogen. The buildup of the hydrogen causes the acidosis.

26. **Correct answer: B**

    Renal infarction can occur with cocaine intoxication. The proteinuria and RBCs in the urine are indicative of the renal infarction. Cocaine abuse can lead to any infarction, including MI.

27. **Correct answer: B**

    Aldosterone is secreted when the extracellular sodium level is low and/or when extracellular potassium is high. Aldosterone is a hormone secreted by the adrenal glands. Aldosterone is also secreted if the blood pressure is too low and when there is extreme physical stress.

28. **Correct answer: C**

    Because of the defective seventh chromosome, patients with cystic fibrosis lose sodium through their skin and mucous membranes. This results in a thickening of the mucous layers, leading to infection and hyponatremia.

29. **Correct answer: A**

    Amelia is at risk for hyponatremia. Large amounts of extracellular fluids are in the peritoneal cavity. If sodium is lost in here, then the calcium is no longer available to be absorbed into the vasculature.

30. **Correct answer: A**

    This patient is suffering from hypernatremia. Because of her diabetes this patient was unable to drink sufficient fluids, leading to dehydration and hemoconcentration. Due to her diabetes she may have additional renal injury. Because of the decreased blood flow through the kidneys from the CHF, the kidneys were unable to filter the excess sodium from her body.

31. **Correct answer: D**
    Sodium is the major extracellular cation, and potassium is the major intracellular cation.

32. **Correct answer: A**
    Approximately 2% of potassium is extracellular, whereas the remaining 98% is intracellular. Intracellular electrolytes cannot be directly measured, but extracellular levels can be measured. Normal extracellular values range from 3.5 to 5.0 mEq/L.

33. **Correct answer: B**
    Regulated excretion (absorption) of potassium is in the distal tubules.

34. **Correct answer: B**
    As aldosterone is secreted, potassium excretion increases. The same is true in reverse: if aldosterone secretion is slowed, potassium excretion is slowed and more potassium is retained.

35. **Correct answer: D**
    Potassium from the vascular circulation will move into the cell. Excessive alcohol intake leads to an alkalotic state. Because potassium has a positive charge and hydrogen moves opposite of potassium, as potassium moves into the cell, hydrogen moves out to correct the alkalosis.

36. **Correct answer: C**
    Potassium and hydrogen move opposite of each other. When a patient is hypokalemic, hydrogen moves into the extracellular fluid, leading to both respiratory and metabolic alkalosis.

37. **Correct answer: A**
    Hypokalemia due to excessive urinary excretion is not caused by oliguria. Oliguria is a result of hyperkalemia. Renal disease, Lasix, and increased adrenal cortical hormones lead to hypokalemia.

38. **Correct answer: B**
    A U wave is seen in hypokalemia. A peaked T wave, a shortened QT interval, and an absent P wave are seen with hyperkalemia.

39. **Correct answer: D**
    The patient will become hyperkalemic as the potassium from the cells is released into the vasculature after the crush injury.

40. **Correct answer: C**
    It is recommended that adults consume approximately 2000 mg of potassium daily.

41. **Correct answer: D**
    Carrots have the lowest amount of potassium at 233 mg. Avocados have about 1484 mg, raisins 751 mg, and potatoes 610 mg.

42. **Correct answer: A**
    Boiling leaches out most of the nutrients into the water. Baking is the best method, allowing the vegetables to retain most of their potassium and other nutrients.

43. **Correct answer: C**
    Potassium should not be infused at any rate greater than 10 mEq/hour to prevent extravasations, pain, or spasms related to rapid electrolyte changes.

44. **Correct answer: C**

    Addison's disease results in a decrease in aldosterone secretion. This leads to hypokalemia.

45. **Correct answer: B**

    Kaon is not a treatment for hyperkalemia. Kaon is another name for potassium gluconate, a common potassium replacement medication. Glucose and insulin, calcium gluconate, and bicarbonate all bind or push the potassium back into the cell from the intravascular space and reduce extracellular potassium levels.

46. **Correct answer: A**

    Maria is exhibiting signs and symptoms of hypokalemia. Hypokalemia is defined as any potassium level under 3.5 mEq/L. It is important to reinforce teaching patients how diuretics impact electrolyte levels and the underlying condition.

47. **Correct answer: C**

    The current recommended serum magnesium level is 2–3 mg/dl. This level may be higher for patients with cardiac disease or in their third trimester of pregnancy to treat pregnancy-induced hypertension and to control premature contractions.

48. **Correct answer: A**

    Magnesium is required for all of the following physiologic functions except acting as an antagonist to calcium. Magnesium is usually synergistic with calcium to control neuromuscular function within all muscle groups.

49. **Correct answer: A**

    The parathyroid controls the calcium level within the body. Magnesium has been found to influence the secretion rate of the parathyroid and, thus, calcium levels.

50. **Correct answer: C**

    Approximately 50% of the body's magnesium is within the bone marrow. The measured serum magnesium reflects only approximately 1% of the body's magnesium and the remaining 49% is found in the intracellular space.

51. **Correct answer: D**

    Currently, the recommended adult intake for magnesium is 350–420 mg per day. For pregnant women the preferred intake is at the higher range. Children's intake should be less, based on age.

52. **Correct answer: A**

    Honey has the lowest amount of magnesium. It is better to recommended foods such as leafy vegetables that have a deep, green color, whole grains, nuts, legumes, seafood, cocoa, and chocolate.

53. **Correct answer: B**

    Because magnesium is absorbed in the small intestines, surgeries such as gastric bypass that remove or alter the small intestines, place the patient at risk for hypomagnesemia. Gastric surgeries also impact water reabsorption, time processing in the intestines, calcium level, and amount of lactose in the diet.

54. **Correct answer: D**

    Edna is exhibiting signs and symptoms of hypomagnesemia. This is related to the high calcium intake. Calcium and magnesium are absorbed in the small intestines.

Calcium consumed in extremely high doses competes with magnesium absorption. Edna needs nutritional teaching to balance her diet.

55. **Correct answer: B**
    Abdominal trauma leads to increased stress on the body and increased aldosterone secretion. This increase in aldosterone secretion leads to an increase in magnesium excretion that contributes to hypomagnesemia. This condition lasts for approximately 24 hours. There is an additional risk with any abdominal injury that impairs small bowel absorption of magnesium.

56. **Correct answer: A**
    Convulsions are an expected symptom in this patient. Ketoacidosis leads to excessive urinary secretion of magnesium as a result of osmotic diuresis caused by the elevated glucose concentration. In addition, insulin therapy used to treat the hyperglycemia forces magnesium into the cells and further drops the extracellular concentration of magnesium. As magnesium levels drop, cellular irritability increases and there is an increased risk of convulsions. You would see an increased overall irritability, positive Babinski sign, and increased reflexes.

57. **Correct answer: A**
    As cancer spreads through bone, calcium is released into the serum. In a hypercalcemic state, magnesium secretion decreases, thus leading to hypomagnesemia.

58. **Correct answer: B**
    Only if a patient is in cardiopulmonary arrest would you infuse 1 to 2 grams of magnesium. IV infusions of magnesium should run no faster than 30 mg per minute. Careful monitoring should be done for possible EKG changes.

59. **Correct answer: D**
    The patient is exhibiting the signs and symptoms of hypermagnesemia. The dose should be held, the physician contacted, and the magnesium level evaluated.

60. **Correct answer: C**
    Renal failure is one of the most common causes of hypermagnesemia. The patient is unable to excrete excess magnesium via the urine. Gastrointestinal bypass and fistulas lead to hypomagnesemia.

61. **Correct answer: B**
    The best answer from the choices listed is, "His magnesium level is a little high and causes his face to look flushed." Magnesium levels greater than 5 mEq/L lead to vasodilation of the facial vessels.

62. **Correct answer: A**
    99% of the body's calcium is stored in the bone.

63. **Correct answer: C**
    If calcium is bonded with protein, the molecule is too large to pass from the extracellular fluid into intracellular due to restrictive capillary permeability. Fifty to 70% of serum calcium is ionized in the serum. Because of the protein binding ability of calcium, albumin and calcium levels can be directly correlated. Calcium plays a role in coagulation.

64. **Correct answer: A**
    Vitamin D increases serum calcium levels.

65. **Correct answer: A**

Parathyroid is the hormone most related to serum calcium management. In response to rising calcium levels, the parathyroid gland decreases secretion to decrease or stabilize calcium levels.

66. **Correct answer: C**

The technique for eliciting a Trousseau's sign is to inflate a blood pressure cuff greater than the systolic blood pressure for 3 minutes. A positive sign is if the carpal nerve spasms, causing the hand to curve inward with all fingers touching.

67. **Correct answer: A**

Beta-blockers may cause an anaphylactic reaction with the membranes or the filter in the CRRT filter. Bradykinins are released as a result, causing the systemic anaphylaxis.

68. **Correct answer: C**

For a nonpumped continuous renal replacement therapy (CRRT) to function appropriately, the minimal mean arterial blood pressure must be 60 mmHg. The patient's blood pressure provides the gradient on which the system functions. If the blood pressure is too low, the system will not filter appropriately.

69. **Correct answer: D**

Some individuals do not tolerate the sight of blood. Because CRRT occurs outside the body, blood is in full sight. To improve communication between both patient and visitors, it is best for the patient to let visitors know when procedures are occurring so they may visit at a time when a CRRT procedure is not occurring. There are some restrictions to how many people may fit in one room with the equipment. This will vary by facility. The more people in a room, the higher the risk that the equipment could be touched and/or disconnected.

70. **Correct answer: B**

CVVH and CVVHD therapies require only venous access and pumping function. The C stands for continuous. The second two letters refer to the access and return sites. CVV types of dilution require a pump function as the blood must be pumped through the system. CAV types of filtration use arterial pressures to drive the flow and the filtration. H, HD, and HDF refer to the type of filtration: hemofiltration, hemodialysis, or hemodiafiltration, respectively. SCUF, or slow continuous ultrafiltration, is used to remove fluid from the patient, and no replacement is given.

71. **Correct answer: C**

Continuous renal replacement therapy results in slower volume regulation to avoid rapid shifts in volume. This method results in continuous removal and/or regulation of solutes and volume.

72. **Correct answer: D**

Urea clearance in the blood is the best indicator for monitoring dialysis effectiveness. Electrolytes may be altered due to fluid shifting and the distillate used. Blood pressure may fluctuate with fluid removal and is not the best measurement method. Urine creatinine clearance indicates residual renal function.

73. **Correct answer: B**

Lack of thrill and/or bruit may indicate that the graft has occluded and dialysis is not possible. It is best to use a Doppler to determine graft patency prior to any calls or administration of any medication. Although you may not hear or feel the thrill and bruit, the graft may still be patent. The surgeon should be notified if the Doppler study is negative. Heparin will not break an existing clot.

74. **Correct answer: C**
Hemodialysis is used to administer phosphate binders for patients with hyperphosphatemia. In addition, it may be used to provide vitamin D and calcium carbonate for osteoporosis, erythropoietin for iron deficiencies (anemia), and glucose for hypoglycemia.

75. **Correct answer: B**
It is imperative that all staff members are made aware of graft site location. This includes lab techs, nursing assistants, student nurses, medical staff, physical therapy, and respiratory therapy. You want to avoid any lab or blood draws, blood pressures, or occlusions in the grafted limb.

76. **Correct answer: C**
2–3 L of dialysate is commonly used for peritoneal dialysis.

77. **Correct answer: B**
The correct sequence for fluid exchange in peritoneal dialysis is to first instill the dialysate, allow the fluid to dwell within the abdomen for a predetermined time, and drain the fluid. The number of exchanges is determined by the physician and the desired outcomes.

78. **Correct answer: D**
Peritoneal dialysis functions by the principles of diffusion and osmosis. Diffusion is the passive movement of solutes across a membrane. The direction of diffusion is based on concentration (from higher to lower), heat, and pressure. The speed at which diffusion occurs is based on the grade or steepness of the differences in concentrations on each side of the membrane and the molecule moving across the membrane (size, polarity). Osmosis is the passive movement of solvents (i.e., water) over a permeable membrane. Movement of the solvent depends on the permeability of the membrane. The more permeable the membrane, the more passive the movement of solutes and solvents. Permeability may impact the type of solutes able to unintentionally cross the membrane.

79. **Correct answer: B**
It is common for patients to have a feeling of abdominal fullness and shortness of breath related to the 2–3 L of dialysate installed in the abdomen and allowed to dwell. Leaking at the insertion site must be reported to the physician as the patient may develop peritonitis and the patient should be monitored closely. Dialysis cannot continue until the insert site is repaired. If fluid is felt or seen in the groin, this indicates a hernia and may lead to strangulation of any bowel that enters the groin during the dwell phase and is trapped there when the dialysate is drained. If a patient feels dizzy or has palpitations during the drain phase, this indicates a too rapid fluid shift or triggering of the vagal nerve. The drain time may need to be lengthened.

80. **Correct answer: B**
Kinking, bends, and cracks in the tubing are the most likely causes of a decreased dialysate return. If that does not correct fluid flow, then reposition the patient, assess for any subcutaneous fluid or fluid within the groin, double check the amount of fluid installed, and complete an assessment before reporting the situation to the physician.

81. **Correct answer: C**

    The dialysate often contains glucose. During diffusion, glucose may cross the membranes and cause hyperglycemia. It is important for the patient to monitor this complication at home. Careful education will assist the family in managing any complications and when to notify the physician. Some smaller emergency departments are performing outpatient peritoneal dialysis or hiring dialysis nurses to perform this function.

82. **Correct answer: A**

    Immunoadsorption is used in the treatment of paraneoplastic neurologic syndromes. Multiple sclerosis is treated with plasma lymphocytes. Cutaneous T-cell lymphoma is treated using a combination of photopheresis and leukopheresis. Heart transplant rejections are treated with a combination of photopheresis and plasmapheresis.

83. **Correct answer: B**

    Apheresis is the general term used for all pheresis techniques and encompasses any selective removal of cells, plasma, and substances from blood with the return of remaining components and volume to the patient. Plasmapheresis is the removal of plasma and/or proteins from the blood or as a plasma exchange. Cytapheresis is the selective removal of cellular components from the blood (i.e., WBC). Leukocytopheresis is the specific removal of WBCs. Erythrocytopheresis is the removal of RBCs. Plateletpheresis is the removal of platelets. Plasma-adsorption/perfusion is the filtering and treatment of plasma via adsorptive fiber filters. Immunoadsorption is the removal of an antigen via an antibody filter. Photopheresis is the removal and return of blood after exposure to ultraviolet light to destroy specific cells (in solid organ transplant rejection).

84. **Correct answer: A**

    Replacement of plasma volume in plasmapheresis is usually at 1:1 or 1.5:1. Replacement fluids include FFP, thawed plasma, albumin, and electrolytes and fluids based on the patient's condition.

85. **Correct answer: D**

    Citrate binds with calcium in the blood and metabolizes into sodium bicarbonate, increasing sodium and phosphate alkaline. ACT, ionized calcium levels, and ABGs show the extent of binding. The tingling is from a decrease in calcium to the tissues.

86. **Correct answer: C**

    Sodium cannot be completely eliminated from the diet. Sodium is a major cation in the extracellular fluid within the body. Sodium plays a key part in the sodium-potassium pump and stabilizing polarization of cells and water balance. The body protects sodium levels by titrating aldosterone and antidiuretic hormone (ADH), and changing filtration within the kidneys. Fresh fruits and vegetables contain minimal amounts of salt. Canned vegetables use sodium to preserve flavor and have the highest sodium levels.

87. **Correct answer: B**

    The daily recommended sodium intake for someone limiting sodium from their diet should be between 1000 and 2000 mg per day. This challenges the body to use sodium efficiently without overstressing the body's systems. A low sodium diet aims for sodium intake less than 1000 mg.

88. **Correct answer: D**
Many water-softening systems filter out calcium and magnesium (these minerals make water hard) and replace them with sodium. The longer the filter has been in place, the greater the sodium content of the water. Not all water softeners use sodium, so recommend to patients to check their system type. Possibly, instead of drinking the tap water, Ben should drink and food should be prepared with distilled or bottled water. He may also consider replacing the water filter with a reverse osmosis system. Ben is following his diet as prescribed and does not exhibit any signs of renal failure. Hypotonic fluids would lead to higher sodium levels. Diabetes insipidus would lead to elevated sodium levels due to the lack of ADH.

89. **Correct answer: D**
Blackberries have 1 mg of sodium per 3.5 ounce serving. Peaches have 2 mg, grapes have 3 mg, and cantaloupe has 12 mg.

90. **Correct answer: C**
Lucas should eat fresh pike. Most fresh fish are low in sodium. Pike has only 51 mg sodium per 3.5 ounce serving compared with chicken at 60–80 mg, canned beef hash at 540 mg, and canned crab at 1000 mg. Any canned or processed meat contains some preservative. If it is not low sodium, the preservative may be sugar. For most people eating fresh or fresh frozen meats, vegetables, and fruits will aid in limiting sodium, fat, and sugar intake.

91. **Correct answer: D**
Parmesan cheese has a sodium level of 1862 mg, whereas Swiss has 260 mg, cheddar has 620 mg, and mozzarella has 373 mg.

92. **Correct answer: A**
With hyponatremia, sodium levels drop below 135 mEq/L. Twitching and seizures are common, as well as apnea (not tachypnea), irritability (lethargy is seen with hypernatremia), and generalized muscle weakness (late sign). Flattened T waves are seen with hypokalemia.

93. **Correct answer: B**
Overhydration is a common cause of hyponatremia. The level is below normal due to dilution and not a disease process or injury. Intake of fluids orally (or intravenously) has caused an artificial drop in sodium. Correction is done through fluid restriction or decreasing IV rates. Other causes of hyponatremia include loss of sodium through sweating or vomiting, shock, bleeding, SIADH, renal failure (inability to save sodium), hypoxia, fresh-water drowning, or an overadministration of hypotonic fluids.

94. **Correct answer: D**
Herpes simplex, either type I or II, can cause this patient's symptoms. The cluster of blisters is seen anywhere boxer shorts fit from the waist to the midthigh, although the genitalia is the most common location for both men and women. Syphilis presents with a single painless lesion in the initial phase. *Molluscum contagiosum* is highly contagious and has flesh-colored dome-shaped papules with an umbilicated center. Herpes zoster is shingles. Blisters along dermatomes are seen with herpes zoster.

95. **Correct answer: A**
A patient presenting with fever, chills, dysuria, frequency, and pain at the costovertebral angle is likely suffering from pyelonephritis. The patient will also likely present

with orthostatic vital signs and pain on palpation or urination that may radiate toward the umbilicus or lower abdomen.

96. **Correct answer: A**

    The primary causative organism for urinary tract infections is *Escherichia coli*. Newer studies have shown that adenovirus-related hemorrhagic cystitis is becoming a more frequently diagnosed cause of UTIs.

97. **Correct answer: C**

    This patient has fever, chills, pain on urination, moderate burning at the supra pubic area, and diarrhea. This patient is most likely suffering from a lower urinary tract infection. Females are more likely to have urinary tract infections than men because they have shorter urethras and bacteria can easily ascend the tract.

98. **Correct answer: D**

    Urinary calculi most often form in the renal pelvis. Patients who consume a diet high in proteins, calcium, or fruit juices are at risk as are patients with a sedentary lifestyle and a history of gout or previous calculi.

99. **Correct answer: B**

    Benign prostatic hyperplasia is common in elderly men. The prostate gland enlarges and impinges on the urethra.

100. **Correct answer: D**

     Genital herpes is the most common sexually transmitted infection, more than the other three diseases combined. The patients may carry the virus for decades before the initial outbreak. Chlamydia is the second most common STI.

101. **Correct answer: A**

     Dysuria, myalgia, and burning pain are common symptoms of genital herpes. Genital herpes (herpes simplex II) may have no symptoms for years. The most common symptoms of an initial outbreak include fever, malaise, dysuria, dyspareunia, and vesicles anywhere boxer shorts fit. Most of the vesicles occur on the labia for a female and the penis, glans, or scrotum for the male.

102. **Correct answer: B**

     Acyclovir (Zovirax), valacyclovir (Valtrex), or famciclovir (Famvir) are the three antiviral medications used for herpes outbreaks.

103. **Correct answer: A**

     Ceftriaxone and doxycycline are the treatment of choice for PID. Metronidazole may also be added twice daily for 14 days. Fluoroquinolones are no longer recommended as treatment for PID due to drug resistance.

104. **Correct answer: B**

     The primary lesion of syphilis is a painless chancre or lesion generally found on the genitalia. Because of the painless nature of the lesion and the pubic hair the lesion may be missed.

105. **Correct answer: A**

     Candida vaginitis discharge is the consistency of ricotta or fine cottage cheese. There is no odor, but the pruritis is intense.

106. **Correct answer: D**
A single oral dose of fluconazole is the most effective agent against candida vaginitis. There are also topical azole medications such as miconazole vaginal cream that are also effective.

107. **Correct answer: A**
The most important initial treatment for a rape victim is to assess and treat any injuries. The psychiatric evaluation, birth control, and the identification of the rapist, although important, are not the priority. The patient may be offered Plan B or other birth control if necessary but that can be delayed up to 72 hours. No Plan B or other birth control should be given until a pregnancy test is performed and the results are negative.

108. **Correct answer: B**
The chain of evidence is extremely important in rape cases. Labeling and placing the victim's clothing in a paper bag and having it in direct observation until it is collected by the police are required. It is also important to document the evidence as accurately as possible. Handling the clothing in any other way may destroy the evidence.

109. **Correct answer: C**
A rape victim may have any of the diagnoses listed above, but the most appropriate one is rape-trauma syndrome.

110. **Correct answer: C**
Injecting phenylephrine 100–500 µg into the corpora cavernosa can resolve priapism in about 65% of the cases. The urologist may also try aspirating 20–30 ml from this area prior to the administration of phenylephrine. A shunt may also be inserted to remove blood from the penis and must be inserted before the blood clots.

111. **Correct answer: A**
A painful erection lasting more than 4 hours is the definition of priapism. It often occurs without sexual stimulation and may be seen in spinal cord–injured patients. Other patient history includes a history of trauma to the penis, hematologic abnormalities, cardiovascular disease, certain medications, recreational drugs, and a history of priapism.

SECTION 10: GENITOURINARY AND RENAL REFERENCES

Ahmed, I., & Beckingham, I. J. (2007). Liver trauma. *Trauma, 9*(3), 171–180.

Allison, S. O., & Lev-Toaff, A. S. (2010). Acute pelvic pain: What we have learned from the ER. *Ultrasound Quarterly, 26*(4), 211–218.

Anderson. B., & Khadra, A. (2006). Acute urinary retention: Developing an A&E management pathway. *British Journal of Nursing, 15*(8), 434–438.

Babel, N., Sakpal, S. V., & Chamberlain, R. S. (2010). The Page kidney phenomenon secondary to a traumatic fall. *European Journal of Emergency Medicine, 17*(1), 24–26.

Betz, T. G., Lee, P., & Victor, J. C. (2008). Hepatitis A vaccine versus immune globulin for postexposure prophylaxis. *New England Journal of Medicine, 358*(5), 531–532.

Bielawska, H., & Epstein, N. L. (2010). A stone down below: a urethral stone causing acute urinary retention and renal failure. *Canadian Journal of Emergency Medical Care, 12*(4), 377–380.

Bisan, S. (2008). How to recognize the top three STDs in women: Elusive and often misleading, these infections can have serious consequences if not caught in time. Here's how to diagnose and treat them. *Clinician Reviews, 18*(8), 39.

Bolmers, M. D. M., Linthorst, G. E., Soeters, M. R., Nio, Y. C., & van Lieshout, J. J. (2009). Green urine, but no infection. *Lancet, 374*(9700), 1566.

Bradway, C., & Rodgers, J. (2009). Evaluation and management of genitourinary emergencies. *Nurse Practitioner, 34*(5), 36–43.

Brown, A. S. (2010). Renal tubular acidosis. *Dimensions of Critical Care Nursing, 29*(3), 112–119.

Burns, S. M. (Ed.). (2007). *American Association of Critical-Care Nurses (AACN): AACN Protocols for practice: Healing environments* (2nd ed.). Sudbury, MA: Jones and Bartlett.

Cohen, M. J., Serkova, N. J., Wiener-Kronish, J., Pittet, J. F., & Niemann, C. U. (2010). 1H-NMR-based metabolic signatures of clinical outcomes in trauma patients beyond lactate and base deficit. *Journal of Trauma-Injury Infection & Critical Care, 69*(1), 31–40.

Davis, A. D., & Calvet, H. M. (2003). Sexually transmitted diseases in the emergency department. *Topics in Emergency Medicine, 25*(3), 247–255.

Desilva, M. B, & Mueller, P. S. (2009). Renal consequences of long-term, low-dose intentional ingestion of ethylene glycol. *Renal Failure, 31*(7), 586–588.

Emergency Nurses Association, Newberry, L., & Criddle, L. M. (2007). *Sheehy's manual of emergency care* (6th ed.). St. Louis, MO: Mosby.

Fisher, E. M., & Brown, D. K. (2010). Hepatorenal syndrome: Beyond liver failure. *AACN Advanced Critical Care, 21*(2), 165–184.

Gadler, T., Keedy, M., & Rivas, N. (2010). A case of hematuria. *Advanced Emergency Nursing Journal, 32*(1), 30–41.

Gasparis Vonfrolio, L., & Noone, J. (1997). *Emergency nursing examination review* (3rd ed.). Staten Island, NY: Power Publications.

Gupta, A., Rohrscheib, M., & Tzamaloukas, A. H. (2008). Extreme hyperglycemia with ketoacidosis and hyperkalemia in a patient on chronic hemodialysis. *Hemodialysis International, 12*(S2), S43–437.

Guthrie, P. S. (2010). Combining herbal remedies and prescription drugs. *American Journal of Nursing, 110*(7), 18–19.

Haase, M., Haase-Fielitz, A., Bellomo, R., & Mertens, P/R. (2011). Neutrophil gelatinase-associated lipocalin as a marker of acute renal disease. *Current Opinion in Hematology, 18*(1), 11–18.

Hardin, S. R., & Kaplow, R. (Eds.) (2004). *Synergy for clinical excellence: The AACN synergy model for patient care*. Sudbury, MA: Jones and Bartlett.

Hardin, S. R., & Kaplow, R. (2010). *Cardiac surgery essentials for critical care nursing*. Sudbury, MA: Jones & Bartlett Learning.

Hernandez, J. O., Norstrom, J., & Wysock, G. (2009). Acyclovir-induced renal failure in an obese patient. *American Journal of Health-System Pharmacy, 66*(14), 1288.

Hickey, J. V. (2002). *The clinical practice of neurological and neurosurgical nursing* (5th ed.). Philadelphia, PA: Lippincott Williams & Wilkins.

Holleran, R. S. (2005). *Emergency transport nursing* (4th ed.). St. Louis, MO: Mosby.

Jacobs, B. B., & Hoyt, K. S. (2007). *Trauma nursing core course provider manual* (6th ed.). Bedford, IL: Emergency Nurses Association.

Jones & Bartlett Learning (2011). *2011 nurse's drug handbook* (10th ed.). Sudbury, MA: Jones & Bartlett Learning.

Joshi, B., Jones, D., Rochford, A., & Giblin, L. (2009). Hypothyroidism and associated acute renal failure. *Journal of the Royal Society of Medicine, 102*(5), 199–200.

Kawamoto, S., Horton, K., & Fishman, E. K. (2008). Detection of renal calculi on late arterial phase computed tomography images: Are noncontrast scans always needed to detect renal calculi? *Journal of Computer Assisted Tomography, 32*(6), 859–864.

King, J., & Rosner, M. H. (2010). Osmotic demyelination syndrome. *American Journal of the Medical Sciences, 339*(6), 561–567.

Koirala, S., Penagaluri, P., Smith, C., & Lippmann, S. (2009). Priapism and risperidone. *Southern Medical Journal, 102*(12), 1266–1268.

Krost, W. S., Mistovich, J. J., & Limmer, D. D. (2009). Beyond the basics: Electrolyte disturbances. *EMS Magazine, 38*(4), 47–50, 52–55.

Kuhn, L., Wang, C., Tsai, W., Wright, T. C., & Denny, L. (2010). Efficacy of human papillomavirus-based screen-and-treat for cervical cancer prevention among HIV-infected women. *AIDS, 24*(16), 2553–2561

Lippincott. (2010). *Professional guide to signs and symptoms* (6th ed.). Philadelphia, PA: Lippincott.

Medina, J., & Puntillo, K. (2006). *AACN protocols for practice: Palliative care and end-of-life issues in critical care*. Sudbury, MA: Jones and Bartlett.

Merchant, R. C., Depalo, D. M., Stein, M. D., & Rich, J. D. (2009). Adequacy of testing, empiric treatment, and referral for adult male emergency department patients with possible chlamydia and/or gonorrhoea urethritis. *International Journal of STD & AIDS, 20*(8), 534–539.

Pace, R. C. (2007). Fluid management in patients on hemodialysis. *Nephrology Nursing Journal, 34*(5), 557–559.

Phillips, E., Kieley, S., Johnson, E. B., & Monga, M. (2009). Emergency room management of ureteral calculi: Current practices. *Journal of Endourology, 23*(6), 1021.

Powell, H. R. F., & Almeyda, J. (2009). An immunocompetent patient presenting with severe nasal herpes simplex: A case report. *Cases Journal, 1*(2), 9079.

Proehl, J. A. (2008). *Emergency nursing procedures* (4th ed.). St. Louis, MO: Saunders.

Seo, W., & Oh, H. (2010). Alterations in serum osmolality, sodium, and potassium levels after repeated mannitol. *Journal of Neuroscience Nursing, 42*(4), 201–207.

Shirey, T. L. (2011). Identification of acute kidney injury. *Critical Care Medicine, 39*(1), 200–201.

Smeltzer, S., & Bare, B. G. (2003). *Brunner and Suddarth's textbook of medical-surgical nursing.* (10th ed.). Philadelphia, PA: Lippincott Williams & Wilkins.

Soper, D. E. (2010). Pelvic inflammatory disease. *Obstetrics & Gynecology, 116*(2), 419–428.

Stroup, S. P., & Auge, B. K. (2008). Important military role for medical expulsion therapy of urolithiasis. *Military Medicine, 173*(4), 393–398.

Urdern, L. D., Stacy, K. M., & Lough, M. E. (2005). *Thelan's critical care nursing* (5th ed.). St. Louis, MO: Mosby.

Venzin, R. M., Cohen, C. D., Maggiorini, M., & Wüthrich, R. P. (2009). Aliskiren-associated acute renal failure with hyperkalemia. *Clinical Nephrology, 71*(3), 326–328.

Watson, S., & Gorski, K. A. (2011). *Invasive cardiology* (3rd ed.). Sudbury, MA: Jones & Bartlett Learning.

Williams, P. T. (2008). Effects of running distance and performance on incident benign prostatic hyperplasia. *Medicine & Science in Sports & Exercise, 40*(10), 1733–1739.

SECTION 11:

Gastrointestinal

1. Assessment of the abdomen should occur in which order?
   A. Inspection, palpation, auscultation, percussion
   B. Auscultation, inspection, palpation, percussion
   C. Percussion, inspection, palpation, auscultation
   D. Inspection, auscultation, percussion, palpation

2. Your patient has acute esophageal and gastric varices. Which esophagogastric tamponade tube is the best choice for differentiating bleeding from the esophagus or the stomach?
   A. Minnesota tube
   B. Sengstaken-Blakemore tube
   C. Linton-Nachlas tube
   D. Standard nasogastric tube

3. Three or more episodes of acute, midline abdominal pain lasting for 2 hours to several days with periods without symptoms is known as
   A. An abdominal migraine
   B. Chronic appendicitis
   C. Functional dyspepsia
   D. Esophagitis

4. Annabel is a 50 year old seen in the emergency department for abdominal pain and vomiting. Her heart rate is 150, respiratory rate is 30, blood pressure is 105/60, and temperature 100.4°F. She indicates that the pain began 6 hours ago with abdominal rigidity, and she has absent bowel tones when assessed. Which of the following symptoms supports a diagnosis of acute mesenteric artery occlusion?
   A. Warm, flushed skin
   B. Bruit noted in the left iliac fossa
   C. Colicky periumbilical pain associated with explosive diarrhea
   D. Pain is intermittent and localized

5. Your patient has been diagnosed with gastroenteritis. The primary causative agent for this condition is
   A. *Clostridium difficile*
   B. *Salmonella typhi*
   C. Cryptosporidium
   D. A rotavirus

6. Stephanie was admitted to the ED after a motor vehicle accident that left her only mildly bruised. Just prior to discharge, Stephanie complains of diffuse abdominal pain and described symptoms she has had during the past week. Which symptom probably indicates an early sign of appendicitis?
   A. Flank pain
   B. Pain while resting
   C. Night waking
   D. Pain after vomiting

7. Which of the following terms describes bleeding that is bright or dark red blood and that is passed from the rectum?
   A. Melena
   B. Occult
   C. Hematemesis
   D. Hematochezia

8. The stage of hepatitis characterized by jaundice, pallor, pale stool, dark urine, and pruritis is called the _____ stage.
   A. Preicteric
   B. Fulminant
   C. Toxic
   D. Icteric

9. Melena stools indicate bleeding from what body area?
   A. Mouth
   B. Upper gastrointestinal
   C. Descending colon
   D. Liver

10. Which of the following methods for measuring intra-abdominal pressures is most commonly used?
    A. Intraperitoneal measuring with a peritoneal dialysis catheter
    B. Measurement of the bladder pressures via indwelling urinary catheter
    C. Intragastric measurement with a nasogastric tube
    D. Rectally with a rectal tube

11. The most common cause of death related to acute hepatic failure is
    A. Pulmonary embolism
    B. Anemia
    C. Brainstem herniation
    D. Pulmonary edema

12. Hepatorenal syndrome is a complication of hepatic failure due to
    A. Vasodilatation
    B. Increased circulating plasma
    C. Increased renal circulation
    D. Release of mediators

13. Cullen's sign presents as
    A. A marbled appearance to the abdomen
    B. Bruising of the scrotum or labia
    C. Bluish discoloration of the flanks
    D. Bluish discoloration of the periumbilical area

14. Marjean is a model and weighs 95 pounds. She was found unconscious in the bathroom. She was admitted for severe dehydration and starvation. Which of the following symptoms would you expect to observe with this patient?
    A. Decreased serum lactate
    B. Normal urinary nitrogen excretion
    C. Conservation of body fluids with third spacing
    D. Decreased serum catecholamines, glucagon, and cortisol

15. Your patient is a recovering anorexic who attends group counseling sessions at your facility. She came to the ED for a cast removal. The ED was busy, so you ordered a lunch for the patient. You are preparing to discharge the patient when you note she has not touched her lunch. Your best therapeutic statement should be
    A. "It's okay. I know that hospital food is not gourmet, but the cafeteria is more appetizing"
    B. "If you don't eat, we will have to put a feeding tube in you"
    C. "You need to eat to regain strength and prevent complications. We will work with you to find foods that you like"
    D. "Food is not your enemy. Eating this is not going to make you fat"

16. Which of the following forms of hepatitis is often misdiagnosed as gastroenteritis?
    A. Hepatitis A
    B. Hepatitis B
    C. Hepatitis C
    D. Hepatitis E

17. Which form of hepatitis originates as a DNA virus?
    A. Hepatitis A
    B. Hepatitis B
    C. Hepatitis C
    D. Hepatitis D

18. Daniela arrived from Hungary 3 weeks ago to attend an advanced language school. She has been suffering for 2 weeks with flu-like symptoms, increased bruising, headaches, pounding pulses, and fever. She was reluctant to seek treatment until this morning when her headache became unbearable. Which diagnosis is the mostly likely cause of Daniela's symptoms?
    A. DIC related to bacterial infection
    B. Acute liver failure related to unintentional overdose of acetaminophen
    C. Vitamin K deficiency related to poor nutritional intake
    D. Anemia related to Gaucher's disease

19. Which of the following lab results would contraindicate administration of peritoneal lavage?
    A. RBC 5.4 million/mm³
    B. PLT 78,000 mm³/ml
    C. PT 12.5 sec and PTT 75 sec
    D. Hgb 14.5 g/dL and Hct 46%

20. You are preparing Frank for a paracentesis. Which of the following actions should be the first step in assisting with a paracentesis?
    A. Have Frank void or insert a Foley catheter
    B. Examine the abdomen for dullness
    C. Order an upright X-ray of the abdomen
    D. Position Frank with the affected side up

21. During gastric lavage for stress-related erosion syndrome (SRES) gastric bleeding, your patient becomes hyperthermic, tachycardic, complains of sudden abdominal pain, and has abdominal rigidity. As an ED nurse, you should
    A. Continue with the lavage; the symptoms are normal
    B. Stop the infusion and contact the physician
    C. Stop the infusion and rewarm the fluid
    D. Slow the infusion and change the fluid

22. Your patient was diagnosed with Barrett's esophagus. Which of the following conditions is your patient at greatest risk for developing?
    A. Esophageal varices
    B. Gastritis
    C. Esophageal cancer
    D. GERD

23. Anastomotic leaks are common after bariatric surgeries. Symptoms can be subtle and may include hyperthermia, tachycardia, tachypnea, abdominal pain, and anxiety. If undiagnosed, all of the following complications may result except
    A. Hyperoxia
    B. Sepsis
    C. MODS
    D. Death

24. Julie was admitted to the ED because of abdominal pain. She recently had knee surgery for which she received Tylenol #3 for pain control. She has no bowel sounds, her abdomen is firmly distended, and she is diffusely tender across the abdomen. What is the probable cause of Julie's symptoms?
    A. Appendicitis from the pain meds
    B. Paralytic ileus from the codeine
    C. Gastroenteritis after eating undercooked chicken
    D. Pancreatitis from lack of exercise

25. Common adverse reactions to cimetidine include
    A. Elevated BUN and creatinine
    B. Rash, nausea, and agitation
    C. Decreased liver enzymes and anorexia
    D. Jitteriness and mottled skin

26. Cimetidine, famotidine, and ranitidine belong to which class of medications?
    A. Proton pump inhibitors (PPIs)
    B. Antacids
    C. H_2 blockers
    D. Antiemetics

27. Medications that are bound to protein may have which of the following effects?
    A. Increased availability
    B. Rapid distribution
    C. Less available drug for the desired effect
    D. Idiosyncrasy

28. Your patient has been diagnosed with chronic liver disease. In addition to a venous hum or murmur, you may also note which of the following findings during abdominal auscultation?
    A. Aortic bruit
    B. Hepatic bruit
    C. Iliac artery bruit
    D. Renal artery bruit

29. Normal portal pressures are in the range of
    A. 5–10 mmHg
    B. 10–20 mmHg
    C. 5 mmHg below the inferior vena cava pressure
    D. 10 mmHg above the inferior vena cava pressure

30. Your patient was involved in a motor vehicle accident with blunt abdominal trauma related to the seatbelt placement. He begins complaining of severe abdominal pain around the epigastric area that is knife-like and twisting. You also note a low-grade fever with diaphoresis, abdominal distention, decreased bowel tones, and rebound tenderness. You suspect this patient may be suffering from
    A. Pancreatitis
    B. Acute liver failure
    C. Gastrointestinal bleeding
    D. Abdominal bruising

31. Nolan is a nonalcohol-abusing patient. He was diagnosed with portal hypertension and direct variceal bleeding. His wedge hepatic venous pressure is less than portal pressure due to portal vein thrombosis. His symptoms may be due to
    A. Chronic active hepatitis
    B. Umbilical vein catheterization as a neonate
    C. Metastatic carcinoma
    D. Congestive heart failure

32. Quinn is a frequent patient to your ED for alcohol-induced comas. Just before transfer to the ICU, he begins projectile vomiting bright red blood. Your first action should be to
    A. Position the patient flat
    B. Obtain and insert a Linton-Nachlas tube
    C. Maintain airway and stop the bleeding
    D. Start dopamine at 5 µg/kg/min

33. Ed, a 20 year old college student, had an appendectomy in another state while on spring break 1 week ago. He is admitted to the ED with fever, nausea and vomiting, and abdominal pain with a red, swollen surgical incision. You anticipate his next treatment to include
    A. Immediate surgery with IV antibiotics
    B. Hydration and antibiotics
    C. Bedside excision of abscess
    D. Bedside wound debridement

34. Greg has chronic pancreatitis and was admitted to the ED for respiratory distress and pulmonary edema. These symptoms are due to
    A. Pulmonary capillary endothelial damage related to phospholipase
    B. Bronchospasms related to stress
    C. Aspiration
    D. Atelectasis

35. Your patient was admitted to the ED for dehydration and malnutrition after collapsing in his bedroom. His wife reports he has been eating very bland, soft foods for 3 weeks because of reflux and difficulty swallowing. You suspect
    A. Partial tongue paralysis
    B. Gastric cancer
    C. Tracheal neoplasm
    D. Esophageal neoplasm

36. Liz just got a tattoo and a lip ring last week. Now she complains of flu-like symptoms. She has increasing lethargy and decreased appetite with weight loss of 10 pounds. Generally a cheerful and active person, she reports overwhelming malaise with a sense of foreboding. Nursing interventions should include
    A. Weight-bearing exercise
    B. Extended teaching sessions regarding her disease process
    C. Diet orders for low fat and high carbohydrates
    D. Admission under strict isolation precautions

37. You are admitting an emergency department patient after a head injury. As you perform your assessment you note a stoma to the right iliac fossa in the lower abdomen. There are soft, scattered bowel tones. Output is loose, brownish tinged without form. You document your findings as a(n)
    A. Sigmoid colostomy
    B. Ileostomy
    C. Loop colostomy
    D. Ascending colostomy

38. Olivia is a postgastric bypass patient experiencing dumping syndrome after eating any type of meal. Which of the following medications should Olivia stop immediately?
    A. Nitroglycerin
    B. Insulin
    C. Pepcid
    D. Reglan

39. When patients have liver failure, fatty nodules may develop subcutaneously due to cholesterol accumulation. These nodules are called
    A. Asterixis
    B. Factor hepaticus
    C. Xanthomas
    D. Telangiectasis

40. Which of the following types of bowel obstructions leads to infarction or strangulation?
    A. Acute
    B. Subacute
    C. Chronic
    D. Intermittent

41. Jacob is an Orthodox Jew who presents with an unintentional weight loss of 20 pounds. Jacob also suffers from fatigue, anorexia, and chronic, watery diarrhea with bloody mucus. He is tachycardic, tachypneic, hyperthermic, with a Hgb of 7 g/dL and Hct of 21%. You suspect Jacob is suffering from
    A. Colonic diverticulitis
    B. Ulcerative colitis
    C. Pancreatitis
    D. Cholecystitis

42. Alex has recurrent gallstones and has been treated medically at home for the last 6 months. He was brought into the ED for severe dehydration, vomiting, and fever. On admission, your assessment reveals abdominal distention, guarding, tympany, absent bowel tones, jaundice, Grey-Turner's sign, and Cullen's sign. Alex's blood pressure is 74/56, heart rate is 136, and respiratory rate is 40 and shallow. You suspect Alex is suffering from
    A. Cholecystitis
    B. Pancreatitis
    C. Cirrhosis
    D. Gastritis

43. Liam has been medically treated for GERD for the past 3 years. He is being treated in the ED for aspiration pneumonia due to increasing difficulty swallowing and vomiting. He admits to noncompliance with his GERD medication regime and was diagnosed with Barrett's esophagus 6 months ago. Liam has also been diagnosed with esophageal cancer. Which surgical procedure will Liam likely have to remove his cancer?
    A. Whipple
    B. Modified Whipple
    C. Esophagectomy
    D. Esophagastrectomy

44. Sandostatin is ordered for your patient with portal hypertension. Which of the following nursing actions is most important to perform when first starting this drug?
    A. Careful monitoring of input and output
    B. Check nerve stimulation
    C. Blood glucose checks
    D. Check blood pressure every 5 minutes

45. What is the drug of choice for treating gastroesophageal reflux?
    A. Metoclopramide
    B. Questran
    C. Regitine
    D. Procan

46. Owen frequently eats at fast-food restaurants. He presented to the ED with severe abdominal pain and diarrhea. The probable causative organism for his condition is
    A. *Giardia lamblia*
    B. *E. coli*
    C. *Staphylococcus aureus*
    D. Norwalk virus

47. The most frequent cause of parasitic gastroenteritis in the United States is
    A. *Giardia lamblia*
    B. *Clostridium difficile*
    C. *Entamoeba histolytica*
    D. *Cryptosporidium*

48. An antimicrobial drug should improve diarrhea caused by
    A. *E. coli*
    B. *Staphylococcus aureus*
    C. *Shigella*
    D. A rotavirus

49. A glycoprotein produced in the stomach that is required for vitamin B_{12} absorption is
    A. Hydrochloric acid
    B. Pepsinogen
    C. Secretin
    D. Intrinsic factor

50. Which of the following statements about splanchnic circulation is true?
    A. Splanchnic circulation supplies blood to the kidneys
    B. Splanchnic circulation receives one fourth of the cardiac output to the body
    C. Splanchnic circulation empties via the hepatic vein to the liver
    D. Splanchnic circulation is the flow from the liver to the duodenum

51. Which of the following medications inhibits gastrin synthesis and gastric acid output and decreases splanchnic circulation?
    A. Vasopressin
    B. Famotidine
    C. Octreotide acetate
    D. Ranitidine

52. Which drug is classified as an ammonia detoxicant and a hyperosmotic laxative?
    A. Lactulose
    B. Cyclosporine
    C. Tacrolimus
    D. Muromonab

53. A contraindication for use of magnesium hydroxide (Milk of Magnesia) is
    A. Intestinal obstruction
    B. Hyperacidity
    C. Bowel evacuation
    D. Depressed immune system

54. A side effect of erythromycin is
    A. Tachycardia
    B. Headache
    C. Eosinophilia
    D. Anemia

55. On the pancreatic injury severity scale, a proximal transaction or parenchymal injury with probable duet injury is known as a
    A. Class I injury
    B. Class II injury
    C. Class III injury
    D. Class IV injury

56. Ruby presented to the ED with recurrent pneumonia and severe dysphagia. You are unable to pass an NG tube. You suspect Ruby is suffering from
    A. Tracheoesophageal fistula
    B. Varices
    C. Intestinal atresia
    D. A diaphragmatic hernia

57. Gabriel presented to the ED with appendicitis. Morphine has controlled his symptoms during his stay in the ED, and the physician plans to try to manage the appendicitis medically. As you are transferring him to a medical-surgical unit, he asks if the pain will ever come back. You tell him
    A. "No. You should not ever have this problem again"
    B. "Yes, but not for several years"
    C. "Yes, but the pain will not be as severe"
    D. "Possibly. About one-third of patients are readmitted and require surgery within 1 year"

58. Carter has cirrhosis, and he came to the ED today after a weekend party with alcohol, drugs, and smoking. His lab results are as follows:
    ALT 245 U/L   AST 147 U/L
    PT 24 sec   PLT 75 × 10^3/mm^3
    Hgb 8.4 g/dl   Hct 31%
    Bilirubin 10 mg/dl
    These results indicate Carter has a high risk for
    A. Variceal bleeding
    B. Peptic ulcer disease
    C. Gastritis
    D. Boerhaave's syndrome

59. Ascites is a common finding in patients with chronic liver failure. Which of the following statements about ascites is true?
    A. Ascites is a result of an increase in albumin
    B. Ascites is the result of decreased hydrostatic pressure and increased oncotic pressures in the portal system
    C. Ascites occurs secondary to aldosteronism
    D. Ascites is due to an increased ventilation/perfusion (V/Q) ratio

60. Caroline has severe Crohn's disease and an ileostomy. Caroline is at greatest risk for which of the following complications?
    A. Dehydration
    B. Hypernatremia
    C. Hemorrhage
    D. Prolapsed stoma due to vigorous exercise once discharged

61. During a Whipple procedure, which of the following organs is removed?
    A. Esophagus
    B. Gallbladder
    C. Ascending colon
    D. Jejunum

62. Jane underwent the Whipple procedure 10 days ago for pancreatic cancer. She was started on clear liquids and then advanced to a soft diet. She is in the ED because of repetitive vomiting. She is sweating profusely, shaking, and confused as to place. On the monitor you note tachypnea and tachycardia. You suspect Jane is experiencing
    A. An anxiety or panic attack
    B. Gastroesophageal reflux disease (GERD)
    C. Dumping syndrome
    D. Hypoglycemia

63. Joseph was hospitalized for a myocardial infarction with an emergency cardiopulmonary artery bypass graft surgery 3 weeks ago and had an uneventful recovery. He has been having recurrent uncontrolled atrial fibrillation intermittently for the last 6 hours. This evening Joseph is complaining of abdominal pain with distension, intolerance for his soft diet, nausea, vomiting, and fever. The ED physician orders a plain film of the abdomen. Which of the following results would you expect to see on Joseph's X-ray?
    A. Air in the biliary tree with signs of small bowel obstruction and calculus in the pelvis
    B. Dilated small bowel loops
    C. Dilation of the entire bowel including the stomach, "thumb printing," pneumatosis intestinalis
    D. Air under the diaphragm on the right upper chest or even the right lobe of the liver

64. Patients considering gastric bypass for weight management control should begin bariatric education
    A. Prior to the decision to have surgery
    B. When the decision to have surgery is made
    C. Bariatric surgery education is not necessary
    D. After surgery

65. Your patient underwent the Roux-en-Y gastric bypass procedure 2 days ago. Which nutritional complication is your patient most at risk for developing?
    A. Hypercalcemia
    B. Vitamin C deficiency
    C. Vitamin B_{12} deficiency
    D. Hyperalbuminism

66. How do proton pump inhibitors (PPIs) work?
    A. PPIs inhibit the release of cytokines
    B. PPIs antagonize the H_2 histamine receptors
    C. PPIs increase gastric emptying, reducing the acid production
    D. PPIs inhibit the release of hydrochloric acid by gastric parietal cells

67. The family of your patient with chronic liver failure would like to know what they can do to make him more comfortable. You tell them that when they visit the patient in his long-term care facility, they can
    A. Provide deep tissue massage every 2 hours
    B. Apply a moisturizing lotion when visiting
    C. Assist with rapid range of motion every 4 hours
    D. Limit visitation to once a day

68. Nicolai was admitted to the ED with vague epigastric discomfort, *vomiting times 1 week*, inability to eat more than a few bites of solid foods, weight loss, weakness, and postprandial fullness. Labs showed a Hgb 10.8 g/dl and a positive stool guaiac. Based on the findings you would expect to see which of the following results after the upper gastrointestinal studies?
    A. "Unitis plastia"—leather bottle stomach
    B. Localized ulcer
    C. Esophageal varices
    D. Pyloric stenosis

69. Robert is visiting his sister in the ED. She was complaining of severe stomach cramping. There is a familial history of polyposis and inflammatory bowel disease. He is worried about his risk of developing cancer, so in a quiet moment he asks you about the possibility of his developing cancer. Which of the following statements is true regarding colorectal cancers?
    A. Adenocarcinomas are the least common cancer
    B. Right colon lesions are rare
    C. Left colon tumors spread, ulcerate, and erode blood vessels
    D. Rectal tumors are associated with localized metastasis

70. What is the most common means of infection with *Giardia lamblia*?
    A. Eating undercooked game such as rabbit
    B. Drinking water from a mountain stream
    C. Teens sharing food and soda
    D. Having venison steak at a restaurant

71. What type of organism is *Giardia lamblia*?
    A. A spirochete
    B. A type of tapeworm
    C. A protozoan
    D. A flagellated bacterium

72. What is the treatment of choice for *Giardia lamblia*?
    A. Amoxicillin
    B. Levofloxacin
    C. Metronidazole
    D. Erythromycin

73. How are tapeworm infestations spread?
    A. Fecal–oral route
    B. Infected animal contact only
    C. Infected meat sources only
    D. Contaminated water only

74. Your patient sustained an abdominal injury 2 hours ago. Now you note a decrease in urine output, an increased CVP, and decreased cardiac output. In addition, the ventilator continuously alarms low volume despite intact circuits. Based on these findings you would expect which of the following intra-abdominal pressure values?
    A. 5 mmHg
    B. 15 mmHg
    C. 25 mmHg
    D. 50 mmHg

SECTION 11: GASTROINTESTINAL ANSWERS

1. **Correct answer: D**
   This is another of those deceptively easy questions. Make absolutely certain you know the correct order for assessment. Inspection to determine landmarks and appearance, auscultation to establish location and quality of bowel tones, percussion notes or tones are different for various internal organs, and palpation to establish wall tone, tenderness, and size of organs. Percussion and palpation prior to inspection or auscultation could affect the assessment findings.

2. **Correct answer: A**
   The Minnesota tube is the best choice for differentiating bleeding from the esophagus or the stomach. The Minnesota tube has separate suction and balloons that can function independently. The Sengstaken-Blakemore tube has only three lumens with only one suction port. The Linton-Nachlas tube is for gastric varices only. The standard nasogastric tube has no balloon function to tamponade bleeding.

3. **Correct answer: A**
   Three or more episodes of acute, midline abdominal pain lasting for 2 hours to several days with periods without symptoms is known as an abdominal migraine.

4. **Correct answer: C**
   A diagnosis of acute mesenteric artery occlusion is supported by a history of colicky periumbilical pain associated with explosive diarrhea. Abdominal pain becomes constant and diffuse. As symptoms progress, the patient will become tachycardic, tachypneic, with fever and hypotension with worsening abdominal pain and rigidity. Skin will become cold and clammy with shunting as compensatory mechanisms fail.

5. **Correct answer: D**
   The primary causative agent for gastroenteritis is a rotavirus.

6. **Correct answer: C**
   An early sign of appendicitis is night waking. The patient has nonspecific discomfort and wakes frequently.

7. **Correct answer: D**
   Hematochezia describes bleeding that is bright or dark red blood that is passed from the rectum.

8. **Correct answer: D**
   The stage of hepatitis characterized by jaundice, pallor, pale stool, dark urine, and pruritis is called the icteric stage.

9. **Correct answer: B**
   Melena is black tarry stool containing blood from the upper gastrointestinal area or ascending colon. Oral bleeding may result in hematemesis. Descending colon bleeding may lead to bright red stools. Iron, bismuth, and other foods may be mistaken for melena, but an occult blood test of the stool rules this out.

10. **Correct answer: B**
    The most commonly used method for measuring intra-abdominal pressure is via the bladder. A specialized catheter with a transducer allows for direct measurement of pressures.

11. **Correct answer: C**

    The most common cause of death related to acute hepatic failure is brainstem herniation. Brainstem herniation is the most common cause of death due to increased coagulation times, intracranial hemorrhaging, and hypoxia leading to cerebral edema. Anemia is a complication of prolonged bleeding times but not the primary cause of death. Pulmonary impairment is the result of hemorrhaging, not embolism or edema.

12. **Correct answer: D**

    Hepatorenal syndrome is a complication of hepatic failure due to the release of mediators. The release of mediators results in vasoconstriction that diverts blood flow to the kidneys. There is a decrease in circulating plasma as the patient develops ascites. Vasoconstriction, not vasodilatation, occurs in end-stage liver failure. There is a decrease in renal circulation due to plasma shifting and vasoconstriction.

13. **Correct answer: D**

    Cullen's sign refers to the bluish discoloration of the periumbilical area as seen in pancreatitis and/or abdominal trauma. Marbled appearance is common with abdominal trauma. Coopernail's sign is bruising of the scrotum or labia. Turner's sign is bruising of the flanks.

14. **Correct answer: C**

    Prolonged starvation and protein loss resulting in fluid shifting and third spacing are symptoms seen in a patient who is suffering from starvation and dehydration. Muscle wasting results in an increase in serum lactate levels, not a decrease. Initially, there is an increased urinary nitrogen excretion followed by a decrease. There is also an increase in serum catecholamine, glucagons, and cortical as the body releases elements to maintain energy and glucose available.

15. **Correct answer: C**

    The goal when working with bulimic and anorexic patients and their families is to support positive nutritional changes while acknowledging and supporting the psychological changes in body and food perception. By acknowledging the difficulties the patient has with food perception and willingness to providing support and counseling with a nutritionist, dietician, and psychologist, the patient will find foods that are both appealing and provide needed nutrition. The remaining answers are abrasive or do not address the physiologic or psychological struggle with eating.

16. **Correct answer: A**

    Hepatitis A is often misdiagnosed initially as gastroenteritis because symptoms are usually self-limiting. Fecal–oral transmission may also be mistaken as food poisoning.

17. **Correct Answer: B**

    Hepatitis B is the only DNA virus listed. The other forms of hepatitis are RNA viruses.

18. **Correct answer: B**

    Acute liver failure related to acetaminophen overdose is consistent with this patient's presentation. Individuals without full command of the English language are at risk for overdose when self-medicating if the medication label is not read and understood correctly. The symptomology is inconsistent with DIC and vitamin K deficiency. Gaucher's disease is a genetic enzyme deficiency disease that is typically diagnosed in childhood. Symptoms are progressive as the glucocerebroside is collected in the spleen and liver. This patient would also present with skeletal weakness, neurologic complications, swollen lymph nodes, and pain not related to just the last 2 weeks.

19. **Correct answer: B**

    A patient with a platelet count of 78,000 mm^3/ml is thrombocytopenic and at risk for coagulation complications. Heparin is normally added to the solution to prevent clotting and can lead to further complications of bleeding. The other lab values are within normal range for either males or females.

20. **Correct answer: A**

    The correct order for these interventions when assisting with a paracentesis is to have the patient void or insert a Foley catheter, order an upright X-ray of the abdomen, position the patient with the affected side up, and examine the abdomen for dullness.

21. **Correct answer: B**

    The patient is exhibiting signs and symptoms of gastric perforation. This is a surgical emergency, and the lavage should be stopped, fluid aspirated, and the physician notified immediately. Additional actions include the placement of at least two large-bore IVs, preparing to administer IV fluid replacement if hypovolemic shock occurs, and prepare the patient for immediate surgery.

22. **Correct answer: C**

    Because of cellular changes in the esophageal lining, the patient is at increased risk for esophageal cancer. Barrett's esophagus is a result of mucosal changes in the esophagus after repeated and prolonged exposure to gastric secretions seen in untreated gastroesophageal reflux disease (GERD).

23. **Correct answer: A**

    Patients who have had bariatric surgery are at risk for hypoxia, not hyperoxia.

24. **Correct answer: B**

    Julie is probably suffering from a paralytic ileus from the codeine. Codeine slows the gastric motility throughout the GI tract. This patient needs a nasogastric tube and motility medications such as metoclopramide.

25. **Correct answer: B**

    Common adverse reactions to cimetidine can include rash, nausea, agitation, vomiting, diarrhea, flushing, neutropenia, elevated liver enzymes, and drowsiness.

26. **Correct answer: C**

    Cimetidine, famotidine, and ranitidine are H_2 blockers. They inhibit gastric acid production by antagonism of the histamine H_2 receptors. They are used for prevention of ulcers and in the treatment of GI bleeding.

27. **Correct answer: C**

    Medications that are bound to protein may have less available drug for the desired effect.

28. **Correct answer: B**

    Hepatic bruits are heard over the liver and may also indicate primary liver cancer, alcoholic hepatitis, or vascular liver metastases. An aortic bruit over the epigastric area indicates a partial aortic occlusion. Iliac artery bruits are heard over the left/right inguinal areas. Renal artery bruits indicate renal artery stenosis.

29. **Correct answer: A**
Normal portal pressures are 5 to 10 mmHg (7 to 14 cm H_2O). Portal pressures should be 4 to 5 mmHg higher than the inferior vena cava pressures. Pressures this high above the inferior vena cava pressures indicate severe portal hypertension.

30. **Correct answer: A**
Acute pancreatitis may occur as a result of seatbelt trauma to the pancreatic duct or abdominal ischemia. Acute liver failure is characterized by flu-like symptoms, jaundice, confusion, and enlarged liver. Gastrointestinal bleeding has a history of ulcers and/or esophageal varices with hemodynamic changes, narrowing pulse pressures, hematemesis, and hyperactive bowel tones. Abdominal trauma does not produce the knife-like and twisting pain, and tenderness and a marbled appearance would be noted.

31. **Correct answer: B**
Nolan may have had an umbilical catheter placed when he was a neonate—a prehepatic factor. Prehepatic (presinusoidal) factors lead to hepatic venous pressures less than portal pressures. Chronic active hepatitis is an intrahepatic (sinusoidal) factor. Wedge hepatic venous pressures are increased or equal to portal pressures. Metastatic carcinoma and cardiac diseases such as CHF can cause portal hypertension and may indirectly cause variceal bleeding.

32. **Correct answer: C**
This patient has likely ruptured varices. Priorities are to maintain airway, stop bleeding, place NPO, and verify venous access for blood replacement, fluid management, and homeostasis. You want to position the patient upright to prevent aspiration, not flat. You would anticipate the placement of a Minnesota tube, not a Linton-Nachlas tube. Dopamine at 5 μg/kg/min would better support renal function and not blood pressure as needed in this patient.

33. **Correct answer: A**
This patient is exhibiting signs and symptoms of an abscess after surgical intervention for appendicitis, which occurs in 5–33% of patients. Surgical debridement of the incision and IV antibiotics are appropriate immediate treatment to prevent sepsis. Hydration and antibiotics alone will not treat the abscess. Bedside excision of the abscess may reduce the amount of infected fluid and tissue at the site but will not prevent further infection. Bedside wound debridement places a high risk of further contamination of the site. In approximately 2% of cases the abscess may be intra-abdominal and may require surgical intervention under anesthesia as well as continued antibiotic treatment.

34. **Correct answer: A**
Chronic pancreatitis results in the release of digestive enzymes into the body. Phospholipase A_2 breaks down the cellular structure of the capillary beds, resulting in tissue injury throughout the body. In the lungs capillary damage is manifested by pulmonary edema and dyspnea, leading to respiratory distress. Although stress may lead to bronchospasms in patients with existing respiratory diseases such as asthma, that finding is not indicated within the information given. Aspiration and atelectasis are occasional complications in PICU patients but do not explain both symptoms as related to the ongoing disease process.

35. **Correct answer: D**

   This patient is exhibiting classic progression of a developing esophageal neoplasm. Complications that coincide with this disease process are related to changes in nutritional intake. Narrowing of the esophageal lumen results in increasing difficulties and pain when swallowing, leading to a softer diet until the patient can swallow only liquids. Partial tongue paralysis would be supported if the patient also had difficulty speaking, but that symptom is not given. Gastric cancer is indicated with indigestion and fullness, not difficulty swallowing. Tracheal neoplasm would be exhibited with more respiratory distress.

36. **Correct answer: C**

   This patient's history and symptomology is consistent with new-onset hepatitis C. Hepatitis C results in a hypermetabolic state. Nursing interventions should focus on minimizing symptoms and reducing stress on the body. A low-fat, high-carbohydrate diet supports an increase in caloric demand and helps prevent weight loss. The greater the liver compromise related to infection, the lower the fat and protein intake as the liver may not be able to assist with effective digestion. This patient should remain on strict bedrest to allow for energy conservation in the acute phase. Light ambulation is permitted as long as the patient is not fatigued with the activity. Although teaching is vital for this patient and her family, extended teaching sessions may tax the patient's ability to concentrate. Teaching should be available in multiple forms that can be referred to at the patient's and family's leisure. Family may be supportive, but planned rest periods should be maintained and supported as patient tolerance allows.

37. **Correct answer: B**

   An ileostomy is located at the right ileac fossa just before the colon. Because most water absorption occurs in the colon, stool from the small intestines is loose and unformed. Sigmoid colostomy stools more closely resemble normal stools as most of the water has been absorbed. Loop, or transverse, and ascending colostomies have loose stools with more formation.

38. **Correct answer: D**

   Olivia is experiencing dumping syndrome after gastric bypass surgery and should stop taking reglan. Reglan increases gastric emptying by increasing peristalsis, thus increasing the effects of dumping syndrome. Reglan may be used after gastrectomy when gastroparesis is present, but once peristalsis has resumed it should be stopped.

39. **Correct answer: C**

   When patients have liver failure, fatty nodules called xanthomas may develop subcutaneously due to cholesterol accumulation.

40. **Correct answer: A**

   Acute bowel obstruction is the only type of obstruction that leads to infarction or strangulation. Obstruction occurs rapidly and may inhibit blood to a portion of the bowel. The other types of obstructions permit limited or intermittent blood flow that sustains but compromises tissue function.

41. **Correct answer: B**

   Based on the presenting symptoms and ethnicity, Jacob probably has ulcerative colitis. He may also have leukocytosis and cachexia. Colonic diverticulitis presents with left upper quadrant pain, hyperthermia, vomiting, chills, diarrhea, and tenderness over the descending colon. Pancreatitis presents with left upper quadrant pain that radiates to the back or chest, hyperthermia, rigidity, rebound abdominal tenderness, nausea and vomiting, jaundice, Cullen's sign, Grey-Turner's sign, abdominal distention, and diminished bowel sounds. Cholecystitis presents with right upper quadrant or epigastric pain, pain that lasts up to 6 hours after a fatty meal, vomiting, and increased white blood cell counts.

42. Correct answer: B
Although Alex's initial symptoms and family history may indicate cholecystitis, his symptoms now are classic for pancreatitis. Abdominal rigidity, Grey-Turner's sign, and Cullen's sign are late indicators of pancreatitis. In addition, he is presenting in severe hypovolemic shock. Immediate fluid resuscitation should be initiated to support cardiovascular function.

43. Correct answer: C
Liam will probably undergo an esophagectomy. This procedure involves removal of the damaged esophagus to the proximal portion of the stomach. The stomach is then resectioned to form a new esophagus. If the stomach is also cancerous, the stomach is removed and the small bowel is resectioned to create a new esophagus.

44. Correct answer: C
Glycemic emergencies may occur with sandostatin, especially in the diabetic patient. It is important to monitor blood glucose to prevent hyperglycemia and/or hypoglycemia. Blood pressure and urinary function may also be impacted but are not as quickly life-threatening as unstable glucose levels.

45. Correct answer: A
Metoclopramide increases gastric emptying and motility, thereby reducing reflux symptoms. The patient should be monitored for diarrhea and neurologic signs such as tremors or muscle twitching.

46. Correct answer: B
E. coli is linked with abdominal pain and diarrhea from fast-food restaurants.

47. Correct answer: A
Giardia lamblia is the most frequent cause of parasitic gastroenteritis in the United States.

48. Correct answer: C
An antimicrobial drug should improve diarrhea caused by *Shigella*.

49. Correct answer: D
Intrinsic factor is a glycoprotein produced in the stomach that is required for vitamin B_{12} absorption.

50. Correct answer: B
Splanchnic circulation receives one-fourth of the cardiac output to the body.

51. Correct answer: C
Octreotide acetate inhibits gastrin synthesis and gastric acid output and decreases splanchnic circulation.

52. **Correct answer: A**

    Lactulose is classified as an ammonia detoxicant and a hyperosmotic laxative.

53. **Correct answer: A**

    Intestinal obstruction is a contraindication for use of magnesium hydroxide (Milk of Magnesia). Additional contraindications include ileostomy, colostomy, and appendicitis.

54. **Correct answer: C**

    Eosinophilia is a side effect of erythromycin. Additional side effects include bradycardia, abdominal pain, nausea, ventricular arrhythmias, and cholestatic jaundice.

55. **Correct answer: C**

    On the pancreatic injury severity scale, a proximal transaction or parenchymal injury with probable duet injury is known as a class III injury.

56. **Correct answer: A**

    When a patient has a tracheoesophageal fistula, the nurse will be unable to pass an NG tube.

57. **Correct answer: D**

    This question requires honest communication with the patient regarding possible reoccurrence of symptoms. Approximately one-third of patients with appendicitis who are treated with antibiotics and pain management are readmitted and require appendectomies within 1 year. These remaining answers are stated as absolutes and are inappropriate for a nurse. If the appendix is not removed, the patient may have a recurrence of symptoms at a later date. There is no way to predict if and when an appendix may become infected or diseased. There is no way to predict the pain level of appendicitis, because pain is perceived differently for each patient.

58. **Correct answer: A**

    These results indicate that Carter has a high risk for variceal bleeding. Fifty percent of deaths of patients with cirrhosis are from variceal bleeding. These lab tests are used to differentiate causes of bleeding. History and lab values lean toward varices. Although the Hgb and Hct are decreased in peptic ulcer disease and gastritis, the other lab changes would not be occurring. Boerhaave's syndrome is a full-thickness rupture or perforation of the esophageal wall due to prolonged and frequent vomiting related to eating disorders.

59. **Correct answer: C**

    Ascites occurs secondary to aldosteronism. Aldosteronism initiates sodium retention, increasing portal hypertension. Low albumin levels with increased hydrostatic pressure and decreased oncotic pressures result in ascites. Because of fluid shifting there would be a decrease in ventilation/perfusion (V/Q) ratio.

60. **Correct answer: A**

    Dehydration is a severe complication in patients with ileostomies. Water reabsorption is normally accomplished by the colon. This patient may have had a large portion or all of the large intestine removed related to the Crohn's disease process. Fluids should be encouraged and IV support maintained to prevent hypovolemic shock. Teaching should include signs and symptoms of shock and preventative home management. Although a stoma prolapse may occur after discharge home, the stoma can be reopened without major complications. Hyponatremia, not hypernatremia, is a serious complication as sodium uptake also occurs in the colon. Hemorrhage is not a concern unless the stoma is scratched or damaged during care. Light pressure should be applied until bleeding stops, but it is not a life-threatening complication.

61. **Correct answer: B**
    The Whipple procedure removes the tip or head of the pancreas, the gallbladder, the duodenum, and part of the bile duct. Occasionally, part of the stomach may also be removed. The extent of the cancerous pancreatic tumor indicates the extent of removal.

62. **Correct answer: C**
    Jane's symptoms are consistent with late dumping syndrome related to the partial gastrectomy during the Whipple procedure. With late dumping syndrome symptoms occur 1 to 3 hours after meals. Additional symptoms include weakness, fatigue, dizziness, anxiety, palpitations, and fainting. Patients may also exhibit early signs of dumping syndrome approximately 15–30 minutes after a meal with nausea, vomiting, cramps or abdominal pain, diarrhea, bloating, tachycardia, dysrhythmias, and dizziness. Although anxiety may be exhibited with dumping syndrome, an alteration in mental status with relation to food consumption and history support a dumping syndrome diagnosis. Hypoglycemia is a greater risk for patients than just gastrectomy or bypass. GERD presents with heartburn and epigastric pain.

63. **Correct answer: B**
    Joseph is exhibiting signs of an early ischemic bowel. At this time there will be some dilation of the bowel with loops behind the ischemic bowel because the ischemic bowel is not performing peristaltic actions. Late signs, if not diagnosed and treated early, include dilation of the entire bowel including the stomach. "Thumb printing" is seen on an X-ray when edema of the bowel wall shows the convex indentations of the lumen, and pneumatosis intestinalis is seen when there is a mottled gas pattern in the bowel wall. Air in the biliary tree is indicative of a gallbladder emergency, and air under the diaphragm is a pneumoperitoneum.

64. **Correct answer: A**
    Patients considering gastric bypass for weight management control should begin bariatric education prior to the decision to have surgery. Gastric bypass surgery can be a lead to permanent gastric changes and places the obese patient at risk for both surgical- and anesthesia-related complications. For many bariatric patients the initial gastric bypass surgery is not necessarily the only surgery required. Often, cosmetic surgery to remove loose skin around the stomach, back, thighs, arms, and chest is required to improve self-image. Each surgery has additional risks. Therefore, complete bariatric education should be provided to any patient considering bariatric surgery. Education should include preoperative changes in diet, nutritional consultation, psychological evaluation, and full medical evaluation including lab work and cardiovascular testing. Education and support for the bariatric surgery patient should continue throughout the surgical process with ongoing education, nutritional support, and physiological support for years after surgery.

65. **Correct answer: C**
Because the gastric size is greatly reduced, there is less intrinsic factor to assist in vitamin B_{12} absorption to prevent pernicious anemia. Oral supplements are not recommended as they may not be absorbed quickly enough. Sublingual or injected vitamin B_{12} may be required. Iron, thiamin, and calcium are all absorbed in the duodenum. In gastric bypass the duodenum is also bypassed greatly, limiting the absorption of these vitamins and minerals. Careful supplementation is mandatory to prevent malnutrition. Protein deficiencies are also common and supplementation is necessary, especially in early postoperative recovery to prevent muscle wasting during the rapid weight loss period.

66. **Correct answer: D**
Proton pump inhibitors work by inhibiting an enzyme that triggers the gastric parietal cells to release hydrochloric acid. This reduction in acid production can reduce the effectiveness of many oral medications such as antifungals. It may increase the absorption of drugs such as digoxin and furosemide.

67. **Correct answer: B**
Skin becomes very dry, and gentle application of a moisturizer may relieve discomfort. Deep tissue massage is contraindicated due to the decreased platelet count and increased bruising. Development of orthostatic hypertension prohibits any rapid movement due to dizziness and risks of fall. Patients and family members are at risk for depression, so visits may decrease the risk and will provide staff the opportunity to assess for and intervene if depression observed.

68. **Correct answer: A**
This patient is exhibiting subjective and objective signs and symptoms of stomach cancer. There is a higher incidence of stomach cancer in males from cultures farthest from the equator. Upper gastrointestinal series would show a "leather bottle" stomach. Symptoms do not support a diagnosis of an ulcer. Radiologic studies would show ulceration or free air with perforation. Radiologic studies for varices would not show any distinct changes. Pyloric stenosis is typically seen in infants and would show as distended abdomen, nonbilious, projectile vomiting.

69. **Correct answer: C**
Left colon (descending) lesions spread, ulcerate, and erode blood vessels within the colon. Obstruction is a very common complication with this type of lesion. Adenocarcinomas are the most common of the neoplasms. Right colon, or ascending colon, lesions are typically polypoid lesions and are associated with a familial history of polyps. Rectal lesions may spread to the vagina or prostate but are known for systemic metastasis.

70. **Correct answer: B**
Drinking water from a mountain stream is not the only way to acquire giardiasis, because any contaminated water can lead to infection.

71. **Correct answer: C**
Giardia lamblia is a protozoan parasite that colonizes the small intestine, causing diarrhea.

72. **Correct answer: C**
    Metronidazole (Flagyl) 250 mg orally every 8 hours is the treatment of choice for *Giardia lamblia*.

73. **Correct answer: A**
    Tapeworms, of which there are several types, are most often spread by the fecal–oral route. This can happen through eating contaminated foods, poor hygiene, and handling animals. *Hymenilepis nana* is the most common tapeworm in humans.

74. **Correct answer: C**
    Intra-abdominal pressures of 5 to 15 mmHg indicate a low to moderate pressure problem. When respiratory function is impaired, values range to about 25 mmHg, and you would expect to see more extensive respiratory distress and compromise. Severe compromise is seen with pressures exceeding 40 mmHg. Thoracic pressures increase as intra-abdominal pressures increase, which inhibits lung expansion and diaphragm movement, resulting in hypoventilation and hypoxia.

SECTION 11: GASTROINTESTINAL REFERENCES

Adusumalli, J., Bonney, E. A., Odenat, L., & Jamieson, D. J. (2004). Hepatitis C virus (HCV): Prevalence in a gynecological urgent care clinic population. *Infectious Diseases in Obstetrics and Gynecology, 12*(1), 9–12.

Albaba, M., & Takahashi, P. Y. (2009). 83-year-old woman with abdominal distention and constipation. *Mayo Clinic Proceedings, 84*(12), 1126.

Allison, S. O., & Lev-Toaff, A. S. (2010). Acute pelvic pain: What we have learned from the ER. *Ultrasound Quarterly, 26*(4), 211–218.

Anonymous. (2005). Sengstaken-Blakemore intrauterine tamponade is indicated for hemorrhage. *Health & Medicine Week*, 1153.

Anonymous. (2010). Compartment syndrome: Studies from Umea University describe new findings in compartment syndrome. *Obesity, Fitness & Wellness Week*, 1412.

Anonymous. (2010). Compartment syndrome: Study results from University of Lubeck broaden understanding of compartment syndrome. *Medical Devices & Surgical Technology Week*, 3159.

Anonymous. (2010). Acute appendicitis: Researchers at American College target acute appendicitis. *Medical Devices & Surgical Technology Week*, 781.

Anonymous. (2011). Crohn disease: Researchers from Medical School, Department of Internal Medicine discuss findings in Crohn disease. *Pediatrics Week*, 164 (1).

Anonymous. (2011). Acute appendicitis: New acute appendicitis study findings have been reported by researchers at B. P. Koirala Institute of Health Sciences, Department of Family Medicine. *Gastroenterology Week*, 128.

Appelboam, R., & Hammond, E. (2004). Viral gastroenteritis—A danger to the patient, a danger to the staff. *Anaesthesia, 59*(3), 293–295.

Aslan, S., Meral, M., Akgun, M., Acemoglu, H., Ucar, E. Y., Gorguner, M., & Mirici, A. (2007). Liver dysfunction in patients with acute pulmonary embolism. *Hepatology Research, 37*(3), 205–213.

Baek, S. K., Kim, Y. H., & Kim, S. P. (2010). Acute lower gastrointestinal bleeding due to appendiceal mucosal erosion. *Surgical Laparoscopy, Endoscopy & Percutaneous Techniques, 20*(3), e110–e113.

Bair, M., Chen, H., Lin, I., & Wu, C. (2010, May). Simultaneous left renal infarction and right iliac artery occlusion in a healthy man. *American Journal of the Medical Sciences, 339*(5), 485.

Basavaraju, K. P., & Wong, T. (2008). Eosinophilic oesophagitis: A common cause of dysphagia in young adults? *International Journal of Clinical Practice, 62*(7), 1096–1107.

Baugh, C. W., Venkatesh, A. K., & Bohan, J. S. (2011). Emergency department observation units: A clinical and financial benefit for hospitals. *Health Care Management Review, 36*(1), 28–37.

Bernal, W., Donaldson, N., Wyncoll, D., & Wendon, J. (2002). Blood lactate as an early predictor of outcome in paracetamol-induced acute liver failure: a cohort study. *Lancet, 359*(9306), 558–563.

Bernal, W., Auzinger, G., Dhawan, A., & Wendon, J. (2010). Acute liver failure. *Lancet, 376*(9736), 190.

Bernd, S., Jochen, G., Veit, P., Roland, M. S., & Wolfgang, H. (2010). Splenic artery embolization in a woman with bleeding gastric varices and splenic vein thrombosis: A case report. *Journal of Medical Case Reports, 4*(2), 247.

Bischoff, S. C. (2010). Food allergy and eosinophilic gastroenteritis and colitis. *Current Opinion in Allergy & Clinical Immunology, 10*(3), 238–245.

Blaivas, M. (2011). Ultrasound and abdominal compartment syndrome: Can we cast the other tools aside yet? *Critical Care Medicine, 39*(2), 411–412.

Brener, Z. Z., Winchester, J. F., Salman, H., & Bergman, M. (2011). Nephrolithiasis: Evaluation and management. *Southern Medical Journal, 104*(2), 133–139.

Brountzos, E. N., Critselis, A., Magoulas, D., Kagianni, E., & Kelekis, D. A. (2001). Emergency endovascular treatment of a superior mesenteric artery occlusion. *Cardiovascular and Interventional Radiology, 24*(1), 57.

Brugger, L., Rosella, L., Candinas, D., & Guller, U. (2011). Improving outcomes after laparoscopic appendectomy: A population-based, 12-year trend analysis of 7446 patients. *Annals of Surgery, 253*(2), 309–313.

Calamia, K. T., Schirmer, M., & Melikoglu, M. (2011). Major vessel involvement in Behcet's disease: an update. *Current Opinion in Rheumatology, 23*(1), 24–31.

Chan, S. S. W., Ng, K. C., Lyon, D. J., Cheung, W. L., Cheng, A. F. B., & Rainer, T. H. (2003). Acute bacterial gastroenteritis: a study of adult patients with positive stool cultures treated in the emergency department. *Emergency Medicine Journal, 20*(4), 335.

Chapman, L. E, Sullivent, E. E, Grohskopf, L. A, Beltrami, E. M., Perz, J. F., Kretsinger, K., . . . Hunt, R. C. (2008). Recommendations for postexposure interventions to prevent infection with hepatitis B virus, hepatitis C virus, or human immunodeficiency virus, and tetanus in persons wounded during bombings and other mass-casualty events—United States, 2008: recommendations of the Centers for Disease Control and Prevention (CDC). *Morbidity and Mortality Weekly Report, 57*(RR-6), 1–21.

Cheatham, M. L. (2009). Nonoperative management of intraabdominal hypertension and abdominal compartment syndrome. *World Journal of Surgery, 33*(6), 1116–1122.

Cheatham, M. L. (2009). Abdominal compartment syndrome. *Current Opinion in Critical Care, 15*(2), 154–162.

Chien, J. Y., & Yu, C. J. (2005). Images in clinical medicine. Malposition of a Sengstaken-Blakemore tube. *New England Journal of Medicine, 352*(8), e7.

Choi, P. C., Kim, H. J., Choi, W. H., Park, D. I., Park, J. H., Cho, Y. K., . . . Kim, B. I. (2009). Model for end-stage liver disease, model for end-stage liver disease-sodium and Child-Turcotte-Pugh scores over time for the prediction of complications of liver cirrhosis. *Liver International, 29*(2), 221–226.

Christensen, T. (2004). The treatment of oesophageal varices using a Sengstaken-Blakemore tube: Considerations for nursing practice. *Nursing in Critical Care, 9*(2), 58–63.

Collyer, T. C., Dawson, S. E., & Earl, D. (2008). Acute upper airway obstruction due to displacement of a Sengstaken-Blakemore tube. *European Journal of Anaesthesiology, 25*(4), 341–342.

Dambrauskas, Z., Parseliunas, A., Gulbinas, A., Pundzius, J., & Barauskas, G. (2009). Early recognition of abdominal compartment syndrome in patients with acute pancreatitis. *World Journal of Gastroenterology, 15*(6), 717–721.

Das, V., Boelle, P., Galbois, A., Guidet, B., Maury, E., Carbonell, N., & Offenstadt, G. (2010). Cirrhotic patients in the medical intensive care unit: Early prognosis and long-term survival. *Critical Care Medicine, 38*(11), 2108–2116.

Dasari, T. W., Hanna, E. B., & Exaire, J. E. (2011). Resolution of anuric acute kidney injury after left renal angioplasty and stenting for a totally occlusive in-stent restenosis of a solitary kidney. *American Journal of the Medical Sciences, 341*(2), 163–165.

Deeter, M. (2009). Recognizing the importance of family history and genetic testing: A young woman with a family history of abdominal scars presents with diarrhea accompanied by persistent hematochezia, diffuse abdominal pain, and anemia. *Journal of the American Academy of Physicians Assistants, 22*(9), 29.

Demirpolat, G., Oran, I., Tamsel, S., Parildar, M., & Memis, A. (2007). Acute mesenteric ischemia: endovascular therapy. *Abdominal Imaging, 32*(3), 299.

Diaz, J. J., Norris, P., Gunter, O., Collier, B., Riordan, W., & Morris, J. A. (2011). Triaging to a regional acute care surgery center: Distance is critical. *Journal of Trauma-Injury Infection & Critical Care, 70*(1), 116–119.

Duchesne, J. C., Baucom, C. C., Rennie, K. V., Simmons, J., & McSwain, N. E. (2009). Recurrent abdominal compartment syndrome: An inciting factor of the second hit phenomenon. *American Surgeon, 75*(12), 1193.

Duchesne, J. C., Howell, M. P., Eriksen, C., Wahl, G. M., Rennie, K. V., Hastings, P. E., . . . Malbrain, M. L. (2010). Linea alba fasciotomy: A novel alternative in trauma patients with secondary abdominal compartment syndrome. *American Surgeon, 76*(3), 312–316.

Duchesne, J., Baucom, C., Rennie, K., Simmons, J., & McSwain, N. (2009). Recurrent abdominal compartment syndrome: An inciting factor of the second hit phenomenon. *American Surgeon, 75*(12), 1193-8.

Emergency Nurses Association, Newberry, L., & Criddle, L. M. (2007). *Sheehy's manual of emergency care* (6th ed.). St. Louis, MO: Mosby.

Fisher, E. M., & Brown, D. K. (2010). Hepatorenal syndrome: Beyond liver failure. *AACN Advanced Critical Care, 21*(2), 165–184.

Fleming, F. J., Kim, M. J., Messing, S., Gunzler, D., Salloum, R., & Monson, J. R. (2010). Balancing the risk of postoperative surgical infections: a multivariate analysis of factors associated with laparoscopic appendectomy from the NSQIP database. *Annals of Surgery, 252*(6), 895–900.

Fox, C. J., Liu, H., & Kaye, A. (2011). The anesthetic implications of alcoholism. *International Anesthesiology Clinics, 49*(1), 49–65.

Freedy, J. R., & Simpson, W. M. Jr. (2007). Disaster-related physical and mental health: A role for the family physician. *American Family Physician, 75*(6), 841–846.

Gao, J. M., Du, D. Y., Zhao, X. J., Liu, G. L., Yang, J., Zhao, S. H., & Lin, X. (2003). Liver trauma: Experience in 348 cases. *World Journal of Surgery, 27*(6), 703–708.

Garner, A. J., & Handa, A. (2010). Screening tools in the diagnosis of acute compartment syndrome. *Angiology, 61*(5), 475–481.

Gartenschlaeger, S., Bender, S., Maeurer, J., & Schroeder, F. J. (2008). Successful percutaneous transluminal angioplasty and stenting in acute mesenteric ischemia. *Cardiovascular and Interventional Radiology, 31*(2), 398.

Gasparis Vonfrolio, L., & Noone, J. (1997). *Emergency nursing examination review* (3rd ed.). Staten Island, NY: Power Publications.

Gong, G., Wang, P., Ding, W., Zhao, Y., & Li, J. (2009). Microscopic and ultrastructural changes of the intestine in abdominal compartment syndrome. *Journal of Investigative Surgery, 22*(5), 362–367.

Gonzalez-Castillo, S., Arias, A., & Lucendo, A. (2010). Treatment of eosinophilic esophagitis: How should we manage the disease? *Journal of Clinical Gastroenterology, 44*(10), 663–671.

Gueant, S., Taleb, A., Borel-Kuhner, J., Cauterman, M., Raphael, M., Nathan, G., & Ricard-Hibon, A. (2011). Quality of pain management in the emergency department: Results of a multicentre prospective study. *European Journal of Anaesthesiology, 28*(2), 97–105.

Hamilton, M., French, W., Rhymes, N., & Collins, P. (2006). Liver haemorrhage in haemophilia—A case report and review of the literature. *Haemophilia, 12*(4), 441–443.

Han, H. Y., Shih, I. T., Huang, M. K., Chong, C. F., & Chen, C. C. (2006). Simple method for inflating and measuring oesophageal balloon pressure of Sengstaken-Blakemore tube. *Internal Medicine Journal, 36*(10), 684–685.

Hardin, S. R., & Kaplow, R. (2010). *Cardiac surgery essentials for critical care nursing*. Sudbury, MA: Jones & Bartlett Learning.

Harold, E. (2010). The early days of appendicectomy. *Journal of Perioperative Practice, 20*(12), 451.

Heiss, P., Zorger, N., Hamer, O., Seitz, J., Muller-Wille, R., Koller, M., . . . Wrede, C. E. (2009). Optimized multidetector computed tomographic protocol for the diagnosis of active obscure gastrointestinal bleeding: A feasibility study. *Journal of Computer Assisted Tomography, 33*(5), 698–704.

Hess, J. R., Zimrin, A. B., & Haycocks, N. G. (2010). A 42-year-old man with fevers, chills and abdominal pain. *American Journal of the Medical Sciences, 340*(5), 395–398.

Hirotaka, A., Takehiko, A., Ryuya, S., & Hitoshi, T. (2005). Emergency balloon-occluded retrograde transvenous obliteration for gastric varices. *Journal of Gastroenterology, 40*(10), 964.

Ho, K. M. (2004). Use of Sengstaken-Blakemore tube to stop massive upper gastrointestinal bleeding from Dieulafoy's lesion in the lower oesophagus. *Anaesthesia and Intensive Care, 32*(5), 711.

Hobolth, L., Krag, A., Malchow-Moller, A., Gancho, V., Jensen, S., Moller, S., & Bendtsen, F. (2010). Adherence to guidelines in bleeding oesophageal varices and effects on outcome: Comparison between a specialized unit and a community hospital. *European Journal of Gastroenterology & Hepatology, 22*(10), 1221–1227.

Hogan, A., & Winter, D. (2011). Management of acute diverticulitis: Is less more? *Diseases of the Colon & Rectum, 54*(1), 126–128.

Holleran, R. S. (2005). *Emergency transport nursing* (4th ed.). St. Louis, MO: Mosby.

Hung, C. W., Wu, W. F., & Wu, C. L. (2009). Rotavirus gastroenteritis complicated with toxic megacolon. *Acta Paediatrica, 98*(11), 1850–1852.

Hwang, J. P., & Hassan, M. M. (2009). Survival and hepatitis status among Asian Americans with hepatocellular carcinoma treated without liver transplantation. *BMC Cancer, 9*, 46.

Hwang, J., Jung, E., Park, W., Kim, Y., & Kim, A. (2011). Balloon-occluded retrograde transvenous obliteration treats hepatic dysfunction and gastric varices. *Journal of Pediatric Gastroenterology & Nutrition, 52*(2), 219–221.

Irani, S., Kowdley, K., & Kozarek, R. (2011). Gastric varices: An updated review of management. *Journal of Clinical Gastroenterology, 45*(2), 133–148.

Jacobs, B. B., & Hoyt, K. S. (2007). *Trauma nursing core course provider manual* (6th ed.). Bedford, IL: Emergency Nurses Association.

Jones & Bartlett Learning (2011). *2011 nurse's drug handbook* (10th ed.). Sudbury, MA: Jones & Bartlett Learning.

Ju, J. H., Park, H. S., Shin, M. J., & Yang, C. W. (2001). Successful treatment of massive lower gastrointestinal bleeding caused by mixed infection of cytomegalovirus and mucormycosis in a renal transplant recipient. *American Journal of Nephrology, 21*(3), 232.

Kamijo, Y., Kondo, I., Kokuto, M., Kataoka, Y., & Soma, K. (2004). Miniprobe ultrasonography for determining prognosis in corrosive esophagitis. *American Journal of Gastroenterology, 99*(5), 851–854.

Kamijo, Y., Kondo, I., Soma, K., Imaizumi, H., & Ohwada, T. (2001). Alkaline esophagitis evaluated by endoscopic ultrasound. *Journal of Toxicology, 39*(6), 623–625.

Kanakala, V., Lamb, C. A., Haigh, C., Stirling, R. W., & Attwood, S. E. (2010). The diagnosis of primary eosinophilic oesophagitis in adults: Missed or misinterpreted? *European Journal of Gastroenterology & Hepatology, 22*(7), 848–855.

Kapadia, F., Latka, M. H., Hagan, H., Golub, E. T., Campbell, J. V., Coady, M. H., . . . Strathdee, S. A. (2007). Design and feasibility of a randomized behavioral intervention to reduce distributive injection risk and improve health-care access among hepatitis C virus positive injection drug users: The Study to Reduce Intravenous Exposures (STRIVE). *Journal of Urban Health, 84*(1), 99–115.

Kaviani, M. J., Pirastehfar, M., Azari, A., & Saberifiroozi, M. (2010). Etiology and outcome of patients with upper gastrointestinal bleeding: a study from South of Iran. *Saudi Journal of Gastroenterology, 16*(4), 253–259.

Kochin, I., Magid, M., Arnon, R., Glasscock, A., Kerkar, N., & Miloh, T. (2010). Variceal bleeding in an adolescent with HIV diagnosed with hepatoportal sclerosis and nodular regenerative hyperplasia. *Journal of Pediatric Gastroenterology & Nutrition, 50*(3), 340–343.

Korley, F. K., Pham, J. C., & Kirsch, T. D. (2010). Use of advanced radiology during visits to U.S. emergency departments for injury-related conditions, 1998–2007. *JAMA, 304*(13), 1465–1471.

Kwon, K. T., Rudkin, S. E., & Langdorf, M. I. (2002). Antiemetic use in pediatric gastroenteritis: A national survey of emergency physicians, pediatricians, and pediatric emergency physicians. *Clinical Pediatrics, 41*(9), 641–652.

Larson, A. M. (2010). Diagnosis and management of acute liver failure. *Current Opinion in Gastroenterology, 26*(3), 214–221.

Lee, J. H., Kim, D. H., Kim, K., Rhee, J. E., Kim, T. Y., Jo, Y. H., . . . Singer, A. J. (2010). Predicting change of hemoglobin after transfusion in hemodynamically stable anemic patients in emergency department. *Journal of Trauma-Injury Infection & Critical Care, 68*(2), 337–341.

Lee, S., Lee, T., Chang, C., Ko, C., Yeh, H., & Yang, S. (2010). Independent factors associated with early outcome in Chinese cirrhotic patients after cessation of initial esophageal variceal hemorrhage. *Journal of Clinical Gastroenterology, 44*(6), e123–e127.

Lee, T., Wang, H., Chiu, H., Lien, W., Chen, M., Yu, L., . . . Wu, M. (2010). Male gender and renal dysfunction are predictors of adverse outcome in nonpostoperative ischemic colitis patients. *Journal of Clinical Gastroenterology, 44*(5), e96–e100.

Leeuwenburgh, M., Lameris, W., van Randen, A., Bossuyt, P. M. M., Boermeester, M. A., & Stoker, J. (2010). Optimizing imaging in suspected appendicitis (OPTIMAP-study): A multicenter diagnostic accuracy study of MRI in patients with suspected acute appendicitis. *BMC Emergency Medicine, 10*, 19.

Levitzky, B. E., & Wassef, W. Y. (2010). Endoscopic management in the bariatric surgical patient. *Current Opinion in Gastroenterology, 26*(6), 632–639.

Liao, C. F., Liu, C. C., Chuang, C. H., & Hsu, K. C. (2010). Obturator hernia: A diagnostic challenge of small-bowel obstruction. *American Journal of the Medical Sciences, 339*(1), 92–94.

Liguori, G., Cortale, M., Cimino, F., & Sozzi, M. (2008). Circumferential mucosal dissection and esophageal perforation in a patient with eosinophilic esophagitis. *World Journal of Gastroenterology, 14*(5), 803–804.

Lippincott. (2010). *Professional guide to signs and symptoms* (6th ed.). Philadelphia, PA: Lippincott.

Lockwood, A. M., Cole, S., & Rabinovich, M. (2010). Azithromycin-induced liver injury. *American Journal of Health-System Pharmacy, 67*(10), 810–814.

Malbrain, M. L., & Wilmer, A. (2007). The polycompartment syndrome: Towards an understanding of the interactions between different compartments. *Intensive Care Medicine, 33,* 1869–1872.

Mao, Y. C., Lin, T. C., & Wang, J. D. (2009). Education and imaging. Gastrointestinal: Benign cause for pneumatosis intestinalis and portomesenteric venous gas. *Journal of Gastroenterology and Hepatology, 24*(5), 927.

McKenzie, R., Fried, M. W., Sallie, R., Conjeevaram, H., Di Bisceglie, A. M., Park, Y., . . . Luciano, C. (1995). Hepatic failure and lactic acidosis due to fialuridine (FIAU), an investigational nucleoside analogue for chronic hepatitis B. *New England Journal of Medicine, 333*(17), 1099–1105.

Mertin, S., Sawatzky, J. V., Diehl-Jones, W. L., & Lee, W. W. R. (2007). Roadblock to recovery: The surgical stress response. *Dynamics, 18*(1), 14.

Milev, B., Mirković, D., Bezmarević, M., Misovic, S., Mitrovic, M., Jovanovic, M., . . . Radenkovic, D. (2010). Intra-abdominal hypertension and abdominal compartment syndrome. *Military-Medical and Pharmaceutical Review, 67*(8), 674–680.

Mills, A. M., Shofer, F. S., Chen, E. H., Hollander, J. E., & Pines, J. M. (2009). The association between emergency department crowding and analgesia administration in acute abdominal pain patients. *Academic Emergency Medicine, 16*(7), 603–608.

Moucari, R., Francoz, C., Lada, O., Abdel Razek, W., Marcellin, P., Valla, D., . . . Durand, F. (2009). Emergency transplantation for acute reactivation of chronic hepatitis B with high viral load: role of antiviral therapy. *Liver International, 29*(5), 775–776.

Nakae, H., Igarashi, T., Tajimi, K., Kusano, T., Shibata, S., Kume, M., . . . Yamamoto, Y. (2007). A case report of hepatorenal syndrome treated with plasma diafiltration (selective plasma filtration with dialysis). *Therapeutic Apheresis and Dialysis, 11*(5), 391–395.

Nübling, M., Hofmann, F., & Tiller, F. W. (2002). Occupational risk for hepatitis A and hepatitis E among health care professionals? *Infection, 30*(2), 94–97.

Okpalugo, C. E., & Oguntibeju, O. O. (2008). Prevalence of human immunodeficiency virus and hepatitis B virus in preoperative patients: Potential risk of transmission to health professionals. *Pakistan Journal of Biological Sciences, 11*(2), 298–301.

Ozdogan, M., & Ozdogan, H. (2006). Balloon tamponade with Sengstaken-Blakemore tube for penetrating liver injury: Case report. *Journal of Trauma-Injury Infection & Critical Care, 60*(5), 1122–1123.

Papagoras, C., Kountouras, J., Brilakis, S., Chatzopoulos, D., Zavos, C., & Topalidis, A. (2007). Rheumatic-like syndrome as a symptom of underlying gastric cancer. *Clinical Rheumatology, 26*(6), 1029–1031.

Patnaik, J. L., Dippold, L., & Vogt, R. L. (2011). Hepatitis A in a food worker and subsequent prophylaxis of restaurant patrons. *Journal of Environmental Health, 69*(1), 16.

Pelosi, P., Quintel, M., & Malbrain, M. L. (2007). Effect of intra-abdominal pressure on respiratory mechanics. *Acta Clinica Belgium Supplimentl, 62,* 78–88.

Peters-Reed, N. (2010). Do not underestimate the "otherwise healthy" patient. *Advanced Emergency Nursing Journal, 32*(3), 216–225.

Prasch, F., Grothaus, J., Mossner, J., Schiefke, I., & Hoffmeister, A. (2010). Differences in bleeding behavior after endoscopic band ligation: A retrospective analysis. *BMC Gastroenterology, 10,* 5.

Proehl, J. A. (2008). *Emergency nursing procedures* (4th ed.). St. Louis, MO: Saunders.

Radeleff, B., Sommer, C. M., Schawo, S., Lopez-Benitez, R., Sauer, P., Schemmer, P., . . . Richter, G. M. (2008). Acute liver failure after a late TIPSS revision. *Cardiovascular and Interventional Radiology, 31*(1), 209–214.

Rocca, L. G., Yawn, B. P., Wollan, P., & Kim, W. R. (2004l). Management of patients with hepatitis C in a community population: diagnosis, discussions, and decisions to treat. *Annals of Family Medicine, 2*(2), 116–124.

Romesburg, J., & Imam, K. (2010). Stump appendicitis. *Applied Radiology, 39*(10), 36.

Rotholtz, N., Bun, M. E., Laporte, M., Sandra, L., Carlos, P., & Mezzadri, N. (2009). Rectal bleeding in Klippel-Trenaunay syndrome: Treatment with laparoscopic ultralow anterior resection with intersphincteric dissection. *Surgical Laparoscopy, Endoscopy & Percutaneous Techniques, 19*(5), e206–e209.

Rubin, R. N. (2000). An elderly woman with painless, large-volume hematochezia. *Consultant, 40*(6), 1075.

Sakorafas, G. H., Mastoraki, A., Lappas, C., Sampanis, D., Danias, N., & Smyrniotis, V. (2011). Conservative treatment of acute appendicitis: Heresy or an effective and acceptable alternative to surgery? *European Journal of Gastroenterology & Hepatology, 23*(2), 121–127.

Sato, O., Okamoto, H., & Matsumoto, H. (2003). Emergency CT scan for the diagnosis of superior mesenteric artery embolism: Report of 2 cases. *International Angiology, 22*(4), 438.

Schutz, J., Babl, F. E., Sheriff, N., & Borland, M. (2008). Emergency department management of gastro-enteritis in Australia and New Zealand. *Journal of Paediatrics and Child Health, 44*(10), 560–563.

Seror, J., Allouche, C., & Elhaik, S. (2005). Use of Sengstaken-Blakemore tube in massive postpartum hemorrhage: a series of 17 cases. *Acta Obstetricia et Gynecologica Scandinavica, 84*(7), 660–664.

Sharma, A., Sachdev, H., & Gomillion, M. (2009). Abdominal compartment syndrome during hip arthroscopy. *Anaesthesia, 64*(5), 567–569.

Sistrom, M. G., & Hale, P. J. (2006). Outbreak investigations: Community participation and role of community and public health nurses. *Public Health Nursing, 23*(3), 256–263.

Smith, M. M. (2010). Emergency: Variceal hemorrhage from esophageal varices associated with alcoholic liver disease. *American Journal of Nursing, 110*(2), 32–39.

Sorodoc, L., Lionte, C., Sorodoc, V., Petris, O., & Jaba, I. (2010). Is MARS system enough for A. phalloides-induced liver failure treatment? *Human & Experimental Toxicology, 29*(10), 823–832.

Speer, A. L., Sohn, H. J., Moazzez, A., Portillo, J., Clarke, T., Katkhouda, N., & Mason, R. (2010). Establishing an acute care surgery service: Lessons learned from the epidemiology of emergent non-trauma patients and increasing utilization of laparoscopy. *Journal of Trauma-Injury Infection & Critical Care, 69*(4), 938–942.

Steiner-Sichel, L., Greenko, J., Heffernan, R., Layton, M., & Weiss, D. (2004). Field investigations of emergency department syndromic surveillance signals—New York City. *Morbidity and Mortality Weekly Report, 53*(Suppl), 184–189.

Sugrue, M., & Buhkari, Y. (2009). Intra-abdominal pressure and abdominal compartment syndrome in acute general surgery. *World Journal of Surgery, 33*(6), 1123–1127.

Thuijls, G., Wijck, K., Grootjans, J., Derikx, J., van Bijnen, A., Heineman, E., . . . Poeze, M. (2011). Early diagnosis of intestinal ischemia using urinary and plasma fatty acid binding proteins. *Annals of Surgery, 253*(2), 303–308.

Toti, L., Manzia, T. M., Romano, P., Lenci, I., Baiocchi, L., Anselmo, A., . . . Tisone, G. (2010). Successful management of a same-day emergency delivery and liver transplant in a 27 weeks pregnant woman with fulminant hepatic failure. *Transplant International: Official Journal of the European Society for Organ Transplantation, 23*(1), 114–115.

Ubee, S. S., Manikandan, R., Athmanathan, N., Singh, G., & Vesey, S. G. (2009). Compartment syndrome in urological practice. *BJU International, 104*(5), 577–578.

Uchiyama, S., Sannomiya, I., Hidaka, H., Oshikawa, S., Ashizuka, S., & Chijiiwa, K. (2010). Meckel diverticulum diagnosed by double-balloon enteroscopy and treated laparoscopically: Case report and review of the literature. *Surgical Laparoscopy, Endoscopy & Percutaneous Techniques, 20*(4), 278–280.

Urden, L. D., Stacy, K. M., & Lough, M. E. (2005). *Thelan's critical care nursing* (5th ed.). St. Louis, MO: Mosby.

Urita, Y., Domon, K., Yanagisawa, T., Ishihara, S., Hoshina, M., Akomoto, T., . . . Miki, K. (2007). Salivary gland scintigraphy in gastro-esophageal reflux disease. *Inflammopharmacology, 15*(4), 141–145.

Vikrama, K. S., Shyamkumar, N. K., Vinu, M., Joseph, P., Vyas, F., & Venkatramani, S. (2009). Percutaneous catheter drainage in the treatment of abdominal compartment syndrome. *Canadian Journal of Surgery, 52*(1), E19–E20.

Wakabayashi, H., Shiode, T., Kurose, M., Moritani, H., Fujiki, S., Morimoto, N., & Kusachi, S. (2004). Emergent treatment of acute embolic superior mesenteric ischemia with combination of thrombolysis and angioplasty: Report of two cases. *Cardiovascular and Interventional Radiology, 27*(4), 389–393.

Watson, S., & Gorski, K. A. (2011). *Invasive cardiology (3rd ed.)*. Sudbury, MA: Jones & Bartlett Learning.

White, S. I., Frenkiel, B. B., & Martin, P. J. (2010). A ten-year audit of perforated sigmoid diverticulitis: Highlighting the outcomes of laparoscopic lavage. *Diseases of the Colon & Rectum, 53*(11), 1537–1541.

Xu, X., Ling, Q., Zhang, M., Gao, F., He, Z., You, J., & Zheng, S. (2009). Outcome of patients with hepatorenal syndrome type 1 after liver transplantation: Hangzhou experience. *Transplantation, 87*(10), 1514–1519.

Yousef, N., Habes, D., Ackermann, O., Durand, P., Bernard, O., & Jacquemin, E. (2010). Hepatorenal syndrome: Diagnosis and effect of terlipressin therapy in 4 pediatric patients. *Journal of Pediatric Gastroenterology & Nutrition, 51*(1), 100–102.

SECTION 12:

Substance Abuse, Toxicologic, and Environmental

1. Hypertonic solutions are used frequently for burn patients. An advantage of using this type of solution is
   A. Lower cost
   B. A decreased chance for sepsis
   C. Elimination of the need for vitamin replacements
   D. Minimization of wound edema

2. The type of burn most likely to cause hemorrhage, thrombus formation, or generalized vascular disruption is a(n)
   A. Chemical burn
   B. Electrical burn
   C. Direct flame burn
   D. Steam burn

3. Acetaminophen overdose may cause hypoglycemia and should be treated with a
   A. Continuous IV infusion of D_5W at 100 cc/hour
   B. Bolus of D_{10}, continuous infusion of 0.45% normal saline
   C. Bolus of D_{50}, continuous infusion of D_5W
   D. Continuous IV infusion of lactated Ringer's

4. Your patient is undergoing alcohol withdrawal and exhibits diplopia, peripheral neuropathy, confusion, recent memory loss, and hyperexcitability. You suspect that this patient is suffering from
   A. Jorn's syndrome
   B. Leucine deficiency
   C. Increased caritine levels
   D. Wernicke-Korsakoff syndrome

5. Phoebe was admitted to the ED with recurrent *Pneumocystis carinii*. She is currently taking protease inhibitors and nonnucleoside reverse transcriptase inhibitor. Which of the following herbals may be contributing to her recurrent *Pneumocystis carinii*?
   A. Ginkgo Biloba
   B. Ginseng
   C. St. John's Wort
   D. Thyme

6. Frank, a victim of a black widow spider bite, became obtunded, bradycardic, apneic, and hypotensive soon after arrival in the ED. Your first action should be to
   A. Administer morphine 2 mg IV
   B. Administer antivenin
   C. Tie a tourniquet around the leg
   D. Prepare to intubate

7. Grace is preparing to go home after treatment with antivenin for a black widow spider bite. Which of the following discharge instructions is appropriate?
   A. "You may experience muscle spasms for only a few days"
   B. "You may experience tingling and weakness for several years"
   C. "Call your doctor immediately if you have joint or abdominal pain or begin to have trouble breathing"
   D. "It is normal to have a rash or fever in the next 3 days"

8. Many people are adding "exotic herbs" and supplements into their food and diets. Many may be very harmful and interact with medicines they are taking or may result in serious or deadly complications of existing diseases. Your patient is experimenting with flavorings. She made a roast with Scotch Broom on it for her parents to try. After ingesting the soup she began to feel lightheaded and experienced palpitations and weakness. She is being treated in your unit after a cardiac arrest at home. A priority of treatment is to
   A. Insert a nasogastric tube and provide gastric lavage with activated charcoal
   B. Insert a Foley catheter
   C. Continue quinidine medications taken at home
   D. Continue the amiodarone infusion started by EMS

9. Michael was helping a friend clean out a garage yesterday. He developed a raised area that initially looked like a mosquito bite but is now red, pus filled, and inflamed. He is admitted to the unit with a necrotizing wound. You suspect a brown recluse spider bite. Michael may also exhibit all the following signs and symptoms except
   A. Dyspnea
   B. Nausea and vomiting
   C. DIC
   D. Hemolysis and thrombocytopenia

10. Ada was admitted to your unit after experiencing abdominal cramping, nausea, and severe diarrhea. Her EKG shows sinus tachycardia with frequent PVCs. She is currently on an amiodarone infusion. The only significant history was that Ada ate at a seafood restaurant 3 days ago. Ada is probably suffering from
    A. Irritable bowel syndrome
    B. Hypokalemia
    C. Celiac disease
    D. Shellfish poisoning

11. Your patient is receiving activated protein C. The actions of this drug include
    A. Profibrinolytic action
    B. Antimicrobial agency
    C. Antiviral agency
    D. Blockade of angiotensin II

12. Acetaminophen overdose may take up to 2 weeks to resolve. From 72 to 96 hours after ingestion symptoms will include
    A. Pallor, lethargy, metabolic acidosis
    B. Jaundice, confusion, coagulation disorders
    C. Right upper quadrant pain, increased serum hepatic enzymes
    D. Increased renal function

13. Which of the following statements about cocaine is false?
    A. Cocaine use, even one time, can cause rhabdomyolysis
    B. Cocaine and tobacco use are associated with spontaneous abortion
    C. Cocaine will not cause premature detachment of the placenta
    D. Specimens should be kept on ice

14. An antidote for ethylene glycol toxicity is
    A. Digoxin
    B. Anisindione
    C. Fomepizole
    D. Narcan

15. GHB (Ecstasy) overdoses can lead to amnesia in approximately what percentage of cases?
    A. 13%
    B. 21%
    C. 24%
    D. 32%

16. Cadmium accumulates in the lungs, liver, and kidneys from exposure to
    A. Cigarette smoke
    B. Asbestos
    C. Lead paint
    D. Fungicide

17. Your patient's prothrombin time has an increased INR. You question the patient and determine the patient had taken one of the following medications that may have affected the INR level. That medication is a(n)
    A. Antacid
    B. Herbal and natural remedy
    C. Antihistamine
    D. Diuretic

18. Factors that may affect results of urine morphine levels include all the following except
    A. Poppy seed ingestion may produce false-positive results
    B. 10 mg MS IV may be detectable in urine up to 84 hours
    C. Use of stealth adulterant will cause negative results in a positive sample
    D. High levels of lymphocytes will mask morphine in urine

19. Your patient is experiencing delirium tremens. Nursing interventions include keeping the room well lit and minimizing stimulation. Staff members continuously reorient the patient to time, place, and person. Haldol has been given as ordered, and the patient is in 4 point restraints. Which of these nursing interventions should be discontinued?
    A. Reorientation
    B. Medication administration
    C. Restraints
    D. Controlling stimulation

20. What is the incubation period for inhalation anthrax?
    A. 7–10 days
    B. 5–7 days
    C. 7–60 days
    D. 20–30 days

21. What are the initial symptoms for inhaled anthrax?
    A. Mild, flu-like symptoms
    B. Severe dyspnea and productive cough
    C. High fever, cough, and stridor
    D. Cutaneous lesions, cough, and high fever

22. Deborah works at a fast-food restaurant. She found an envelope that was torn and had white powder falling out of the tear. She and her fellow employees were sent to the hospital and are being evaluated for possible inhalation anthrax. What is the treatment of choice for Deborah?
    A. Penicillin G 2 million units intravenously every 6 hours
    B. Ciprofloxacin 400 mg intravenously every 12 hours
    C. Doxycycline 500 mg intravenously every 12 hours
    D. Augmentin 875/125 mg intravenously every 12 hours

23. How long is antibiotic therapy continued after inhalation anthrax exposure?
    A. 10 days of intravenous antibiotics
    B. 14 days of intravenous and then oral antibiotics
    C. 30 days of intravenous and then oral antibiotics
    D. 60 days of combined intravenous and oral antibiotics

24. What form of isolation should be used for the patient with inhalation anthrax?
    A. Full isolation with laminar air flow
    B. Droplet precautions
    C. Standard contact precautions
    D. Reverse isolation

25. Your hospital is put on an external disaster notice after a ricin poisoning incident at a local train station. Your ED prepares to accept casualities. What makes ricin so toxic to humans?
    A. Ricin causes respiratory failure
    B. Ricin causes renal failure
    C. Ricin inhibits protein synthesis, leading to cell death
    D. Ricin destroys the mitochondria in the cell, causing cell death

26. Your patient is a young woman with diffuse abdominal pain and confusion. Just after admission she had generalized seizures and bradycardia. Opioid overdose was suspected and she was given naloxone with only minimal effect. The patient is now lethargic but does tell you she is a "body packer" to help pay for beauty school. She becomes hypotensive and bradycardic. Appropriate therapy includes
    A. Bowel irrigations, intubation, mechanical ventilation, anticonvulsants
    B. Sodium bicarbonate activated charcoal, hemodialysis
    C. Antiemetics, gastric lavage, bronchodilators
    D. Activated charcoal, sodium bicarbonate, vasopressors

27. A male patient was pumping gas when a spark ignited the fumes. He suffered full thickness burns of the right arm. During your initial assessment you note that eschar is present and the right radial pulse is not palpable. A Doppler pulse is also not discernible. Which of the following actions is appropriate at this time?
    A. Move arm away from torso and elevate it on a pillow
    B. Escharotomy
    C. Morphine 4 mg IV
    D. Ice packs to reduce swelling

28. Dallas was admitted to your ED after a burn injury. He was helping his friend barbeque in the back yard and a sudden flame-up burned his chest, right shoulder, and chin. What finding would be indicative of smoke inhalation in this patient?
    A. PaO_2 81, met HgB level of 2%
    B. PaO_2 76, pCO_2 26
    C. Increased CO_2
    D. Carboxyhemoglobin of 18%, burned chin

29. During the immediate postburn period, which of the following fluids would be most beneficial?
    A. Normal saline
    B. 0.45% normal saline
    C. Lactated Ringer's
    D. Albumin

30. Gladys suffered severe respiratory depression after ingestion of a large amount of diazepam. She has now developed atrial fibrillation. Anticipated treatment would include
    A. Amiodarone
    B. Lidocaine
    C. Adenosine
    D. Prostaglandin

31. Your patient was burned over the anterior chest, both arms, anterior neck, and the lateral aspect of the right leg. The burns on his chest and right arm have a white, leather-like appearance, and the patient has no sensation in that area. What classification of burn are these injuries?
    A. First degree
    B. Second-degree partial thickness
    C. Third-degree full thickness
    D. Fourth-degree full thickness

32. If muscle is burned, what classification is this type of burn?
    A. First degree
    B. Second-degree partial thickness
    C. Third-degree full thickness
    D. Fourth-degree full thickness

33. Your patient has burns on the right arm that are circumferential (all the way around the arm). What is a potential risk with this type of burn?
    A. Infection into the bone
    B. Difficulty removing dead tissue
    C. Compartment syndrome
    D. Escharotomy

34. This morning a fire broke out in your patient's home. Because it is a cold environment, the patient was surrounded by wool blankets and wool clothing was in the closet. She did not suffer any burns but did inhale large quantities of smoke. What would be the most potent toxin she might have inhaled?
    A. Carbon monoxide
    B. Smoke
    C. Inhaled nitrates
    D. Cyanide

35. Your patient lived in the country at a camp all summer and ate large quantities of deer and fish. He was admitted to the ED for respiratory distress, weight loss, vomiting, and numbness around the mouth. He is also suffering from mouth sores and he drools constantly. His probable diagnosis is
    A. Botulism
    B. Chlamydia infection
    C. *Difficile* infection
    D. Mercury poisoning

36. Your patient was very anxious prior to a bronchoscopy. He received an IM injection of versed. His blood pressure dropped from 142/80 to 88/56 and he became bradycardic. To counter this reaction, he should be given
    A. Xanax
    B. Ativan
    C. Valium
    D. Romazicon

37. Which of the following vasodilators should not be mixed with Ringer's lactate?
    A. Nesiritide
    B. Captopril
    C. Cardene
    D. Epinephrine

38. Joe lives on a ranch. Yesterday he complained of a stiff neck and was very lethargic. Last night he was found unconscious and had apparently vomited and possibly aspirated. Joe was immediately transported to your ED. He was intubated and is being evaluated. Joe probably has
    A. Pneumonia
    B. West Nile virus
    C. Western equine encephalitis
    D. A brain tumor

39. Which statement about plague is incorrect?
    A. Plague is caused by *Yersenia pestis*
    B. Aerosal droplets may spread plague person to person
    C. Plague is usually transmitted by rats
    D. Plague is seen on a Gram stain as a gram-positive rod

40. Which of the following choices is not a form of anthrax?
    A. Nonspecific
    B. Cutaneous
    C. Pulmonary
    D. Gastrointestinal

41. The type of chemical agent that can cause blistering is called a
    A. Vesicant
    B. Contaminant
    C. Intoxicant
    D. Nerve agent

42. The type of device made by combining radioactive materials and an explosive is known as a(n)
    A. Improved nuclear device
    B. Radiologic dispersal device
    C. Simple radiological device
    D. Improved explosive device

43. When treating salicylate overdose, which of the following goals is appropriate for this condition?
    A. A hypocalcemic state
    B. Urine pH of 7 to 8
    C. Resolution of jaundice
    D. Entry of salicylate into the CNS

44. Your patient is irritable, confused, and has paresthesias around the mouth. He is having watery, rice-like diarrhea, nausea, and vomiting. These symptoms are indicative of
    A. Arsenic poisoning
    B. Digoxin toxicity
    C. Methanol poisoning
    D. Insecticide poisoning

45. A blast injury that occurs when a body is hurled though the air and struck by another object is known as
    A. A primary blast injury
    B. A compound blast injury
    C. A secondary blast injury
    D. A tertiary blast injury

46. An example of a primary blast injury is
    A. Hemorrhagic contusion
    B. Fractured femur
    C. An arm impaled by a stick
    D. Gunshot wound

47. A burn that involves muscle, fat, or bone is classified as a
    A. First-degree partial thickness burn
    B. Second-degree partial thickness burn
    C. Third-degree full thickness burn
    D. Fourth-degree full thickness burn

48. Use of 0.5% silver nitrate solution is a good treatment for burns because of its broad-spectrum antibacterial action. As an ED nurse you know a disadvantage of using this medication is
    A. Metabolic acidosis
    B. Hypochloremia and hyponatremia
    C. Transient leucopenia
    D. Limited penetration of eschar

49. The area of a burn that has the closest contact with the heat source and sustains the most damage is the
    A. Zone of stasis
    B. Zone of hyperemia
    C. Zone of erythema
    D. Zone of coagulation

50. After a patient ingests toxic levels of iron, there is a latent asymptomatic phase. This phase may cause caregivers to underestimate the continuing risk to the patient. This latent phase usually occurs _____ hours after ingestion
    A. 1–4
    B. 2–12
    C. 8–16
    D. 12–24

51. The toxic ingredient in automobile antifreeze is
    A. Freon
    B. Ethanol
    C. Methanol
    D. Ethylene glycol

52. An acid that is absorbed even through intact skin, causing local and systemic effects, is
    A. Hydrochloric acid
    B. Hydrofluoric acid
    C. Carbonic acid
    D. Acetic acid

53. Which statement is true regarding alkaline substances?
    A. The pH is lower than 2
    B. Vascular thrombosis may result
    C. Eschar forms over the burn
    D. Alkalines dehydrate tissues

54. Which of the following substances contain large amounts of alkali?
    A. Toilet bowl cleaners
    B. Swimming pool chemicals
    C. Oven cleaners
    D. Metal cleaners

55. Symptoms of salicylate poisoning include
    A. Respiratory acidosis and bradycardia
    B. Lethargy and hypotension
    C. Abdominal cramping and hyperglycemia
    D. Tachycardia and hyperthermia

56. Which of the following drugs has a half-life of approximately 24 hours and requires continuous doses of naloxone?
    A. Demerol
    B. Heroin
    C. Cocaine
    D. Methadone

57. The triad of symptoms usually associated with opioid overdose is
    A. Respiratory depression, meiosis, and coma
    B. Obtundation, hypotension, and ventricular arrhythmias
    C. Confusion, slurred speech, and seizures
    D. Stupor, respiratory alkalosis, and hypotension

58. The antidote for iron poisoning is
    A. No antidote is available, treat symptoms only
    B. Chelation
    C. Deferoxamine
    D. Activated charcoal

59. The acid-base imbalance likely to be seen with an iron overdose is
    A. Respiratory acidosis
    B. Metabolic alkalosis
    C. Metabolic acidosis
    D. Respiratory alkalosis

60. The specific antidote for a benzodiazepine overdose is
    A. Calcium chloride
    B. Flumazenil
    C. Atropine
    D. Calcium gluconate

61. You just discovered your patient is being treated at home for MRSA. She has been receiving vancomycin. You are able to check a trough level and the result was > 20 µg/ml. This level
    A. May cause ototoxicity
    B. May cause nephrotoxicity
    C. Is therapeutic
    D. Indicates the current dosage is too low

62. The specific antidote for methamphetamine is
    A. Desipramine
    B. Alkalinizing agents
    C. There is no antidote
    D. Naloxone

63. Poisoning by arsenic may cause which of the following symptoms?
    A. Pneumonia, renal dysfunction
    B. Tachycardia, hypertension
    C. Paresthesia, cerebral edema
    D. Convulsions

64. Your patient was admitted for severe flank pain and hematuria. He is scheduled for a kidney biopsy later today, but the pain was unbearable so he came to the ED. Your patient and family teaching should include
    A. Report any pain in the flank or abdomen post-procedure
    B. A small kidney stone may be passed after the procedure
    C. The patient will be on bed rest for 24 hours
    D. No teaching is necessary

65. Following a lung scan (V/Q), you should observe your patient for
    A. Sixty minutes after the study for possible reaction to the nucleotides
    B. Signs and symptoms of pneumonia
    C. Twenty-four hours to measure urine output and maintain strict I & O
    D. No observation is necessary

66. Your patient overdosed on metoprolol. As an ED nurse you know an appropriate nursing action would be to
    A. Prepare for cardioversion
    B. Administer activated charcoal
    C. Have a pacer at the bedside
    D. Prepare to administer beta-blockers

67. Patients who are undergoing alcohol withdrawal are frequently hypoglycemic. Treatment should include
    A. Bolus of $D_{10}W$, q 2 hour blood glucose monitoring
    B. TPN with high concentrations of sugars, q 2 hour blood glucose monitoring
    C. Maintenance fluids of $D_{25}W$ at 125 ml/h peripherally
    D. Thiamine, then bolus with D_{50}, then infusion of D_5W

68. The burn on your patient's right arm is pink and blistered. When touched the patient screams with pain. This classification of burn is
    A. First degree
    B. Second-degree partial thickness
    C. Third-degree full thickness
    D. Fourth-degree full thickness

69. Initially, a burned area can be estimated by the Rule of Nines, or using the palm as 1% of the body surface area. There are many ways to calculate the body surface area involved. If your patient was burned over 30% of his body and weighs 70 kg, calculate the total fluid requirements during the first 24 hours using the Parkland formula for burn resuscitation.
    A. 2100 ml
    B. 6300 ml
    C. 4500 ml
    D. 8400 ml

70. Using the Parkland formula for burn resuscitation, calculate the fluid requirements (first 24 hours) for a patient who weighs 65 kg and is burned over 45% of his body
    A. 29,250 ml
    B. 11,700 ml
    C. 26,000 ml
    D. 10,300 ml

71. When utilizing the Parkland formula to calculate fluid needs, the preferred fluid for burn resuscitation is
    A. Normal saline
    B. D_5/Isolyte M
    C. Lactated Ringer's
    D. D_5W

72. To minimize inflammation in burns, which of the following therapies may be used?
    A. Vitamin C
    B. Hyperbaric therapy
    C. Prednisone
    D. Burns open to air

73. The antidote for digoxin overdose is
    A. Calcium gluconate
    B. Digoxin immune Fab
    C. Glucagon
    D. Potassium chloride

74. Rocky Mountain spotted fever is caused by
    A. A parasite
    B. Fleas
    C. Rotavirus
    D. Fungi

75. Nathan was a spectator at a soccer tournament when he was struck by lightning. He was thrown about 10 feet into a tree. Nathan suffered a fractured left radius and ulna, a concussion, and burns on his left arm, chest, and right leg. He has been somewhat confused since the accident. Which of the following statements about lightning injuries is true?
    A. Internal burns are common
    B. Barotrauma is rare
    C. Myoglobinuria is rarely seen
    D. DC current will most likely cause ventricular fibrillation

76. Kathy lives on a farm. She frequently helps her sister home-prepare meat and vegetables and preserve them by canning. Kathy is admitted to the ED with profound weakness, double vision, slurred speech, and dysphagia. Her initial diagnosis is Guillain-Barré syndrome. While you are interviewing her sister you learn that a few days ago Kathy ingested some home-canned green beans that were several years old. No other family members ate the beans because the color was odd. What do you do with this information?
    A. Do nothing, it is of no consequence
    B. Notify the physician immediately, Kathy may have botulism
    C. Tell the physician the patient may have had a stroke
    D. Continue the interview

77. A possible adverse effect with the use of fentanyl is
    A. Neutropenia
    B. Chest wall rigidity
    C. Hyperthyroidism
    D. Tachypnea

78. A possible adverse effect of morphine is
    A. Ileus
    B. Hyperactive bowel tones
    C. Ototoxicity
    D. Increased venous capacitance

79. Fentanyl administered intravenously is incompatible with
    A. Piperacillin
    B. Phenytoin
    C. Esmolol
    D. Morphine

80. A contraindication for the use of fentanyl is
    A. Asthma
    B. A urinary tract infection
    C. Concomitant use of penicillin
    D. Open heart surgery

81. Your patient tells you she smokes pot. How is today's marijuana different from the marijuana of 10 years ago?
    A. Pot today is purer than pot was 10 years ago
    B. There is no difference
    C. Pot 10 years ago was safer
    D. Pot has delayed effects of 3 hours

82. Addiction and abuse are terms often used interchangeably in conversation with parents and family members. Which statement best defines these terms?
    A. They are the same terms
    B. Addiction is when the user cannot stop using with mild systems of withdrawal, and abuse is when the user cannot live without the substance or drug
    C. Addiction is when a user cannot live or function without the substance or drug and abuse is when the user uses the drug or substance in amounts or functions not intended
    D. Addiction is when the user uses the drug or substance in a way not intended, and abuse is when the user uses without the knowledge of other people

83. Which of the following illegal drugs is the most commonly abused?
    A. Marijuana
    B. Toluene
    C. Cocaine
    D. Heroin

84. Mary tells you she uses witch hazel. Your first question after hearing this should be
    A. "Why did you take witch hazel?"
    B. "How did you obtain the witch hazel?"
    C. "How much and how often did you use witch hazel?"
    D. "Does your family know you use witch hazel?"

85. Maria was brought into the emergency room after collapsing at a party. Maria's cardiac and neurologic work-up is negative. Her urine drug screen is negative. What do you suspect caused her collapse?
   A. GHB
   B. Dehydration
   C. Ecstasy
   D. Toxic ingestion

86. You are assessing a 25 year old patient named Carla. Carla appears euphoric and confused. While looking around the room you note a chewed-up pacifier on the gurney. Why would the pacifier be significant?
   A. It was from a previous patient
   B. Carla may have been using the pacifier prior to your entering the room
   C. The pacifier was caught in the railing and torn
   D. Carla's children were in the room just before you arrived

87. Which of the following statements is false regarding the use of activated charcoal for suspected or confirmed poisoning?
   A. Activated charcoal adsorbs most poisons
   B. Activated charcoal adsorbs metals
   C. Activated charcoal cannot be mixed with ice cream
   D. Single doses of activated charcoal are indicated for serious poison exposures

88. Multiple doses of activated charcoal should be used for ingestions of
   A. Theophylline
   B. Gentamicin
   C. Aspirin
   D. Acetaminophen

89. Acetaminophen is metabolized by the
   A. Spleen
   B. Kidneys
   C. Liver
   D. Lungs

90. A side effect of ethanol is to
   A. Cause supraventricular tachycardia
   B. Suppress the liver's ability to produce glucose
   C. Cause corneal burns
   D. Cause hyperglycemia

91. Your patient was admitted to the ED for intractable cyanosis. The cyanosis does not improve with oxygen, and the patient's blood appears brown when placed on white paper. You suspect this individual is suffering from
   A. Tricyclic overdose
   B. Gentamicin overdose
   C. Methemoglobinemia
   D. GI bleeding

92. Methemoglobinemia may be treated with
    A. Sodium bicarbonate
    B. Packed RBCs
    C. Methylene blue
    D. Whole blood

93. The drug of choice for the treatment of tricyclic antidepressant overdose is
    A. Atropine
    B. Imipramine
    C. Doxepin
    D. Sodium bicarbonate

94. A cyclic antidepressant that may cause cardiovascular effects and will probably cause status epilepticus is
    A. Amoxapine
    B. Amitriptyline
    C. Desipramine
    D. Doxepin

95. The specific antidote for a benzodiazepine overdose is
    A. Calcium chloride
    B. Flumazenil
    C. Atropine
    D. Calcium gluconate

96. A patient intoxicated with methamphetamine would exhibit which of the following conditions?
    A. Elevated liver enzymes
    B. Bradycardia
    C. Hypothermia
    D. Hypotension

97. Lithium is used as an antipsychotic medication to treat bipolar disorder. Lithium toxicity is deadly. Which of the following statements is true regarding lithium toxicity?
    A. Toxicity may occur if blood levels reach 1 mEq/L
    B. Signs of lithium toxicity include constipation, hypertonicity, and giddiness
    C. Untreated lithium toxicity may lead to seizures, coma, and cardiac dysrhythmias
    D. Lithium toxicity may be treated safely on a medical-surgical floor

98. Cheryl gave birth 2 months ago to a healthy baby boy. She has been suffering from postpartum depression. She presented to the ED with hallucinations, agitation, ventricular arrhythmias, and a possible seizure (witnessed by her husband). She has been taking a tricyclic antidepressant. Which of the following drugs is classified as a tricyclic antidepressant?
    A. Amitriptyline
    B. Gentamicin
    C. Clonidine
    D. Fluvastatin

99. Sally's husband said the last time Sally took one of the prescribed doses of her amitriptyline was last evening. A blood level was drawn in the ED and considered a trough level. Sally's treatment should include
    A. Hemodialysis
    B. Sodium bicarbonate
    C. Syrup of Ipecac
    D. Trazodone

100. Ketamine is contraindicated in a patient with
    A. Bronchospasm
    B. Altered intracranial pressure
    C. Barbiturate overdose
    D. Opioid overdose

101. Which of the following statements is true regarding the administration of propofol?
    A. Propofol is used for long-term procedures
    B. Propofol is not indicated for use in a patient with bronchospasm
    C. Propofol is made from eggs and soybeans
    D. Propofol increases cerebral blood flow

102. Methamphetamine is officially classified as a(n)
    A. Stimulant
    B. Euphoric
    C. Hallucinogen
    D. Antidepressant

103. The use of alkalinizing agents for the treatment of methamphetamine overdose is
    A. Not necessary
    B. Only to be used if seizures are present
    C. Contraindicated
    D. The only method to treat the resultant muscle spasms

104. The primary symptoms of cocaine toxicity include hyperthermia, hyperactivity, tachycardia, and hypertension. These symptoms may be managed by administration of
    A. Morphine
    B. Fentanyl
    C. Codeine
    D. Ativan

105. Your patient will be undergoing a cardiac catheterization. Your patient admits to cocaine use and appears to have suffered an anterior wall myocardial infarction. An anticipated treatment for this patient would include
    A. Evaluation for stroke
    B. A toxicology screen
    C. A stress test
    D. Hypothermia

106. Which of the following statements about superficial frostbite is true?
    A. Use heavy blankets to help rewarm the entire patient
    B. The skin will be bright pink and feel cold to the touch
    C. Rewarm the affected part using warm water at 104 degrees to 110 degrees F
    D. Keep the affected part dependent

107. Your patient was admitted with deep frostbite. Which of the following actions should not be performed ASAP for this patient?
    A. Remove the patient's wet clothing
    B. Administer warm, noncaffeinated fluids
    C. Administer narcotic analgesics
    D. Amputate tissue that is black in color

108. After exposure to radioactive iodine following a nuclear accident, which of the following substances would be appropriate to administer to a patient to help prevent thyroid cancer?
    A. Ciproflaxin
    B. Potassium iodide
    C. Calcium chloride
    D. Desipramine

SECTION 12: SUBSTANCE ABUSE, TOXICOLOGIC, AND ENVIRONMENTAL ANSWERS

1. **Correct answer: D**
   Hypertonic solutions minimize wound edema in burn patients.

2. **Correct answer: B**
   Electrical burns are insidious and follow the path of least resistance. Muscle tissue breaks down and causes rhabdomyolysis from the myoglobin that was released into the circulation.

3. **Correct answer: C**
   Acetaminophen overdose may cause hypoglycemia and should be treated with a bolus of D_{50} and a continuous infusion of D_5W. Hypoglycemia occurs because of the hepatotoxic effects of acetaminophen. Infusions must also be based on blood glucose results.

4. **Correct answer: D**
   The patient undergoing alcohol withdrawal and who exhibits diplopia, peripheral neuropathy, confusion, recent memory loss, and hyperexcitability has Wernicke-Korsakoff syndrome. Wernicke-Korsakoff syndrome is a thiamine deficiency and a metabolic encephalopathy.

5. **Correct answer: C**
   St. John's Wort is contraindicated in patients with HIV/AIDS because the herb interferes with the metabolism of protease inhibitors and nonnucleoside reverse transcriptase inhibitors.

6. **Correct answer: D**
   Frank is apneic and bradycardic. Priorities are to maintain the airway to provide ventilation and oxygen therapy. The next step is to administer antivenin as soon as available. Morphine may help with pain but will worsen the bradycardia and hypotension. It is a myth that tying a tourniquet around the affected limb will stop the venom from reaching the bloodstream or lymphatic system. At this point the venom is already systemic. In minor cases involving healthy patients, symptoms may be managed with pain control, muscle relaxants, and comfort measures. Symptoms should dissipate during the first 3 days after exposure.

7. **Correct answer: C**
   Grace suffered a black widow spider bite. Her discharge instructions should include contacting her physician immediately if she has joint or abdominal pain or difficulty breathing. Joint and abdominal pain (pain related to splenomegaly), as well as dyspnea, may be signs of anaphylaxis or serum sickness up to 2 to 4 weeks after antivenin administration. Patients should be taught to contact their physicians immediately so early treatment can be initiated to prevent complications. Administration of corticosteroids and antihistamines will aid in combating the inflammatory response to the animal proteins in the antivenin. The neurotoxin may cause residual muscle spasms, tingling, weakness, and nervousness for weeks to months after the exposure to the venom. Patients may need to slowly increase activity during their recovery.

8. **Correct answer: A**
The priority of care is to insert a nasogastric tube and provide gastric lavage with activated charcoal. Scotch Broom contains sparteine, which has very powerful cardiovascular effects. Arrhythmias, blood pressure changes (increased or decreased), coagulation changes, and vision changes are possible side effects of this herb. The best action listed is to lavage the stomach to remove any un- or partially digested Scotch Broom. You will need to insert a Foley catheter as Scotch broom does have diuretic properties, but it is not a priority. Quinidine and amiodarone should be stopped immediately because they will interact with the Scotch Broom to cause further cardiovascular collapse by increasing the toxicity of the Scotch Broom.

9. **Correct answer: A**
Patients presenting after recluse spider bites will not present with dyspnea. Patients may not initially know they where bitten and will seek medical help 12 to 36 hours after the initial bite. Because treatment is delayed, symptoms may be difficult to treat. Most patients may present with flu-like symptoms such as nausea and vomiting. DIC, hemolysis, and thrombocytopenia are severe symptoms. Treatment includes ice to control inflammation, keeping the area clean and protected, and treating symptoms. No specific treatment has been proven to be 100% effective. Dapsone has limited support for preventing necrosis. Nitroglycerin patches counter the vasoconstrictive properties of the venom and lead to hemodilution in the bloodstream and increased bleeding at the site to wash the venom out.

10. **Correct answer: D**
Shellfish poisoning can exhibit symptoms days after ingestion. The toxin contained in shellfish, clams, and oysters is called saxotoxin and is not affected by steaming or cooking. It inhibits sodium channels of membranes, blocking propagation of nerve and muscle action potentials. If the nerves are involved, there may be parasthesias of the lips, tongue, gums, and face. The parasthesias may spread to the trunk and lead to paralysis and respiratory arrest. There is no definite treatment, so care is driven by treating symptoms and psychological support.

11. **Correct answer: A**
Activated protein C (Xigris) is a profibrinolytic that inhibits factors Va and VIIIa. It inhibits human tumor necrosis factor production by monocytes. It also limits thrombin-induced inflammatory responses.

12. **Correct answer: B**
From 72 to 96 hours after acetaminophen ingestion, symptoms will include jaundice, confusion, and coagulation disorders. Renal function is possibly decreased, and the patient may have increased ALT and AST. At about 4 days to 2 weeks the symptoms abate.

13. **Correct answer: C**
Cocaine will indeed cause the placenta to detach prematurely. Cocaine is a schedule II central nervous system stimulant and is used as a local anesthetic. It is also used as a bronchodilator and vasoconstrictor. Cocaine compromises the heart's antioxidant defense system and an overdose can cause an MI. Cocaine can also cause aortic dissection, stroke, intestinal ischemia, hallucinations, and adverse effects on fetuses.

14. **Correct answer: C**

    An antidote for ethylene glycol toxicity is fomepizole. Ethylene glycol is a compound found in antifreeze. After ingestion it is converted to oxalic acid, which is excreted by the kidneys. This causes crystals in the urine, acidosis, tetany, and renal failure. Hemodialysis and peritoneal dialysis will remove ethylene glycol.

15. **Correct answer: A**

    GHB (Ecstasy) overdoses can lead to amnesia in approximately 13% of cases. Ecstasy can also cause ataxia, central nervous system depression, coma, bradycardias, hypothermia, hypotension, hypothermia, respiratory depression, and respiratory acidosis.

16. **Correct answer: A**

    Cadmium accumulates in the lungs, liver, and kidneys by exposure to cigarette smoke. Cadmium is actually a heavy metal with a half-life of 15–20 years. It is a respiratory irritant and can produce pulmonary edema, interstitial pneumonia, and cardiovascular collapse if inhaled. It is used in the manufacture of storage batteries, alloys, and in electroplating. If cadmium is ingested, the individual will have severe gastrointestinal symptoms within 30 minutes. Most cadmium collects in erythrocytes and kidney tissues. It is not metabolized in the body.

17. **Correct answer: B**

    Many herbs and natural remedies affect the INR because they are oral anticoagulants. They are dan shen, dang gui, dong quai, ginkgo biloba, garlic, ginseng, and ginger.

18. **Correct answer: D**

    Factors that may affect results of urine morphine levels include all the following except high levels of lymphocytes. The stealth adulterant masks morphine in the urine. When heroin is taken, it breaks down into morphine. Ten milligrams of morphine is detectable in urine for 84 hours and can be measured in corpses for about a week.

19. **Correct answer: C**

    Restraints should be used only if alternative methods for behavioral correction are ineffective. There is no indication that the patient is violent or has caused any threat to staff or self. Restraints should be used only as a last resort to prevent injury to self and staff. Reorientation, medication, and controlling external stimulation are all effective methods for controlling behavior.

20. **Correct answer: C**

    Inhalation anthrax has an incubation period of 7 days to as long as 60 days after exposure. Symptoms are initially vague and flu-like such as malaise, low-grade fever, and nausea. These symptoms quickly progress to profound diaphoresis, chest discomfort, and rhonchi. The mild symptoms occur in the first 5 days of the illness followed by a brief rally. There is then an abrupt onset of high fever and severe respiratory distress. Death occurs as early as 24–36 hours after symptoms begin.

21. **Correct answer: A**

    Inhalation anthrax starts with mild, nonspecific symptoms such as malaise, low-grade fever, fatigue, and cough. Untreated, death occurs within 24–36 hours from respiratory failure.

22. **Correct answer: B**
Ciprofloxacin, a fluorquinolone antibiotic, is the drug of choice for inhalation anthrax. Doxycycline, a tetracycline derivative, may also be used, but the dosage in response C is incorrect. Pencillin G is not an option as the bacteria, *Bacillus anthracis*, becomes beta-lactamase positive, making the penicillin ineffective. Augmentin is not used for this situation, and it is only given orally.

23. **Correct answer: D**
Antibiotics for inhalation anthrax are continued for 60 days after exposure, even if the exposure is only suspected. Treatment is initially intravenous and then changed to oral dosing for the remaining time. The two most common antibiotics given are ciprofloxacin and doxycycline.

24. **Correct answer: C**
The CDC states that contact precautions are all that is required for inhalation anthrax. Standard precautions may include the use of a face mask if the patient is having a productive cough.

25. **Correct answer: C**
Ricin is made from castor beans and is one of the most toxic substances known. It interferes with protein synthesis and causes cell death. Chewing castor beans may cause some symptoms, but the most lethal form is inhaled. The toxin is not spread by casual contact. The most likely victims would be seen in enclosed areas such as subway trains, buses, or small rooms. It is usually aerosolized with some liquid like water or a weak acid.

26. **Correct answer: A**
"Body packer" is the term used for people who transport narcotics in body cavities. In this case it is probable that a packet may have ruptured. Bowel irrigations, intubation, mechanical ventilation, and anticonvulsants may be required as treatments for this patient. More doses of naloxone may be necessary, along with supportive treatment for opioid overdose. Be alert for bradycardia, hypotension, respiratory depression, and hypothermia.

27. **Correct answer: B**
This is an emergency and pressure must be relieved via an escharotomy, an incision through multiple layers of tissue. Any circumferential burn of the body may lead to impaired function and necessitate an escharotomy.

28. **Correct answer: D**
Carboxyhemoglobin of 18% and a burned chin is indicative of smoke inhalation in this patient. When a sudden flame-up comes near the face, the first instinct is to gasp. This inhalation of superheated air will cause swelling of the tissues in the air passages. Dallas was probably very near the flame as his chin was burned, and he is at great risk of a compromised airway and may need intubation.

29. **Correct answer: C**
Lactated Ringer's is used for burn patients because it is used for a variety of reasons with many of the formulas for burn resuscitation. It is preferred for large volume resuscitation because LR contains 130 mEq/L of sodium compared with normal saline that has 154 mEq/L. LR has a higher pH (6.5) compared to normal saline (5.0). The pH of

the LR is close to a normal pH. The patient will be in metabolic acidosis, so the metabolized lactate will buffer the acidosis. LR is also an isotonic crystalloid.

30. **Correct answer: A**
    Amiodarone is useful in treatment of atrial fibrillation because the drug decreases sinus rate, increases PD and QT intervals, and results in the development of U waves.

31. **Correct answer: C**
    Third-degree full thickness burns destroy nerve endings because they extend into subcutaneous tissue. The tissue may have a whitish color and will be somewhat firm with a leather-like appearance. Sometimes you can see clotted vessels through the eschar.

32. **Correct answer: D**
    This is a fourth-degree burn. Not many people are familiar with this classification. This is a burn that not only involves muscle but it extends through muscle and bone.

33. **Correct answer: C**
    A circumferential burn may lead to compartment syndrome. Escharotomy is a procedure, not a direct risk. The highest risk at this time is compartment syndrome. As a nurse you must constantly assess for quality of pulses. Edema may be so great as to completely cut off circulation in a limb and cause a myoglobin-related renal failure. Elevating the limb may help drain fluid and mitigate further edema. If the pulse is lost, it still may not mean compartment syndrome is the cause. It could be due to not replacing lost volume secondary to the burn.

34. **Correct answer: D**
    Wool and silk give off cyanide gas. Nitriles, like the gloves we wear, will burn and give off cyanide. Household plastics like melamine dishes, plastic cups, polyurethane foam in furniture cushions, and many other synthetic compounds may produce lethal concentrations of cyanide when burned under appropriate circumstances. Cyanide inhibits cellular respiration, even with enough oxygen stores. Cellular metabolism changes from aerobic to anaerobic and produces lactic acid. The organs with the highest oxygen requirements are the most affected by cyanide inhalation.

35. **Correct answer: D**
    The probable diagnosis for this patient is mercury poisoning. Fish can contain large amounts of mercury. The concentration in fish can be more than 1,000 times greater in the fish than in the surrounding water. People who eat fish as a main component of their diet may be at risk. Organic mercury compounds are very toxic. They are taken into the body by ingestion, inhalation, skin, and eye contact. These mercury compounds can attack all body systems. They can cause nausea, lack of appetite, abdominal pain, kidney failure, swollen gums and mouth sores, numbness and tingling in the lips, mouth, tongue, hands and feet, tremors, and seizures. The patient can become very uncoordinated and feel disconnected from his surroundings. He may lose part or all of his vision and hearing. Additional neurologic issues may include memory loss, personality changes, and headache. Organic mercury can pass to a baby via breast milk. Methyl mercury may cause serious birth defects.

36. **Correct answer: D**
    Romazicon is a benzodiazepine antagonist and should be given to counteract the effects of versed. Xanax, valium, and Ativan are also benzodiazepines.

37. **Correct answer: C**
    Cardene cannot be mixed with Ringer's lactate or sodium bicarbonate infusions. According to studies, although the combination does not cause a precipitate, the Ringer's lactate inactivates 15% to 42% of the drug.

38. **Correct answer: C**
    Western equine encephalitis is a type of encephalitis caused by an arbovirus (togovirus). An arbovirus means it is carried by arthropods. A horse or small mammal was probably infected and the virus was vectored by a mosquito. This type of encephalopathy is not directly transmitted human to human. This patient is at high risk for aspiration pneumonia and ARDS.

39. **Correct answer: C**
    Plague is not transmitted by rats. Plague is transmitted by fleas, and aerosol droplets may spread the disease from person to person.

40. **Correct answer: A**
    Nonspecific is not a form of anthrax. Cutaneous, pulmonary, and gastrointestinal are all forms of anthrax.

41. **Correct answer: A**
    The type of chemical agent that can cause blistering is called a vesicant.

42. **Correct answer: B**
    The type of device made by combining radioactive materials and an explosive is known as a radiologic dispersal device.

43. **Correct answer: B**
    A urine pH of 7 to 8 is an appropriate goal for a patient treated for salicylate overdose.

44. **Correct answer: A**
    Watery, rice-like diarrhea, nausea, vomiting, irritability, confusion, and paresthesias around the mouth are symptoms of arsenic poisoning. Additional symptoms include headache, a metallic taste, palpitations, and EKG changes.

45. **Correct answer: D**
    A tertiary blast injury is a blast injury that occurs when a body is hurled though the air and struck by another object.

46. **Correct answer: A**
    Hemorrhagic contusion is an example of a primary blast injury. A blast injury occurs after an explosion that causes sudden changes in atmospheric pressure.

47. **Correct answer: D**
    A fourth-degree full thickness burn involves muscle, fat, fascia, or bone. This type of burn usually occurs as a result of deep thermal or electrical burns.

48. **Correct answer: B**
    Hypochloremia and hyponatremia are disadvantages of using 0.5% silver nitrate solution for burn patients.

49. **Correct answer: D**
    The area of a burn that has the closest contact with the heat source and sustains the most damage is the zone of coagulation. Coagulation necrosis is usually the result of most burn injuries.

50. **Correct answer: B**

    After a patient ingests toxic levels of iron, there is a latent asymptomatic phase that occurs 2–12 hours after ingestion. After about 12 hours the patient may enter the next phase, which is an abrupt cardiovascular collapse.

51. **Correct answer: D**

    Ethylene glycol is the toxic ingredient in automobile antifreeze.

52. **Correct answer: B**

    Hydrofluoric acid is absorbed even through intact skin, causing local and systemic effects. Hydrofluoric acid is used as a rust remover, metal cleaner, and to etch glass.

53. **Correct answer: B**

    Vascular thrombosis may result from alkaline substances, and liquefaction necrosis will occur. Serious injury results from products with a pH higher than 12.

54. **Correct answer: C**

    Oven cleaners contain large amounts of alkali. Additional alkaline substances include dishwasher detergent, laundry detergent, drain openers, and ammonia capsules.

55. **Correct answer: D**

    Symptoms of salicylate poisoning include tachycardia and hyperthermia. Additional symptoms include tinnitus, tachypnea, LOC changes, respiratory alkalosis, metabolic acidosis, or mixed acid-base abnormalities. Occult GI tract bleeding may occur.

56. **Correct answer: D**

    Methadone has a half-life of approximately 24 hours and requires continuous doses of naloxone. The continuous doses prevent respiratory depression until the methadone is eliminated from the patient's system.

57. **Correct answer: A**

    Respiratory depression, meiosis, and coma are the triad of symptoms associated with opioid overdose.

58. **Correct answer: C**

    Deferoxamine is used to treat iron poisoning by chelation. It is also possible the patient may have to be treated with GI tract decontamination, which may include gastric lavage or whole bowel irrigation.

59. **Correct answer: C**

    Metabolic acidosis is likely to be seen with an iron overdose. After iron is metabolized, free hydrogen is released and leads to metabolic acidosis.

60. **Correct answer: B**

    Flumazenil is a specific antidote for benzodiazepine overdose. This drug should not be used on patients who overdose on tricyclic antidepressants because of an increased risk of seizures.

61. **Correct answer: B**

    A trough vancomycin level > 20 μg/ml is actually a panic level and if not addressed will cause nephrotoxicity. Ototoxicity usually occurs if levels are prolonged at > 30 μg/ml. Vancomycin may cause hypertension, thrombocytopenia, tubular necrosis, colitis, and deafness. The patient may require hemodialysis, hemofiltration, or peritoneal dialysis. Note: charcoal hemofiltration does not remove vancomycin.

Substance Abuse, Toxicologic, and Environmental | 319

62. **Correct answer: C**
    There is no specific antidote for methamphetamine. It is only possible to treat symptoms as they appear. Desipramine may cause sustained activity of amphetamines in the brain. Alkalinizing agents may potentiate the actions of amphetamines.

63. **Correct answer: D**
    Arsenic poisoning may cause convulsions. Arsenic is found in all human tissues as a trace element. The levels may become elevated with exposure. About 60% of ingested arsenic is excreted in the urine. Arsenic may be found in well water, pesticides, paints, cosmetics, treated wood, and coal. Chronic exposure can lead to various types of cancers.

64. **Correct answer: A**
    The biopsy may cause bleeding from highly vascular tissue. Flank pain may be the first sign, so the patient should be told to report any pain in the flank or abdomen after his procedure.

65. **Correct answer: A**
    After a lung scan (V/Q), you should observe your patient for 60 minutes for possible reaction to the nucleotides. An additional consideration is that when you are discarding urine, wear gloves. You must also wash the gloves with soap and water before removing the gloves. Then, wash your hands again. Many nurses have needlessly exposed themselves to radiation because in their haste to empty fluids for I & Os or at shift change, they forget to don gloves.

66. **Correct answer: C**
    A pacer should be kept at the bedside for a patient with metoprolol overdose because bradycardia, AV block, and hypotension will probably occur.

67. **Correct answer: D**
    Patients who are undergoing alcohol withdrawal are frequently hypoglycemic. Treatment should include thiamine, then bolus with D_{50}, and then start an infusion of D_5W.

68. **Correct answer: B**
    This type of burn may be a superficial or a deep second-degree partial thickness burn. The nerve endings are still intact, and this burn is very painful. Sometimes burns can be deceptive. A reddened area can be diagnosed as a first-degree burn may be overlooked when staff is calculating requirements for fluid and nutrient resuscitation. After a few hours these areas can develop blisters and are only then recognized as dermal burns. There is a new way of assessing burn levels by using a laser Doppler during the first week of treatment.

69. **Correct answer: D**
    The Parkland formula was developed by Dr. Charles Baxter at Parkland Hospital in Dallas, Texas in the 1960s and is still utilized today. It is used nationwide as a standard for fluid resuscitation. There are many other formulas in use, but this one is widely known and will probably be on the CEN examination. The formula is 4 ml fluid × patient's weight (in kg) × % of burn, so 4 × 70 = 280 × 30 = 8400 ml fluid requirement for the first 24 hours. Half the calculated volume is given in the first 8 hours, and then the remaining volume is given over the next 16 hours. Remember to calculate from the time the burn occurred.

70. **Correct answer: B**
    The formula is 4 × 65 = 260 × 45 = 11,700.

71. **Correct answer: C**
    Ringer's lactate is used for a variety of reasons with many of the formulas for burn resuscitation. It is preferred for large volume resuscitation because LR contains 130 mEq/L of sodium compared with normal saline that has 154 mEq/L. LR has a higher pH (6.5) compared to normal saline (5.0). The pH of the LR is close to a normal pH. The patient will be in metabolic acidosis, so the metabolized lactate will buffer the acidosis. LR is also an isotonic crystalloid.

72. **Correct answer: A**
    This will probably not be on the exam, but it may show up as a question within the next year or so. The vitamin C is an antioxidant and it is used to counter oxidant-mediated effects on the inflammatory cascade. Animal studies have shown that if the vitamin C is given within 6 hours of the burn, up to 50% of the fluid needed for resuscitation can be eliminated. Always remember that if you have a burn patient you should start at least two large-bore IVs. Another new treatment involves the use of sub-atmospheric pressure dressings. These dressings may aid in removing excess fluid and help save areas that would otherwise have to be grafted or removed.

73. **Correct answer: B**
    The antidote for digoxin overdose is digoxin immune Fab. Digoxin immune Fab reverses hyperkalemia and most dysrhythmias. Patients in renal failure may require dialysis to remove the digoxin immune Fab.

74. **Correct answer: C**
    Rocky Mountain spotted fever is spread by ticks that carry a rotavirus. Symptoms include a sudden onset fever for 2 to 3 weeks and a rash that may cover the entire body. Treatment must include both chloramphenicol and tetracycline.

75. **Correct answer: C**
    Myoglobinuria is rarely seen with lightning burns. AC current usually causes ventricular fibrillation and DC current usually causes asystole. In some cases arrhythmias are delayed for up to 12 hours. The mechanism of lightning strikes is quite complex. There are five ways lightning can injure a person:
    - A side splash from another object is probably the cause of this patient's injuries. The lightning hits something like a tree and then bounces off.
    - A direct strike may also have occurred.
    - Another type of strike can occur when the person is touching an object that is struck.
    - Ground current effect occurs when energy spreads out across the surface of the earth.
    - Lightning has two strokes, upward and downward. If they do not meet, energy can be directed outward.

    Internal burns are rare. Myoglobinuria rarely occurs. Generally, lightning causes cardiac and respiratory arrest, burns from metals touching the victim (watches, necklaces, earrings), and neurologic damage.

76. **Correct answer: B**
    Sometimes, families do not have enough education to make proper decisions or understand the nature of a disease. Attempting to elicit an appropriate history can be challenging. It is likely this patient has botulism.

77. **Correct answer: B**
Possible adverse effects of fentanyl include respiratory depression, chest wall rigidity, apnea, laryngospasm, abdominal distension, loss of bowel sounds, and generalized muscle rigidity.

78. **Correct answer: A**
Possible adverse effects of morphine include respiratory depression, ileus, abdominal distension, delayed gastric emptying, hypotension, bradycardia, and urine retention.

79. **Correct answer: B**
Fentanyl administered intravenously is incompatible with phenytoin, azithromycin, and pentobarbital.

80. **Correct answer: A**
Contraindications for the use of fentanyl include increased intracranial pressure, severe respiratory disease or depression including acute asthma (unless the patient is mechanically ventilated), and seizures. Additional contraindications include CNS depression, paralytic ileus, severe liver or renal insufficiency, and hyperglycemia (fentanyl may elevate blood glucose). Fentanyl is used in open heart surgery.

81. **Correct answer: C**
Pot (marijuana) produced 10 years ago was more natural with fewer additives. Pot grown and sold in today's market contains 20 times more ammonia and 5 times more hydrogen cyanide, formaldehyde, and PCP. The goal of today's brand of pot is to obtain a more profound, faster, and sustained high. Within a few minutes of ingestion or inhalation, the heart rate may increase from 20 to 80 beats per minute above baseline, and memory loss occurs. There will also be failure of the ability to concentrate, confusion, dry mouth, and an increased appetite. The effects may be compounded and varied if other drugs are cut or mixed with the marijuana.

82. **Correct answer: C**
The correct definition of addiction is when the user cannot live or function without the use of a substance or drug. Addiction withdrawals can be severe or life threatening. Abuse is when the user uses a substance or drug in an amount or function that was not originally intended. An individual who abuses a drug might not be an addict. For example, an individual who uses Benadryl to fall asleep when no allergy symptoms are present is abusing the drug. An addict is usually an abuser by both function and amount of the substance or drug used. Substances or drugs abused range from the obvious (alcohol, marijuana, oxycodone, heroin, and cocaine) to the unexpected (glue, spray paint, nail polish remover, energy drinks, ibuprofen, and cough syrups).

83. **Correct answer: A**
Marijuana is the most commonly abused illegal drug in the world. In many countries and some states medicinal marijuana has been legalized and closely regulated. For more information regarding statistics for a specific area and current ranking, the U.S. government websites at www.dea.gov and www.nida.nih.gov are updated frequently. Toluene is the addictive chemical in glue.

84. **Correct answer: A**
Although you may ask all these questions, the first question should be used to determine if Mary was using actual witch hazel for acne or facial cleaning or if she is

using the slang term "witch hazel" for heroin. Many street drugs may present with innocuous names. Heroin may also be referred to as smack, nose drops (liquid heroin), dragon rock (mixed with cocaine), A-bomb (mixed with marijuana), big H, brown sugar, brown tape, diesel, and old navy. Monitor for additional signs and symptoms of heroin abuse such as venous tracks, bruising, and burnt fingertips from holding a roll lighter to smoke the heroin.

85. **Correct answer: A**

    The sudden collapse of a young woman at a party without explanation is suspicious for gamma hydroxybutyrate (GHB) or ketamine ingestion. These are known date or party rape drugs. Due to the anesthetic and amnesic effects of the drug, an affected female may be unable to describe events leading up to the collapse. To determine exposure the drug screen should be repeated, looking specifically for gamma hydroxybutyrate and/or ketamine.

86. **Correct answer: B**

    A chewed-up pacifier and presentation of euphoria and confusion should lead the staff to consider ecstasy addiction and abuse. Ecstasy, or methylenedioxymethamphetamine (MDMA), causes trismus, or teeth grinding. Users may chew on pacifiers to preserve teeth and hide the grinding from others.

87. **Correct answer: B**

    Activated charcoal does not adsorb metals. Activated charcoal adsorbs most poisons. Activated charcoal cannot be mixed with ice cream or syrups because the charcoal adsorbs many of these agents, rendering it less effective. Single doses of activated charcoal are indicated for serious poison exposures.

88. **Correct answer: A**

    Multiple doses of activated charcoal should be used for ingestions of theophylline. Additional drugs for which multiple doses are indicated include digoxin, phenobarbital, and amitriptyline.

89. **Correct answer: C**

    Acetaminophen is metabolized by the liver. There is some renal metabolism of acetaminophen, so renal injury is a possibility. FYI: In children younger than 10 years, a different metabolic pathway may be followed.

90. **Correct answer: B**

    The effect of ethanol is to suppress the liver's ability to produce glucose. Other symptoms include hypoglycemia, altered mental status, hypothermia, respiratory depression, slurred speech, gastric irritation with vomiting, bradycardia, and vasodilation.

91. **Correct answer: C**

    Patients with methemoglobinemia present with intractable cyanosis unresponsive to oxygen administration, and the blood appears brown when placed on white paper. Methemoglobin is the amount of normal hemoglobin that has been converted and cannot carry oxygen.

92. **Correct answer: C**

    Methylene blue is used to treat methemoglobinemia. Toxicity and other symptoms are treated as they occur.

93. **Correct answer: D**
    Sodium bicarbonate is used to treat tricyclic overdose. Imipramine and doxepin are both tricyclics.

94. **Correct answer: A**
    Amoxapine is a cyclic antidepressant that may cause cardiovascular effects and will probably cause status epilepticus. The patient often requires intubation and muscular paralysis because of seizures.

95. **Correct answer: B**
    Flumazenil is a specific antidote for benzodiazepine overdose. This drug should not be used on patients who overdose on tricyclic antidepressants because of an increased risk of seizures.

96. **Correct answer: A**
    A patient intoxicated with methamphetamine exhibits elevated liver enzymes, tachycardia, hyperthermia, and hypertension.

97. **Correct answer: C**
    Untreated lithium toxicity may lead to seizures, coma, and cardiac dysrhythmias when levels reach greater than 2.5 mEq/L. Toxicity usually occurs with levels of 2 mEq/L, but symptoms may be noted at even lower blood levels with certain body chemistries. Initial toxicity is noted when the patient experiences diarrhea, vomiting, drowsiness, muscular weakness, and disorientation. As toxicity and symptoms worsen, nystagmus, ataxia, giddiness, tinnitus, confusion, and blurred vision may be present. Patients must be managed in the ED by close monitoring and immediate intervention of dysrhythmias and electrolyte imbalances.

98. **Correct answer: A**
    Amitriptyline is classified as a tricyclic antidepressant. A tricyclic antidepressant acts by blocking norepinephrine and serotonin uptake in the central nervous system. They also have anticholinergic properties. The really interesting thing about this group of drugs is that they metabolize in the liver to one of the other tricyclics. You must test for levels of all the tricyclics because the one you are testing for may have metabolized and exacerbated the effect on the patient.

99. **Correct answer: B**
    Sally's treatment should include sodium bicarbonate. ABG results should guide the amount to be given. Hemodialysis will not remove amitriptyline from the system. Syrup of Ipecac is not indicated, especially because the patient ingested the medication last evening. You may give hypertonic saline for hypotension.

100. **Correct answer: B**
    Ketamine is contraindicated in a patient with altered intracranial pressure because it increases ICP and cerebral blood flow.

101. **Correct answer: C**
    Propofol is made from egg phosphates and soybeans. It is incumbent on the nurse to determine if the patient has allergies or sensitivities to these ingredients.

102. Correct answer: C

Methamphetamine is officially classified as a hallucinogen by *The Diagnostic and Statistical Manual of Mental Disorders*. The World Health Organization (WHO) published a list that shows methamphetamine as the second most abused chemical substance. The drug may be ingested, smoked, injected, inserted into the anus or urethra, or snorted. Street names include crystal meth, big blue, base, and ice. The base of the drug is pseudoephedrine or ephedrine mixed with common ingredients. The mixture is often highly explosive and the first warning a meth lab is nearby is when it blows up.

103. Correct answer: C

Alkalinizing agents may potentiate the actions of amphetamines, so their use is contraindicated. As mentioned previously there is no specific antidote for methamphetamine. It is only possible to treat symptoms as they appear.

104. Correct answer: D

Ativan may be used to control the symptoms of cocaine toxicity.

105. Correct answer: D

An anticipated treatment for this patient includes hypothermia. Evaluation for stroke, a toxicology screen, and a stress test are all procedures, not treatments. Additional possible causes of sudden death due to cocaine toxicity include stroke, subarachnoid hemorrhage, and an agitated delirium state.

106. Correct answer: C

Rewarm the affected part using warm water at 40 to 43.3°C (104–110° F). Keep the affected part elevated and do not place heavy blankets over the area. The skin will be a waxy, whitish color. The patient may also have numbness, tingling, or a burning sensation of the affected area.

107. Correct answer: D

Amputations are not an emergency. An amputation may be performed days or weeks after the injury. Priorities are to remove wet clothing, rewarm the patient, administer warm noncaffeinated fluids (if the patient has an intact gag reflex), administer analgesics, and consider tetanus prophylaxis.

108. Correct answer: B

Potassium iodide is helpful to give after exposure to radioactive iodine. The thyroid gland cannot distinguish between regular iodine and radioactive iodine. Potassium iodide can be readily absorbed by the thyroid, saturate it and prevent uptake of radioactive iodine. The body can then excrete the radioactive iodine via other routes. After the earthquake and resultant tsunami in Japan, many people panicked and took potassium iodide needlessly. Side effects of the drug may outweigh any benefit.

SECTION 12: SUBSTANCE ABUSE, TOXICOLOGIC, AND ENVIRONMENTAL REFERENCES

Abanades, S., Farré, M., Segura, M., Pichini, S., Barral, D., Pacifici, R., . . . De La Torre, R. (2006). Gamma-hydroxybutyrate (GHB) in humans: Pharmacodynamics and pharmacokinetics. *Annals of the New York Academy of Sciences, 1074*(1), 559–576.

Ahmadi, J., Kampman, K., Dackis, C., Sparkman, T., & Pettinati, H. (2008). Cocaine withdrawal symptoms identify "Type B" cocaine-dependent patients. *The American Journal on Addictions / American Academy of Psychiatrists in Alcoholism and Addictions, 17*(1), 60–64.

Akdur, O., Durukan, P., Ozkan, S., Avsarogullari, L., Vardar, A., Kavalci, C., & Ikizceli, I. (2010). Poisoning severity score, Glasgow coma scale, corrected QT interval in acute organophosphate poisoning. *Human and Experimental Toxicology, 29*(5), 419–426.

Alexandropoulou, C. A., & Panagiotopoulos, E. (2010). Wound ballistics: Analysis of blunt and penetrating trauma mechanisms. *Health Science Journal, 4*(4), 225–237.

Ameisen, O. (2008). Are the effects of gamma-hydroxybutyrate (GHB) treatment partly physiological in alcohol dependence? *The American Journal of Drug and Alcohol Abuse, 34*(2), 235–236.

Astorino, T., Genrich, I., MacGregor, L., Victor, C. S., Eckhouse, D. R., & Barbour, L. (2009). Necrotizing fasciitis: Early detection may save your patient's limb. *Orthopaedic Nursing, 28*(2), 70–79.

Beletsky, L., Ruthazer, R., Macalino, G. E., Rich, J. D., Tan, L., & Burris, S. (2007). Physicians' knowledge of and willingness to prescribe naloxone to reverse accidental opiate overdose: Challenges and opportunities. *Journal of Urban Health: Bulletin of the New York Academy of Medicine, 84*(1), 126–136.

Benhalim, S., Leggett, G. E., Jamie, H., & Waring, W. S. (2008). Proteinuria is unrelated to the extent of acute acetaminophen overdose: a prospective clinical study. *Journal of Medical Toxicology: Official Journal of the American College of Medical Toxicology, 4*(4), 232–237.

Berg, R., Talving, P., & Inaba, K. (2011). Cardiac rupture following blunt trauma. *Trauma: London, 13*(1), 35–46.

Bernal, W., Auzinger, G., Dhawan, A., & Wendon, J. (2010). Acute liver failure. *The Lancet, 376*(9736), 190.

Beynon, A. (2010). Gunshot wounds. *Nursing Standard, 25*(3), 59.

Brier, M. (2010). Brown recluse spider bite. *The Clinical Advisor: For Nurse Practitioners, 13*(1), 57–59.

Buechler, C., Schäffler, A., Johann, M., Neumeier, M., Köhl, P., Weiss, T., . . . Hellerbrand, C. (2009). Elevated adiponectin serum levels in patients with chronic alcohol abuse rapidly decline during alcohol withdrawal. *Journal of Gastroenterology and Hepatology, 24*(4), 558–563.

Carter, M. R., & Gaskins, S. W. (2010). Incorporating bioterrorism content in the nursing curriculum: A creative approach. *Journal of Nursing Education, 49*(7), 406.

Cauchy, E., Cheguillaume, B., & Chetaille, E. (2011). A controlled trial of a prostacyclin and rt-PA in the treatment of severe frostbite. *The New England Journal of Medicine, 364*(2), 189.

Chan, B., Whyte, I., Dawson, A., & Downes, M. (2005). Use of neostigmine for the management of drug induced ileus in severe poisonings. *Journal of Medical Toxicology: Official Journal of the American College of Medical Toxicology, 1*(1), 18–22.

Chan, G. M., Stajic, M., Marker, E. K., Hoffman, R. S., & Nelson, L. S. (2006). Testing positive for methadone and either a tricyclic antidepressant or a benzodiazepine is associated with an accidental overdose death: Analysis of medical examiner data. *Academic Emergency Medicine, 13*(5), 543–547.

Chen, C. Y., & Anthony, J. C. (2004). Epidemiological estimates of risk in the process of becoming dependent upon cocaine: Cocaine hydrochloride powder versus crack cocaine. *Psychopharmacology, 172*(1), 78–86.

Coentrao, L., & Moura, D. (2011). Acute cyanide poisoning among jewelry and textile industry workers. *American Journal of Emergency Medicine, 29*(1), 78–81.

Emergency Nurses Association, Newberry, L., & Criddle, L. M. (2007). *Sheehy's manual of emergency care* (6th ed.). St. Louis, MO: Mosby.

Eyer, F., Stenzel, J., Schuster, T., Felgenhauer, N., Pfab, R., von Bary, C., & Zilker, T. (2009). Risk assessment of severe tricyclic antidepressant overdose. *Human & Experimental Toxicology, 28*(8), 511–519.

Eyer, F., Steimer, W., Muller, C., & Zilker, T. (2010). Cases of note: Free and total digoxin in serum during treatment of acute digoxin poisoning with fab fragments: case study. *American Journal of Critical Care, 19*(4), 387–391.

Fung, H. T., Lai, C. H., Wong, O. F., Lam, K. K., & Kam, C. W. (2008). Two cases of methemoglobinemia following zopiclone ingestion. *Clinical Toxicology, 46*(2), 167–170.

Gagnon, D., Lemire, B. B., Casa, D. J., & Kenny, J. P. (2010). Cold-water immersion and the treatment of hyperthermia: Using 38.6°C as a safe rectal temperature cooling limit. *Journal of Athletic Training, 45*(5), 439–545.

Gasparis Vonfrolio, L., & Noone, J. (1997). *Emergency nursing examination review* (3rd ed.). Staten Island, NY: Power Publications.

Gillman, K. (2010). Interaction of temperature regulation mechanisms. *The Lancet, 376*(9737), 233–235.

Goodman, R., & Hollimon, D. (2010). Allergic contact dermatitis: Poison ivy. *Dermatology Nursing, 22*(4), 26–29.

Hall, A. H., Saiers, J., & Baud, F. (2009). Which cyanide antidote? *Critical Reviews in Toxicology, 39*(7), 541–552.

Hardin, S. R., & Kaplow, R. (2010). *Cardiac surgery essentials for critical care nursing.* Sudbury, MA: Jones & Bartlett Learning.

Hayes, P. C., Faestel, P. M., Shimamoto, P. L., & Holland, C. (2007). Alcohol withdrawal requiring massive prolonged benzodiazepine infusion. *Military Medicine, 172*(5), 556–559.

Holleran, R. S. (2005). *Emergency transport nursing* (4th ed.). St. Louis, MO: Mosby.

Jacobs, B. B., & Hoyt, K. S. (2007). *Trauma nursing core course provider manual* (6th ed.). Bedford, IL: Emergency Nurses Association.

Jagodzinski, N. A., Weerasinghe, C., & Porter, K. (2010). Crush injuries and crush syndrome—a review. Part 1: the systemic injury. *Trauma: London, 12*(2), 69–89.

Jagodzinski, N. A., Weerasinghe, C., & Porter, K. (2010). Crush injuries and crush syndrome—a review. Part 2: the local injury. *Trauma, 12*(3), 133–149.

Järvinen, K. M. (2009). Allergic reactions to stinging and biting insects and arachnids. *Pediatric Annals, 38*(4), 199–210.

Jones & Bartlett Learning (2011). *2011 nurse's drug handbook* (10th ed.). Sudbury, MA: Jones & Bartlett Learning.

Kuzak, N., Brubacher, J. R., & Kennedy, J. R. (2007). Reversal of salicylate-induced euglycemic delirium with dextrose. *Clinical Toxicology, 45*(5), 526–529.

Lee, S., Ryu, S., Lee, J. W., Kim, S. W., Yoo, I. S., & You, Y. H. (2011). Hyperthermia occurred after hyperbaric oxygen therapy for carbon monoxide poisoning. *American Journal of Emergency Medicine, 29*(2), 235.

Lippincott. (2010). *Professional guide to signs and symptoms* (6th ed.). New York, NY: Lippincott.

Mazer, M., & Perrone, J. (2008). Acetaminophen-induced nephrotoxicity: Pathophysiology, clinical manifestations, and management. *Journal of Medical Toxicology: Official Journal of the American College of Medical Toxicology, 4*(1), 2–6.

McLafferty, E. (2010). Prevention and management of hyperthermia during a heatwave. *Nursing Older People, 22*(7), 23–28.

Nanau, R. M., & Neuman, M. G. (2010). Ibuprofen-induced hypersensitivity syndrome. *Translational Research, 155*(6), 275–293.

Napoli, M. (2006). Overdose of acetaminophen, A. K. A. Tylenol, the leading cause of acute liver failure in the U.S. *HealthFacts, 31*(4), 6.

Nelson, L., & Schwaner, R. (2009). Transdermal fentanyl: Pharmacology and toxicology. *Journal of Medical Toxicology: Official Journal of the American College of Medical Toxicology, 5*(4), 230–241.

Nyamathi, A. M., Casillas, A., King, L., Gresham, L., Pierce, E., Farb, D., & Wiechmann, C. (2010). Computerized bioterrorism education and training for nurses on bioterrorism attack agents. *The Journal of Continuing Education in Nursing, 41*(8), 375.

Otto-Duessel, M., Brewer, C., & Wood, J. C. (2011). Interdependence of cardiac iron and calcium in a murine model of iron overload. *Translational Research, 157*(2), 92–99.

Page, C., Hacket, L. P., & Isbister, G. K. (2009). The use of high-dose insulin-glucose euglycemia in beta-blocker overdose: A case report. *Journal of Medical Toxicology: Official Journal of the American College of Medical Toxicology, 5*(3), 139–143.

Pakravan, N., Waring, W. S., Sharma, S., Ludlam, C., Megson, I., & Bateman, D. N. (2008). Risk factors and mechanisms of anaphylactoid reactions to acetylcysteine in acetaminophen overdose. *Clinical Toxicology, 46*(8), 697–702.

Parks, T., Gkrania-Klotsas, E., & Nicholl, C. (2010). Treatment with monoclonal antibodies against clostridium difficile toxins. *The New England Journal of Medicine, 362*(15), 1444.

Phillips, K., Luk, A., Soor, G. S., Abraham, J. R., Leong, S., & Butany, J. (2009). Cocaine cardiotoxicity: A review of the pathophysiology, pathology, and treatment options. *American Journal of Cardiovascular Drugs: Drugs, Devices, and Other Interventions, 9*(3), 177–196.

Pizon, A. F., Riley, B. D., LoVecchio, F., & Gill, R. (2007). Safety and efficacy of crotalidae polyvalent immune fab in pediatric crotaline envenomations. *Academic Emergency Medicine, 14*(4), 373.

Proehl, J. A. (2008). *Emergency nursing procedures* (4th ed.). St. Louis, MO: Saunders.

Rehman, H., & Seguin, A. (2009). Frostbite. *The New England Journal of Medicine, 361*(25), 2461.

Riddle, E., Bush, J., Tittle, M., & Dilkhush, D. (2010). Alcohol withdrawal: Development of a standing order set. *Critical Care Nurse, 30*(3), 38–48.

Rollin, A., Maury, P., Guilbeau-Frugier, C., & Brugada, J. (2011). Transient ST elevation after ketamine intoxication: A new cause of acquired Brugada ECG Pattern. *Journal of Cardiovascular Electrophysiology, 22*(1), 91–94.

Sam, A. H., & Beynon, H. L. (2010). Wound botulism. *The New England Journal of Medicine, 363*(25), 2444.

Schier, J. G., Schurz Rogers, H., Patel, M. M., Rubin, C. A., & Belson, M. G. (2006). Strategies for recognizing acute chemical-associated foodborne illness. *Military Medicine: Bethesda, 171*(12), 1174–1181.

Schroeter, M., Alpers, K., VanTreeck, U., Frank, C., Rosenkoetter, N., & Schaumann, R. (2009). Outbreak of wound botulism in injecting drug users. *Epidemiology and Infection: Cambridge, 137*(11), 1602–1609.

Shepherd, G. (2006). Treatment of poisoning caused by beta-adrenergic and calcium-channel blockers. *American Journal of Health-System Pharmacy: Official Journal of the American Society of Health-System Pharmacists, 63*(19), 1828–1835.

Sorbie, C. (2009). Explosions and Blast Injuries. *Orthopedics (Online), 32*(11), 804–806.

Spain, J. K., Liotta, C., Terrell, T., & Branoff, R. (2010). Heat-related illness in athletes: Recognition and treatment. *Athletic Training & Sports Health Care, 2*(4), 152–155.

Stapenhorst, L., Hesse, A., & Hoppe, B. (2008). Hyperoxaluria after ethylene glycol poisoning. *Pediatric Nephrology, 23*(12), 2277–2279.

Stolbach, A. I., Hoffman, R. S., & Nelson, L. S. (2008). Mechanical ventilation was associated with acidemia in a case series of salicylate-poisoned patients. *Academic Emergency Medicine: Official Journal of the Society for Academic Emergency Medicine, 15*(9), 866–869.

Sztajnkrycer, M. D., Mell, H. K., & Melin, G. J. (2007). Development and implementation of an emergency department observation unit protocol for deliberate drug ingestion in adults: Preliminary results. *Clinical Toxicology, 45*(5), 499–504.

Thanacoody, H. K., & Thomas, S. H. (2005). Tricyclic antidepressant poisoning: Cardiovascular toxicity. *Toxicological Reviews, 24*(3), 205–214.

Tobalem, M., Modarressi, A., Elias, B., Harder, Y., & Pittet, B. (2010). Frostbite complicating therapeutic surface cooling after heat stroke. *Intensive Care Medicine, 36*(9), 1614.

Urdern, L. D., Stacy, K. M., & Lough, M. E. (2005). *Thelan's critical care nursing* (5th ed.). St. Louis, MO: Mosby.

Waring, W. S., Stephen, A. F., Malkowska, A. M., & Robinson, O. D. (2008). Acute ethanol coingestion confers a lower risk of hepatotoxicity after deliberate acetaminophen overdose. *Academic Emergency Medicine: Official Journal of the Society for Academic Emergency Medicine, 15*(1), 54–58.

Warrell, D.A. (2010). Snake bite. *The Lancet, 375*(9708), 77–89.

Watson, S., & Gorski, K. A. (2011). *Invasive cardiology* (3rd ed.). Sudbury, MA: Jones & Bartlett Learning.

Wilkes, J. M., Clark, L. E., & Herrera, J. L. (2005). Acetaminophen overdose in pregnancy. *Southern Medical Journal, 98*(11), 1118–1122.

Williams, G., & Williams, E. (2010). A nursing guide to surviving a radiological dispersal device. *British Journal of Nursing, 19*(1), 24.

Wurst, F. M., Dürsteler-MacFarland, K. M., Auwaerter, V., Ergovic, S., Thon, N., Yegles, M., . . . Wiesbeck, G. A. (2008). Assessment of alcohol use among methadone maintenance patients by direct ethanol metabolites and self-reports. *Alcoholism, Clinical and Experimental Research, 32*(9), 1552–1557.

Zeilig, G., Weingarden, H. P., Zwecker, M., & Rubin-Asher, D. (2010). Civilian spinal cord injuries due to terror explosions. *Spinal Cord: Houndsmills, 48*(11), 814–819.

SECTION 13:

Medical Emergencies

1. Which of the following is not considered a direct source of energy that would lead to a patient's injury?
   A. Electrical
   B. Oxygen deprivation
   C. Chemical
   D. Thermal

2. If a patient sustains an injury from electromagnetic waves such as those from an x-ray, the type of energy involved is
   A. Mechanical
   B. Electrical
   C. Chemical
   D. Radiant

3. When energy is transferred from a bullet to an individual, the type of energy transferred is called
   A. Mechanical energy
   B. Kinematic energy
   C. Physical energy
   D. Thermal energy

4. Which of the following statements is true about mechanical energy, external forces, and moving objects?
   A. Mass and velocity are important to the amount of energy a moving object has, and mass is the most important component
   B. If mass is doubled, then the energy is tripled
   C. All inanimate objects do not have speed. It is the impact of the victim that transfers energy
   D. If velocity is doubled, energy is quadrupled

5. The force that decreases or stops the velocity of a moving person is called
   A. Terminal force
   B. Tensile force
   C. Deceleration
   D. Acceleration

— 329 —

6. When energy is loaded onto the body, the tissues change dimensions. These changes are known as stress and strain. Which of the following is not considered to be a type of stress?
   A. Shearing
   B. Deformative
   C. Tensile
   D. Compressive

7. If your patient was an unrestrained driver and his car was T-boned by another vehicle, given the type of impact (lateral), what injuries is your patient likely to suffer?
   A. Chest
   B. Same side, clavicle
   C. Upper abdomen
   D. Posterior dislocation of the hip

8. Which of the following components is not considered part of a secondary survey of a trauma patient?
   A. History
   B. Comfort measures
   C. Vital signs
   D. Disability

9. When assessing bilateral breath sounds, it is best to place the stethoscope at the
   A. Second intercostal space midclavicular line and fifth intercostal space, anterior axillary line
   B. Fifth intercostal space, midclavicular line and second intercostal space, anterior axillary line
   C. Third intercostal space, midaxillary line and third intercostal space, midaxillary line
   D. Fifth intercostal space, midclavicular line, second intercostal space, midaxillary line

10. When obtaining a history from a trauma patient, some ED nurses use the mnemonic MIVT. These letters stand for
    A. Mechanism, injury, vitals, and treatment
    B. Mental, injury, verbalization, and time
    C. Mentation, injury, vitals, and tensile
    D. Mechanism, injury, verbalization, and time

11. When palpating the abdomen, which of the following responses is considered a subjective sign?
    A. Rigidity
    B. Guarding
    C. A mass
    D. A statement of pain

12. When inspecting the posterior surfaces of a trauma victim, it is important to remember to
    A. Avoid palpation of the vertebral column so as not to displace a possible fracture
    B. Always order chest, C-spine, and pelvic x-rays for patients
    C. Avoid palpation of the anal sphincter as autonomic dysreflexia may occur
    D. Maintain cervical stabilization and logroll the patient away from the inspector

13. The Revised Trauma Score is a physiologic scoring system and has been shown to be a reliable predictor of death. Components of this scoring system include
    A. Location of injuries, level of consciousness, and estimated blood loss
    B. Glasgow coma scale, systolic blood pressure, and respiratory rate
    C. Level of consciousness, motor response, and eye opening
    D. Vital signs, level of consciousness, and blood loss

14. Which of the following injuries is not considered a secondary brain injury?
    A. A fractured skull
    B. Cerebral edema
    C. Hypoxemia
    D. Increased ICP

15. A diffuse brain injury that results from both acceleration and deceleration forces and produces shearing and tensile stresses with axonal damage is called a
    A. Concussion
    B. Brain contusion
    C. Diffuse axonal injury
    D. Subdural bleed

16. The most common cause of blunt chest trauma is
    A. Falls
    B. Gunshot wounds
    C. Automobile accidents
    D. Stabbings

17. A needle thoracentesis should be performed
    A. At the fifth intercostal space, midaxillary line, affected side
    B. At the third intercostal space, midclavicular line, affected side
    C. At the fifth intercostal space, midaxillary line, affected side
    D. At the second intercostal space, midclavicular line, affected side

18. What are the most common presenting symptoms of myxedema coma?
    A. Facial swelling, ptosis, altered mental status, alopecia
    B. Ptosis, goiter, tachycardia, hypertension
    C. Altered mental status, hypertension, bradycardia
    D. Hypothermia, altered mental status, tachycardia

19. There are no intensive care unit beds for your patient with myxedema coma, so initial treatment will be done in the ED until a bed is available. What treatments do you anticipate for this patient?
    A. Tapazole, fluid and electrolyte replacement
    B. Levothyroxine, fluids and electrolyte replacement, correction of cause of myxedema
    C. Fluids and electrolytes, levothyroxine, methimazole
    D. Levothyroxine, beta-blockers, fluids and electrolyte replacement

20. If a patient suffers loss of autonomic function with loss of thermoregulation, the patient is said to be
    A. Poikilothermic
    B. Odontoid
    C. Hypothermic
    D. Hyperthermic

21. Diaphragmatic function is impaired with spinal injury at the level of
    A. C3 to C5
    B. C5 to T3
    C. T3 to T5
    D. T5 to T8

22. Which of the following actions is not required to be performed prior to transfer of an ED patient to another facility?
    A. Provide an appropriate medical screening exam
    B. Certification by the physician that the patient is able to be transferred
    C. Notification of the patient's significant other
    D. Send all medical records with the patient

23. Your hospital has just received word of a mass casualty incident. You are called from home to report to the ED and assist with triage of patients. The preliminary report is that you will be receiving as many as 40 patients. The first patient you see is a male, with multiple lacerations. He is awake and alert and complaining of pain in the right chest and right upper quadrant. There is no rebound tenderness. You confirm that ribs 7–9 are fractured. You suspect which of the following underlying conditions/injuries?
    A. Spleen laceration
    B. Liver laceration
    C. Pneumothorax
    D. Mesenteric infarction

24. The second patient you see during a mass casualty incident is a female who was trapped in her car for almost 2 hours by the steering column. She complains of left shoulder pain, left upper quadrant rebound tenderness, and she presents with an obviously fractured lower leg that was splinted by paramedics. The paramedics had listed her as stable and stated she had no rebound tenderness or guarding at the accident scene. She is tachycardic at 128, BP is 82/50, and has fractures of ribs 9–10. You suspect this patient has a
    A. Ruptured pancreas
    B. Diaphragm rupture
    C. Spleen injury
    D. Lacerated liver

25. The third patient you triage from a mass casualty is a female. She is confused but complains of back pain at the level of L3. She is hypotensive and has swelling at the level of L1-3. You suspect which of the following type of injury?
    A. Splenic rupture
    B. Kidney laceration
    C. Large bowel rupture
    D. Retroperitoneal liver injury

26. The ED unit director has tasked you with representing the emergency department in a risk management task force. The purpose of risk management is to
    A. Identify healthcare staff who are negligent
    B. Collect and store records regarding potential and actual injuries in the hospital
    C. Monitor staff competency
    D. Determine scope of practice within the hospital based on financial liability

27. To provide consistent and complete transfer of care from one healthcare professional to another, regulating bodies recommend standardized report-off or hand-off documentation or reports. An example of this is
    A. RBAR
    B. SOAR
    C. SBAR
    D. DBAR

28. Which type of isolation is required for vancomycin-resistant enterococci (VRE) infections?
    A. Standard or universal precautions
    B. Reverse isolation
    C. Contact isolation
    D. Droplet isolation

29. You are caring for a 45 year old woman in the ED with mononucleosis. What symptoms do expect this patient to exhibit?
    A. Fever, chills, sore throat, cough
    B. Sore throat, lymphadenopathy, maculopapular rash
    C. Hepatosplenomegaly, nasal congestion, maculopapular rash
    D. Lymphadenopathy, fever, cough

30. What teaching should be done for the patient with infectious mononucleosis when discharging them from the ED?
    A. There are no special precautions
    B. Avoid contact sports and activities that increase intra-abdominal pressure
    C. Antibiotics will cure the mononucleosis
    D. Expect to feel better in 7–10 days

31. What treatment do you anticipate for the ED patient with infectious mononucleosis?
    A. Supportive therapy for most patients
    B. Intravenous antibiotics and contact isolation
    C. Acyclovir 400 mg orally every 8 hours for 10 days
    D. High-dose intravenous steroids

32. What is the causative agent in infectious mononucleosis?
    A. *Streptococcus pyogenes*
    B. *Streptococcus mutans*
    C. Epstein-Barr virus
    D. Herpes simplex I

33. The major immunoglobulin of serum and interstitial fluid is
    A. IgG
    B. IgA
    C. IgE
    D. IgM

34. A decrease in the available number of erythrocytes caused by bone marrow production failure is known as
    A. Chronic anemia
    B. Hemolytic anemia
    C. Aplastic anemia
    D. Pernicious anemia

35. What is the purpose of testing $HgbA_{1c}$ in patients with diabetes mellitus?
    A. It is of little help in managing diabetes mellitus
    B. It measures blood sugars over a 6-month period
    C. It measures the effectiveness of diabetes mellitus therapy
    D. It measures red blood cell activity in diabetes mellitus

36. The patient you are caring for has been diagnosed with central diabetes insipidus. The anticipated treatment for this condition is
    A. Thyroid-stimulating hormone
    B. Aldosterone
    C. Sliding scale insulin
    D. DDAVP

37. Your patient was admitted to the ED for low H and H secondary to epistaxis and bleeding into the diaphragm. She bleeds from the gums, even with only the lightest stimulus. Petechiae are noted on her chest and arms. Her platelet count is < 100,000. Her probable diagnosis is
    A. ITP
    B. Pernicious anemia
    C. Aplastic anemia
    D. Hemolytic anemia

38. The anterior pituitary gland controls which of the following glands?
    A. Parathyroid, adrenal medulla, gonads
    B. Thyroid, adrenal cortex, gonads
    C. Parathyroid, thyroid, gonads
    D. Thyroid, adrenal medulla, gonads

39. Which of the following conditions inhibits the release of thyroxine?
    A. Hypocalcemia
    B. Hyperthermia
    C. Hypernatremia
    D. Hypokalemia

40. High blood viscosity and low oxygen tension are the cause of which of the following types of anemia?
    A. Pernicious anemia
    B. Aplastic anemia
    C. Sickle-cell anemia
    D. Hemolytic anemia

41. Your patient has been prescribed Epogen. As an ED nurse, you know adverse effects of Epogen include
    A. Decreased thrombosis
    B. Increased iron
    C. Hypertension
    D. Decreased BUN

42. Cellular humoral immunity is mediated by which of the following types of cells?
    A. Eosinophils
    B. B lymphocytes
    C. T Lymphocytes
    D. Killer cells

43. What is the function of ADH (antidiuretic hormone)?
    A. Aldosterone production
    B. Sodium balance
    C. Water balance
    D. Potassium balance

44. Signs and symptoms of heat stroke include
    A. Slow pulse
    B. Hot dry skin
    C. Muscle cramps
    D. Fatigue

45. All the clotting factors in blood are synthesized in the liver except
    A. VIII and XII
    B. VII and IX
    C. IX and III
    D. IIa and IXa

46. Your patient has a tumor on her anterior pituitary gland. As an ED nurse, you know stimulation of the anterior pituitary gland is from the hypothalamus by way of the
    A. Sympathetic nervous system
    B. Feedback mechanism
    C. Vascular system
    D. Parasympathetic nervous system

47. Calcitonin is released by the
    A. Thyroid gland
    B. Adrenal medulla
    C. Hypothalamus
    D. Anterior pituitary gland

48. The synthesis of hemoglobin is regulated by
    A. A myeloid stem cell
    B. Erythropoietin
    C. Thromboplastin
    D. Thrombopoietin

49. A function of a red blood cell is
    A. Cell humoral mediation
    B. To function as a macrophage
    C. To initiate hemostasis
    D. Carbonic acid dissociation

50. The physician has ordered an MCH test for your patient. This test evaluates
    A. The average concentration of RBCs in a single sample
    B. The average amount (by weight) of hemoglobin in each RBC
    C. The average size and volume of a single RBC
    D. The average concentration of hemoglobin per single RBC

51. Which of the following statements regarding ABO incompatibilities is true?
    A. ABO incompatibility is more frequent in mothers with type O blood
    B. ABO incompatibility is more severe in mothers with type AB blood
    C. ABO incompatibility is more severe than Rh incompatibility
    D. ABO incompatibility does not protect against fetal Rh disease

52. Josh's serum calcium level is high. An increase in serum calcium, glucagon, or magnesium will stimulate the release of
    A. Parathyroid hormone
    B. Calcitonin
    C. Endogenous epinephrine
    D. Aldosterone

53. Georgia has been diagnosed with SIADH. What is the most common presentation of a patient with SIADH (syndrome of inappropriate antidiuretic hormone)?
    A. Excessive, dilute urine output
    B. Seizures
    C. Hypotension
    D. Tetany

54. Your patient has been diagnosed with DIC. Which of the following drugs is useful in the treatment of DIC to inhibit fibrinolysis?
    A. Heparin
    B. Cryoprecipitate
    C. Prednisone
    D. Amicar

55. Ida has a history of hemolytic anemia. She was admitted today for chest pain, fever, and heart failure. These symptoms indicate Ida is probably suffering from
    A. A hemolytic crisis
    B. Pulmonary edema
    C. DIC
    D. A myocardial infarction

56. Immune-mediated HITT usually begins about _____ after the initiation of heparin therapy
    A. 24 hours
    B. 72 hours
    C. 3 days
    D. 5–7 days

57. Which of the following statements is true regarding glucagon?
    A. Glucagon promotes glycolysis
    B. Glucagon enables glucose to move into the cells
    C. Glucagon helps the body store glycogen
    D. Glucagon is released from the alpha cells in the pancreas

58. An increase in catecholamines and amino acids with a decrease in serum glucose stimulates the release of
    A. Calcitonin
    B. Insulin
    C. Aldosterone
    D. Glucagon

59. A high serum magnesium or phosphate level, low serum calcium, with catecholamine release results in secretion of
    A. Aldosterone
    B. Parathyroid hormone
    C. Glyceride
    D. Phosphates

60. Your patient requires an exchange transfusion. A major side effect of an exchange transfusion is
    A. ABO incompatibility
    B. Air embolism
    C. Urticaria
    D. Hematoma

61. A partial thromboplastin time (PTT) is used to assess
    A. Intrinsic and common portions of the coagulation cascade
    B. The number of fibrin degradation products present
    C. The number of platelets
    D. The increased use of clotting factors

62. The extrinsic system of the coagulation cascade is initiated by
    A. Exposure of cell membrane tissue factor
    B. Vascular endothelial injury
    C. Irritation of the intimal lining of blood vessels
    D. Factor X activation

63. Which of the following tests is used to assess the extrinsic and common pathways of the coagulation cascade?
    A. Split fibrin product
    B. Prothrombin time
    C. Partial thromboplastin time
    D. Activated clotting time

64. The most important nursing consideration in the infant patient with HHNS is
    A. To prevent dysrhythmias
    B. The administration of insulin
    C. To prevent aspiration
    D. To monitor electrolytes

65. The most common cause of hypothyroidism is
    A. Graves' disease
    B. Acromegaly
    C. Hashimoto's disease
    D. Decreased cortisol levels

66. A transfusion reaction that usually occurs within 5–30 minutes of the start of the transfusion is known as
    A. An allergic reaction
    B. A febrile reaction
    C. An acute intravascular hemolytic reaction
    D. An acute extravascular hemolytic reaction

67. Pernicious anemia results from a lack of
    A. Vitamin B_6
    B. Vitamin A
    C. Vitamin B_{12}
    D. Vitamin E

68. Which of the following conditions must be present for calcium to be optimally utilized by the body?
    A. Increased oral calcium intake
    B. Increased phosphorus
    C. A euthyroid state
    D. Adequate vitamin D levels

69. Your patient is having aldosterone levels monitored daily. Which of the following is a primary effect of aldosterone?
    A. Aldosterone promotes sodium loss
    B. Aldosterone increases renal potassium excretion
    C. Aldosterone decreases potassium excretion
    D. Aldosterone increases water loss

70. Aldosterone is secreted by the
    A. Zona reticularis of the adrenal cortex
    B. Zona glomerulus of the adrenal cortex
    C. Posterior pituitary gland
    D. Adrenal medulla

71. Aldosterone secretion is regulated by
    A. Anterior hypothalamus
    B. Potassium ions in intracellular fluid
    C. Angiotensin II
    D. Hypercalcemia

72. A pharmacologic antagonist to vitamin K is
    A. Neostigmine
    B. Digoxin
    C. Amiodarone
    D. Phenobarbital

73. Your patient's aldosterone levels are low. As his nurse you know a factor that suppresses aldosterone production is
    A. Hypocalcemia
    B. Hyperkalemia
    C. Stress
    D. Atrial natriuretic hormone

74. Ethan is being treated in the ED for respiratory difficulty. He has been increasingly restless and now has petechiae on the trunk, arms, and legs. His abdomen is slightly distended, and he demonstrates increased respiratory effort. Ethan is now obtunded. During your assessment you note pink-tinged urine in the Foley bag, generalized ecchymosis, and oozing from the IV line insertion point. You suspect Ethan may have
    A. DIC
    B. Pulmonary emboli
    C. A fat embolism
    D. Meningitis

75. Cyclosporine has significant adverse effects that include
    A. Hepatotoxicity
    B. Hypertension
    C. Acute pancreatitis
    D. Hypokalemia

76. An antirejection drug classified as antimetabolite is
    A. Cyclosporine
    B. Terralimus
    C. Prednisolone
    D. Imuran

77. Functions of the thyroid gland, adrenal gland, and male and female reproductive glands are regulated by the
    A. Thyroid gland
    B. Pineal gland of the brain
    C. Pineal–pituitary axis
    D. Hypothalamic–pituitary axis

78. Where is the pituitary gland located?
    A. Superior to the hypothalamus gland near the optic chiasm
    B. Inferior to the hypothalamus and sits in the sella turcica of the skull
    C. Between the thalamus and hypothalamus in the midbrain
    D. Superior to the pons and brainstem

79. Cortisol is a glucocorticoid. A major effect of cortisol in the body is to
    A. Increase the loss of sodium from small intestines
    B. Lower blood pressure in times of stress
    C. Raise the level of free amino acids in the serum
    D. Stimulate urine loss

80. An absolute contraindication for a single-lung, double-lung, or heart-lung transplant is
    A. Liver diseases
    B. Psychiatric illness
    C. Previous cardiothoracic surgery
    D. Kidney disease

81. Factor VIII deficiency is also known as
    A. Hemophilia B
    B. Sickle-cell anemia
    C. Von Willebrand's disease
    D. Aplastic anemia

82. The blood component that contains factor VIII is
    A. FFP
    B. PRBCs
    C. Salt-poor albumin
    D. Cryoprecipitate

83. How does hyperglycemic, hyperosmolar, nonketotic syndrome (HHNS) differ from diabetic ketoacidosis (DKA)?
    A. HHNS has the same onset, higher blood sugars, more dehydration than DKA
    B. HHNS has slower onset, lower blood sugars, less dehydration than DKA
    C. HHNS has a slower onset, much higher blood sugar, more profound dehydration than DKA
    D. HHNS has the same onset, lower blood sugar, no dehydration than DKA

84. Tyrone has been diagnosed with HHNS. What lab results would you anticipate for this patient?
    A. Glucose 550, positive ketones, serum osmolality 280 mOsm/L
    B. Glucose 1258, negative ketones, serum osmolality 375 mOsm/L
    C. Glucose 700, negative ketones, serum osmolality 270 mOsm/L
    D. Glucose 600, positive ketones, serum osmolality 240 mOsm/L

85. Ramon has congenital hypothyroidism. Congenital hypothyroidism is manifested by
    A. A decreased TSH and a decreased T_4
    B. A euthyroid state
    C. An elevated TSH and a decreased T_4
    D. A decreased TSH and an elevated T_4

86. A fluid that causes decreased platelet aggregation and possible allergic reactions is
    A. Hetastarch
    B. Dextran
    C. Lactated Ringer's
    D. D_5/Isolyte M

87. Your patient is to receive two units of packed cells over the next 2 hours. When patients receive multiple transfusions, they are susceptible to increased
    A. Bilirubin and amylase levels
    B. BUN and creatinine levels
    C. Serum potassium levels
    D. Sodium and magnesium retention

88. Signs of vitamin D toxicity include
    A. Seizures
    B. Increased susceptibility to respiratory diseases
    C. Azotemia
    D. Hypocalcemia

89. Kayexalate is given as a treatment for hyperkalemia. What is the mechanism of action of this drug?
    A. Kayexalate exchanges sodium ions for potassium ions
    B. Kayexalate preserves the sodium pump
    C. Kayexalate permanently exchanges 1 gram of medication for 1 mEq of potassium
    D. Kayexalate moves potassium into the intracellular space

90. Nick has a crush injury to his right thigh from falling off his motorcycle. Why does this put Nick at risk for hyperkalemia?
    A. There is more risk for hypokalemia
    B. He is at no risk for hyperkalemia
    C. Cellular destruction leads to increased circulating potassium levels.
    D. Wound infection decreases potassium levels

91. A medication that may cause hemolytic anemia is
    A. Phenobarbital
    B. Furosemide
    C. Quinidine
    D. Captopril

92. Your patient has been diagnosed with decompression illness. The fluid of choice to help resuscitate this patient is
    A. D_5W
    B. $D_{10}W$
    C. Lactated Ringer's solution
    D. D_5/Isolyte M

93. Which of the following conditions contribute to the development of acute hypoglycemia?
    A. Insulinoma
    B. Glucose consumption exceeds glucose production
    C. Oral antihyperglycemic agents
    D. Alcoholism

94. Randall has recurrent episodes of acute hypoglycemia and is a frequent patient in your ED. What therapies may be used to treat acute hypoglycemia (blood sugar less than 50 mg/dl)?
    A. Small, frequent meals, increased carbohydrate consumption
    B. Intravenous D_{50} administration, oral glucose, and treat the cause
    C. Increased carbohydrate diet, intravenous glucose
    D. Treat the cause, increased carbohydrate consumption

95. Joel is admitted to the ED with a diagnosis of diabetic ketoacidosis. As his nurse you know his insulin drip will be titrated by sliding scale and his anion gap. What does the anion gap measure?
    A. An estimate of cations and anions
    B. An estimate of unmeasured anions
    C. An estimate of potassium in the blood
    D. Estimate of the correction of the acid-base balance

96. Your patient was admitted with a factor VIII deficiency. In addition to specific factor VIII, the blood component that carries factor VIII, factor XIII, and fibrinogen is
    A. FFP
    B. PRBC
    C. Salt-poor albumin
    D. Cryoprecipitate

97. Possible causes of thrombocytopenia could include
    A. Alcoholism
    B. Portal hypertension
    C. Latex sensitivity
    D. A low protein diet

98. Your patient with diabetic ketoacidosis has a HCO_3 level of 10 mEq/L. In addition to an insulin drip, you should anticipate which of the following orders?
    A. Increase the insulin drip to hasten the resolution of the metabolic acidosis
    B. Sodium bicarbonate bolus and repeat every 4–6 hours
    C. Sodium bicarbonate drip with frequent HCO_3 levels
    D. Decrease the insulin drip as the acidosis is resolving

99. Your patient is suffering from myxedema coma. He is receiving intravenous thyroid replacement therapy when he suddenly develops hypotension, hypoglycemia, nausea, and vomiting. What has happened to this patient?
    A. An allergic response to the thyroid medication
    B. He needs an increased dose of thyroid medication
    C. He needs a lower dose of thyroid medication
    D. He is experiencing an Addisonian crisis

100. Connie has end-stage renal disease (ESRD) stage IV and is on hemodialysis every Monday, Wednesday, and Friday. During her treatment today she became very confused and was transported to the ED. Her calcium is 6.3 mg/dL and PTH is 70 mg/mL. What is happening to this patient?
    A. Hypoparathyroidism
    B. Secondary hyperparathyroidism
    C. Secondary hyperthyroidism
    D. Hypothyroidism

101. Nursing interventions should include which of the following to minimize risk to a patient with HIT?
    A. Avoid the use of heparin flushes
    B. Assess the need for manual blood pressure measurements
    C. Monitor platelet counts
    D. Observe for petechiae

102. Type II HIT patients are at great risk for developing
    A. Generalized bleeding
    B. Pericarditis
    C. Thrombosis
    D. Limb amputation

103. Which glands regulate thyroid function?
    A. Posterior pituitary and hypothalamus
    B. Anterior pituitary and thalamus
    C. Anterior pituitary and hypothalamus
    D. Posterior pituitary and thalamus

104. Sid was admitted to the ED in hypertensive crisis. You notice large fluctuations in his blood pressure without changing his nitroprusside drip. The physician orders a plasma catecholamine level. Sid's fractional epinephrine level is very high. What does this high level probably indicate?
    A. Cocaine use
    B. A pheochromocytoma
    C. An adrenal cortex tumor
    D. Hyperthyroidism

105. What is the treatment of choice once a diagnosis of pheochromocytoma is made?
    A. Diet changes
    B. Antihypertensive medications
    C. Surgical removal of the tumor
    D. Diuretics

106. Part of your patient education for the family of a patient with pheochromocytoma should include dietary restrictions. Which of the following foods should the patient avoid?
    A. Cream cheese
    B. Red meat
    C. Chocolate
    D. Aged cheddar cheese

107. Your patient was evenomated by a rattlesnake on the right lower leg this morning while crawling under a neighbor's porch. The entire right lower leg is ecchymotic. The best course of treatment would be to provide
    A. Clotting factors and antivenin
    B. Clotting factors and heparin
    C. IV at 100 ml/hour and antivenin
    D. IV at 100 ml/hour and heparin

108. A snake bite results in activation of which of the following responses to physiologic insult to the body?
    A. Fibrinolytic system
    B. Antithrombin system
    C. Intrinsic cascade
    D. Extrinsic cascade

109. With which of the following conditions would you expect to see hypoparathyroidism develop?
    A. Trauma
    B. With hypercalcemia
    C. With hypophosphotemia
    D. After parathyroid or neck surgery

110. Your patient's calcium level is 11.9 mg/dl. This value may be the result of which of the following conditions?
    A. Hypoparathyroidism
    B. Hyperparathyroidism
    C. Excessive calcium intake
    D. Recent fracture of a long bone

111. Treatment for a thyrotoxic crisis includes
    A. No need for treatment, the crisis will resolve spontaneously
    B. Symptomatic care and wait for symptoms to subside
    C. Synthroid administration and supportive care
    D. Administration of PTH and symptomatic care

112. What is an important teaching point for a patient with hypothyroidism?
    A. Take the medication at the same time every day, no need to fast
    B. Take thyroid medication at the same time every day 30 minutes before breakfast
    C. Take the thyroid medicine each evening before bed
    D. Take daily with food

113. Your patient's TSH (thyroid-stimulating hormone) level is 0.001. What condition does this value indicate?
    A. Hypoactive anterior pituitary function
    B. Hyperactive anterior pituitary function
    C. Hypothyroidism
    D. Hyperthyroidism

114. Your patient was thrown from the back of a truck onto a road and suffered abdominal trauma with a splenic rupture and a fractured right humerus. While in the ED awaiting surgery, because the operating rooms were full, he received 6 units of PRBCs. As his nurse you know that this patient should also receive
    A. FFP
    B. Platelets
    C. Whole blood
    D. Heparin

115. A fellow nurse asks you to explain the differences between the Somoygi effect and the Dawn phenomenon. What are the major differences between Somoygi effect and the Dawn phenomenon?
    A. They are essentially the same process
    B. The Dawn phenomenon is nocturnal hypoglycemia, and the Somoygi effect is greatly increased blood sugars in the early morning
    C. The Somoygi effect is nocturnal hypoglycemia with rebound hyperglycemia, and the Dawn phenomenon is increased morning glucose without nocturnal hypoglycemia
    D. The Dawn phenomenon is morning hypoglycemia, and the Somoygi effect is nocturnal hyperglycemia

116. Drake was found unconscious in his backyard by his brother. His blood sugar is 1545, he has negative serum ketones, and his serum osmolality is 340. What fluids do you anticipate for medical treatment of this condition?
    A. D_5½NS intravenous fluids 300 ml/hour and an insulin drip with sliding scale coverage
    B. Normal saline at 100 ml/hour, subcutaneous insulin with sliding scale coverage every 4 hours, and monitor potassium
    C. Intravenous fluids with normal saline in high volumes, insulin drip with sliding scale coverage, monitor electrolyte levels
    D. Normal saline intravenously, bicarbonate drip, monitor electrolytes

117. What changes are seen on the EKG tracing of a patient with hyperkalemia?
    A. Widening QRS, peaked T waves
    B. Narrow QRS, peaked T waves and U waves
    C. Wide QRS, normal T waves, U waves
    D. Narrow QRS, normal T waves, rapid rate

118. Which of the following statements is true about hepatitis D?
    A. Hepatitis D is detectable only with a concurrent HBV infection
    B. IgM rises late in infection
    C. IgG rises slowly and limited only to the acute phase
    D. It is an RNA virus able to self-replicate when present with HBV

119. What is the correct order of response of the renin-angiotensin mechanism when there is a decrease in blood flow to the kidneys?
    A. Renin, aldosterone, angiotensin I, angiotensin I converting enzyme, angiotensin II
    B. Increased ADH, renin, angiotensin I, angiotensin II
    C. Renin, angiotensinogen, angiotensin I, angiotensin I converting enzyme, angiotensin II, aldosterone
    D. Renin, ACTH, angiotensin I

120. What conditions can trigger the renin-angiotensin mechanism?
    A. Aldosterone, diuretics
    B. Diuretics, decreased renal blood flow
    C. Diuretics, adrenergic blockers
    D. Increased renal blood flow, diuretics

121. Where is renin stored in the body?
    A. Renal tubule
    B. Loop of Henle
    C. Juxtoglomerular cells of the nephron
    D. Adrenal cortex

122. Winona has a history of acute lymphoblastic leukemia. During your assessment you note she is confused, hypotonic, and starts having generalized seizures. You would anticipate receiving orders for which of the following tests?
    A. A spinal tap
    B. CT scan
    C. MRI
    D. PET scan

123. Laurie was treated in the ED for new onset of diabetic ketoacidosis. You have referred her to a diabetic educator and are now teaching her about diabetes mellitus and $HgbA_{1c}$. Which of the following $HgbA_{1c}$ test results should be Laurie's goal for good control of her diabetes mellitus?
    A. 7–8%
    B. 4–5%
    C. 6–7%
    D. 8–9%

124. Temperature regulation is controlled by the hypothalamus with the release of which of the following hormones?
    A. Dopamine
    B. Norepinephrine
    C. Cortisol
    D. Epinephrine

125. Which of the following diabetic patients is most likely to develop DKA?
    A. Type 1 well controlled on 70/30 insulin
    B. Type 1 who is noncompliant with cellulitis of his left leg
    C. Type 2 with an $HgbA_{1c}$ of 6.5 and minor surgery
    D. Type 2 who is noncompliant with a mild upper respiratory tract infection

126. Ryan is 23 years old and presented with chest pain and respiratory distress. He weighs approximately 150 pounds. During your assessment you note he is short of breath and has a dry cough. On Ryan's chest you find irregularly shaped lumps near the left infraclavicular border. Based on these findings, which of the following questions should you ask Ryan?
    A. "Have you suddenly gained weight in the last 2 months?"
    B. "Have you noticed skin patches that are itchy and with a green cast?"
    C. "Have you noticed any stomach pain or swelling?"
    D. "Has your appetite increased over the last few months?"

127. Which of the following conditions can cause a thyroid storm in a patient with hyperthyroidism?
    A. An overdose of PTU (propylthyrouricil)
    B. Increased iodine intake
    C. Trauma or infection
    D. Decreased iodine intake

128. Your patient is having a thyrotoxic crisis. Which medication would you give to reduce symptoms?
    A. Propranolol
    B. Levophed
    C. Adenosine
    D. Digoxin

129. What symptoms are to be expected when a patient is having a thyrotoxic crisis?
    A. Hyperthermia, bradycardia
    B. Hypotension, bradycardia
    C. Flushing, hypoventilation
    D. Hypertension, hyperthermia

130. Blood component replacement therapy for DIC may include all but which of the following?
    A. FFP
    B. Cryoprecipitate
    C. Amicar
    D. Platelets

131. Trousseau's sign is seen with which of the conditions listed below?
    A. Increased serum calcium
    B. Decreased serum calcium
    C. Decreased serum phosphorus
    D. Hypothyroidism

132. Which of the following signs may be elicited in a patient with hypocalcemia?
    A. Short QT interval
    B. Hyperparathyroidism
    C. Chvostek's sign
    D. Cullen's sign

133. Which of the following hormones is responsible for the symptoms of hypothyroidism?
    A. Low levels of T_4 (thyroxine)
    B. Low levels of T_3 (thriothyroxine)
    C. Decreased thyrocalcitonin
    D. Increased thyrocalcitonin

134. Where in the body are the catecholamines produced?
    A. Liver
    B. Kidneys
    C. Adrenal cortex
    D. Adrenal medulla

135. What is the origin of microvascular disease associated with diabetes mellitus?
    A. Vasoconstriction from hyperglycemia
    B. Changes in the capillary basement membrane causing hypoxia on the cellular level
    C. Increased atherosclerotic plaques on the intima
    D. Repeated hypoglycemic events

136. Your patient has not been eating correctly for about 2 weeks because he is stressed out about potentially losing his job. He eats a diet of toaster pastries, pastas, and high caloric, high sugar foods. He collapsed at home today after becoming dyspneic. His EKG shows sinus tachycardia without ectopy, and he is pale, somewhat irritable, and complains of a headache. His initial diagnosis is folic acid deficiency. Tomorrow he is scheduled for more tests to determine if there is an underlying disease process. You suspect he simply has a dietary deficiency and prepare to instruct him about foods that contain high amounts of folic acid. These foods include
    A. Green beans
    B. Peanut butter
    C. Oranges
    D. Fish

137. What are the three major problems associated with macrovascular disease in a patient with diabetes mellitus?
    A. Diabetic peripheral neuropathy, peripheral vascular disease, cerebral vascular accident
    B. Peripheral neuropathy, coronary artery disease, cerebral vascular accident
    C. Coronary artery disease, cerebral vascular accident, peripheral vascular disease
    D. Retinopathy, coronary artery disease, cerebral vascular accident

138. What is NASH (nonalcohol steatohepatitis)?
    A. Fatty liver from a poor diet
    B. Fatty liver from a hepatitis B infection
    C. Fatty liver infiltrates seen as a precursor to diabetes mellitus type 2
    D. Fatty liver with obesity and excess consumption of dietary fats

139. What is the role of glucophage in the body?
    A. Glucophage acts on the liver to decrease blood sugar
    B. Glucophage acts on the liver to increase blood sugar
    C. Glucophage acts on the pancreas to decrease blood sugar
    D. Glucophage acts on the pancreas to increase blood sugar

140. Your patient has been diagnosed with anemia. She will be receiving Epogen. Adverse effects of Epogen include
    A. Iron depletion
    B. Hypokalemia
    C. Decreased creatinine
    D. Decreased ability to clot

141. Clopidogrel may interfere with the metabolism of which of the following drugs?
    A. Phenobarbital
    B. Phenytoin
    C. Cimetidine
    D. Estrogen

142. How is insulin secretion regulated?
    A. Hormonal, exocrine gland secretion, glucose controls
    B. Hormonal, insulin and neuronal controls
    C. Chemical, glucagon and insulin controls
    D. Chemical, hormonal and neuronal controls

143. Which of the following are risk factors for the development of diabetes mellitus?
    A. Obesity (BMI of 42), blood pressure 160/95, HDL 28, brother with diabetes mellitus
    B. Obesity (BMI of 27), blood pressure 120/70, HDL 42, no family history of diabetes mellitus
    C. Obesity (BMI of 26), Caucasian ancestry, blood pressure 190/100, family history of diabetes mellitus
    D. Obesity (BMI of 40), blood pressure 100/50, HDL 50, no family history of diabetes mellitus

144. Why are hyperglycemia and hyperlipidemia seen concurrently in patients with diabetes mellitus?
    A. VLDL (very-low-density lipoproteins) production increases in response to increased insulin production
    B. Insulin resistance promotes VLDL (very-low-density lipoproteins) production
    C. Lipid breakdown is hindered by hyperinsulinemia
    D. Glucose increases cause the liver to increase lipid production

145. How does low-molecular-weight heparin (LMWH) differ from unfractionated heparin?
    A. It is more difficult to administer
    B. More side effects with LMWH
    C. LMWH is more stable
    D. Unfractionated heparin is easier to administer

146. Hemoglobin is primarily phagocytized in the
    A. Liver
    B. Gallbladder
    C. Spleen
    D. Pancreas

147. Where is the pancreas located in the abdomen?
    A. Right lower quadrant of the abdomen
    B. Left upper quadrant of the abdomen
    C. Right upper quadrant of the abdomen
    D. Left lower quadrant of the abdomen

148. Where are the parathyroid glands located?
    A. Anterior to the thyroid
    B. Posterior to the thyroid gland
    C. They sit atop the thyroid gland
    D. Below the thyroid gland

149. Where is the thyroid gland located?
    A. Just below the hyoid bone
    B. In the throat on either side of the trachea
    C. Above the larynx
    D. Sits on top of the thymus gland

150. What physical symptoms do you expect a patient to exhibit if diagnosed with Cushing syndrome?
    A. Moon facies, edema, weight loss
    B. Moon facies, acne, weight loss
    C. Moon facies, purple striae on trunk, buffalo hump
    D. Moon facies, easy bruising, weight loss

151. Which of the following hormones are produced by the anterior pituitary gland?
    A. Vasopressin and oxytocin
    B. FSH, LH, TSH, ACTH
    C. ADH, TSH, FSH
    D. GRF, TSH, substance P

152. Ginger has been diagnosed with an oat cell carcinoma. Oat cell carcinomas are primarily found in the
    A. Central airways
    B. Genital area
    C. Bronchial wall
    D. Pancreas

153. Why is DIC usually fatal if untreated?
    A. Exsanguination
    B. Intracranial hemorrhage
    C. Myocardial infarction
    D. Cerebral thrombosis

154. Janice has been preliminarily diagnosed with Cushing syndrome. What diagnostic tests do you anticipate the physician ordering for Janice?
    A. Computerized tomography of the brain, chest, and abdomen, 24-hour urine cortisol levels, ACTH serum concentrations
    B. Computerized tomography of the brain, chest, and abdomen, thyroid levels, basic metabolic panel
    C. Serum and urine cortisol levels, thyroid panels, beta-natriuretic peptide levels
    D. Urine ACTH concentrations, thyroid panel, C-reactive protein level

155. Your patient has DKA. She has a blood glucose level of 460 mg/dl and also has a potassium level of 6.2. You have started an insulin drip. You know that the insulin drip will
    A. Move potassium back into the intracellular space
    B. Not change potassium levels
    C. Draw more potassium from the intracellular space
    D. Draw more potassium from the extracellular space

156. Your patient had a previous transplant 2 years ago. She is now experiencing severe back pain. Back pain or abdominal pain with itching can be indicators of acute rejection in which of the following organs?
    A. Pancreas
    B. Lung
    C. Liver
    D. Kidney

157. What are some of the signs and symptoms associated with DKA (diabetic ketoacidosis)?
    A. Polyuria, polydipsia, polyphagia, dilute urine
    B. Polyuria, polydipsia, polyphagia, fruity breath, dehydration, marked fatigue
    C. Hyperactivity, confusion, nausea, vomiting
    D. Kussmaul's respirations, dilute urine

158. The ACT (activated coagulation time) is more sensitive to _____ and _____ than whole blood clotting time
    A. Oxygenation, hemofiltration
    B. Factor VIII, heparin
    C. Warfarin, leukemia
    D. Liver disease, calcium

159. What is the most common cause of a fatal transfusion reaction?
    A. Immune compromised recipient
    B. Volume overload
    C. Mismatched blood
    D. Severe hyperkalemia

160. Rejection of a transplanted organ usually occurs as a result of
    A. Cellular immunity
    B. Humoral immunity
    C. Delayed hypersensitivity reaction
    D. Compliment cascade

161. Organ rejection that occurs 3–5 days after transplant that is antibody mediated, with fever and oliguria is known as
    A. A chronic rejection
    B. An acute rejection
    C. An accelerated acute rejection
    D. A hyperacute rejection

162. What is the most common precipitating factor in the development of diabetic ketoacidosis (DKA)?
    A. Hypoglycemia only
    B. Hypoglycemia with obesity and family history
    C. Hyperglycemia with concurrent illness or injury
    D. Hyperglycemia only

163. Your patient had a renal transplant about 1 year ago. She is now being seen for severe flu-like symptoms. What sign or symptom would lead you to suspect that this patient is having an acute rejection episode?
    A. Hypotension
    B. Pelvic pain
    C. Increased urine output
    D. Decreased urine osmolality

164. A mnemonic often used to help assess a patient's pain level is
    A. TIPPS
    B. PQRST
    C. AEIOU
    D. RRST

165. Which of the following is not an expected finding with Graves' disease?
    A. Hyperthyroidism
    B. Goiter
    C. Hypothyroidism
    D. Exophthalmos

166. What is the medication of choice for treatment of Graves' disease?
    A. Methimazole
    B. Levothyroxine
    C. Tapazole
    D. Radioactive iodine

167. Which of the following patients is most likely to develop myxedema coma?
    A. 40 year old man with mild hypothyroidism
    B. 69 year old woman with hypothyroidism and pneumonia
    C. 79 year old man with hypothyroidism and an enlarged prostate gland
    D. 52 year old woman with Graves' disease

168. A patient was admitted in full arrest to your ED. The patient had been forced to make a rapid ascent from a SCUBA dive. Within 2 minutes of reaching the surface the diver collapsed and arrested. Your team was unsuccessful after attempting to resuscitate this patient. What is the probable cause of this patient's death?
    A. Stroke
    B. The bends
    C. Myocardial infarction
    D. Arterial gas embolism

169. Which of the following people are least likely to suffer injury related to decompression illness?
    A. SCUBA diver
    B. Pilot
    C. Astronaut
    D. Welder

170. A risk factor for the development of decompression illness would include
    A. Warm water
    B. Obesity
    C. Age
    D. Slow ascent from depth

171. Your patient just returned from diving in the ocean near your facility. He presents with fatigue, a rash over his torso, pruritis, pain in his joints, and muscle weakness. You suspect this patient is suffering from
    A. Caisson disease
    B. Venous gas embolism
    C. Nitrogen toxicity
    D. Arterial gas embolism

SECTION 13: MEDICAL EMERGENCIES ANSWERS

1. **Correct answer: B**
   Oxygen deprivation is not considered a direct source of energy that would lead to a patient's injury. It would be considered a cause of injury or death because of the resultant lack of oxygen.

2. **Correct answer: D**
   If a patient sustains an injury from electromagnetic waves such as those from an x-ray, the type of energy involved is radiant. Other sources of radiant energy are sunlight, sound waves, and radioactive emissions.

3. **Correct answer: A**
   When energy is transferred from a bullet to an individual, the type of energy transferred is called mechanical energy. Energy is loaded onto the patient, and if the load overcomes the body's ability to tolerate it, injury to one or more of the body's tissues occurs.

4. **Correct answer: D**
   If velocity is doubled, energy is quadrupled. This means that the faster the victim or the object is moving, the greater the amount of energy on impact. For example, bullets made to travel faster will likely cause more tissue destruction.

5. **Correct answer: C**
   The force that decreases or stops the velocity of a moving person is called deceleration. When any type of moving object decreases velocity or stops, the energy is dissipated around the impact site. Unfortunately, human tissue is likely to suffer injury. Different parts of the body decelerate at different rates. The type and strength of the tissue involved also affects the severity and location of injuries. Acceleration injuries occur when the body is set in motion or the speed is increased. For example, if you are driving at car at 20 miles per hour, then are struck from behind by a car traveling at 60 miles per hour, your body accelerates. You may be propelled into the steering column where you would decelerate. You could suffer injuries from both acceleration and deceleration. That is why it is critical to obtain as much information as possible about an accident or situation to help determine extent and severity of injuries.

6. **Correct answer: B**
   Deformative is not considered to be a type of stress. Shearing (tangential force), tensile (separation of tissue), and compressive (tissues pressed together) are types of stress. Sprain is the deformation or tissue damage that results from the stress.

7. **Correct answer: B**
   If your patient was an unrestrained driver and his car was T-boned by another vehicle, given the type of impact (lateral), your patient is likely to suffer same-side shoulder or clavicle injuries. In addition, the patient may suffer cervical spine injury, splenic injury, femur fracture, and injuries to the head and face if forced somewhat forward.

8. **Correct answer: D**
   Disability (neurologic status) is not considered part of a secondary survey of a trauma patient. Airway, breathing, circulation, and disability are parts of the primary survey. Exposure, vital signs, comfort measures, history, and inspection of posterior surfaces are part of the secondary survey.

9. **Correct answer: A**
   When assessing bilateral breath sounds, it is best to place the stethoscope at the second intercostal space midclavicular line and fifth intercostal space, anterior axillary line.

10. **Correct answer: A**
    When obtaining a history from a trauma patient, some ED nurses use the mnemonic MIVT. These letters stand for mechanism of injury, injuries sustained, vital signs, and treatment.

11. **Correct answer: D**
    When palpating the abdomen, a statement of pain is considered a subjective sign. Objective signs include rigidity, guarding, and a mass.

12. **Correct answer: D**
    When inspecting the posterior surfaces of a trauma victim, it is important to remember to maintain cervical stabilization and logroll the patient away from the inspector (if possible).

13. **Correct answer: B**
    The Revised Trauma Score is a physiologic scoring system and has been shown to be a reliable predictor of death. Components of this scoring system include the following components and parameters. Currently, the standard is to transport patients to a trauma center if the score is less than 4, however even this number may be too low in cases of head or multisystem trauma.

Glasgow Coma Scale	Systolic Blood Pressure	Respiratory rate	Coded
13–15	> 89	10–29	4
9–12	76–89	> 29	3
6–8	50–75	6–9	2
4–5	1–49	1–5	1
3	0	0	0

14. **Correct answer: A**
    A fractured skull is a primary brain injury, not a secondary brain injury. Secondary brain injuries include conditions like cerebral edema, hypoxemia, increased ICP, hypercarbia, and hypotension.

15. **Correct answer: C**
    A diffuse brain injury that results from both acceleration and deceleration forces and produces shearing and tensile stresses with axonal damage is called a diffuse axonal injury. The patient suffers microscopic hemorrhagic lesions and the injury may involve the brainstem and reticular activating system. Concussions have no identifiable lesions.

16. **Correct answer: C**
    The most common cause of blunt chest trauma is automobile accidents. Rib fractures are the most common result of blunt chest trauma. Blunt chest trauma is also usually associated with other life-threatening conditions.

17. **Correct answer: D**
    A needle thoracentesis should be performed at the second intercostal space (over the third rib), midclavicular line, affected side.

18. **Correct answer: A**
    There are numerous symptoms of myxedema coma that include facial swelling, altered mental status, alopecia, hypotension, bradycardia, hypothermia, ptosis, periorbital edema, and macroglossia. The symptoms that are not seen with myxedema are tachycardia, hypertension, and goiter. These symptoms are seen with hyperthyroidism.

19. **Correct answer: B**
    Intravenous administration of levothyroxine and replacement of fluids and electrolytes are initial therapy for myxedema coma. The patient must also be supported from potential cardiopulmonary collapse, sometimes requiring mechanical ventilation.

20. **Correct answer: A**
    If a patient suffers loss of autonomic function with loss of thermoregulation, the patient is said to be poikilothermic. The patient is not vasoconstricted and cannot shiver or sweat, so the patient assumes the temperature of the surrounding environment.

21. **Correct answer: A**
    Diaphragmatic function is impaired with spinal injury at the level of C3 to C5.

22. **Correct answer: C**
    The Emergency Medical Treatment and Active Labor Act (EMTALA) does not require the ED staff to notify a significant other about a transfer. However, it is a courtesy when possible.

23. **Correct answer: B**
    The liver may be lacerated by either blunt or penetrating trauma. In blunt trauma there are often fractures of the 7th to 9th ribs overlying the liver. You do not have a history of the mechanism of injury for this patient. Right upper quadrant tenderness will be present with a liver laceration. Rebound sensitivity and guarding will not be present because blood has not been in the abdomen at least 2 hours (long enough to cause peritoneal irritation). Suspect liver laceration when penetrating trauma involves the right lower chest or right upper abdomen or when right upper quadrant tenderness accompanies blunt trauma. The patient needs a CT scan after he is stabilized.

24. **Correct answer: C**
    Splenic injury should be suspected when the 9th to 10th ribs on the left are fractured or when left upper quadrant tenderness and tachycardia are present. This patient has complained of pain in the left shoulder, and it is a common complaint with this type of injury. Peritoneal signs such as rebound sensitivity and guarding are delayed until the blood has had time to cause local irritation of the peritoneum. This patient was trapped in her car for almost 2 hours. Hypotension is a sign of an active bleed.

25. **Correct answer: B**
    The kidneys are in the retroperitoneal space at the level of T12 to L3. Kidneys can be damaged by shearing or compression forces and cause laceration or contusion. Renal injuries must be suspected with fractures to the posterior ribs or lumbar vertebrae. Rupture of the renal artery with a deceleration injury like a crash may cause hypovolemia. There is little collateral circulation to the kidney, and damage to the

renal artery may lead to acute tubular necrosis and intrarenal failure. Sometimes, the signs of a kidney injury can be confused with a pancreatic injury. However, you do not generally have hematuria with a pancreatic injury. You have common signs such as Grey-Turner's sign (flank ecchymosis), Cullen's sign (periumbilical bruising), and flank pain. This patient also is exhibiting confusion, which could be a simple concussion to an acute brain injury. The patient needs immediate evaluation.

26. **Correct answer: B**
Risk management plays a role in the collection, analysis, and storage of records regarding potential and actual injuries in the hospital, as well as court filings. It also identifies situations or actions of potential liability and analyzes techniques to prevent future injuries, medication errors, and accidents.

27. **Correct answer: C**
SBAR is an acronym for Situation, Background, Assessment, and Recommendation for use when reporting patient care to another healthcare professional. SBAR is used to organize information succinctly to provide rapid report and recommendations for actions to physicians, advanced practice personnel, another nurse, social services, and ancillary departments. Situation refers to what information is most important or critical to patient care at the time. Background provides the necessary history that has brought the patient into the unit. Assessment includes objective and subjective data relevant to patient situation. Recommendation refers to the course of action that the reporting staff member believes should occur to improve a patient situation.

28. **Correct answer: C**
Vancomycin-resistant enterococci requires contact isolation. The VRE can survive on surfaces for 1 hour on your stethoscope to 6 days on countertops.

29. **Correct answer: B**
Infectious mononucleosis presents with severe sore throat, lymphadenopathy, maculopapular rash, and, at times, hepatosplenomegaly. The patient may also experience mild to moderate abdominal discomfort and fatigue. In severe cases the spleen may rupture. It is important to teach the patient the importance of rest and to follow up with their primary care provider to prevent relapse. It can take several weeks to months to recover from infectious mononucleosis.

30. **Correct answer: B**
It is important to tell a patient with infectious mononucleosis to avoid strenuous activities that increase intra-abdominal pressure, such as heavy lifting, overexertion, minor trauma, and contact sports. These activities may lead to splenic rupture. The patient must be taught to return to the ED if severe abdominal pain develops.

31. **Correct answer: A**
For most patients with infectious mononucleosis, supportive therapy is all that is necessary. NSAIDs may be prescribed for pain or fever along with increased oral fluids and rest. Steroids are sometimes necessary to manage more severe cases. Acyclovir is not indicated and has no value for these patients even though the Epstein-Barr virus is the causative agent.

32. **Correct answer: C**
The Epstein-Barr virus is the causative agent in infectious mononucleosis. It is spread by contact with body fluids—most often saliva. This disease is predominantly seen

in teens and 30 year olds, but people of any age may become infected. *Streptococcus pyogenes* causes strep throat. *Streptococcus mutans* causes tooth decay. Herpes simplex I causes cold sores and is one form of genital herpes.

33. **Correct answer: A**
The major immunoglobulin of serum and interstitial fluid is immunoglobulin G (IgG). This immunoglobulin provides immunity against viral and bacterial pathogens.

34. **Correct answer: C**
A decrease in the available number of erythrocytes caused by bone marrow production failure is known as aplastic anemia. About 50% of all the cases of aplastic anemia are caused by toxins. The other 50% have an unknown cause. Some of the known causes are radiation (x-rays, radioactive isotopes, radium), benzene, streptomycin, carbon tetrachloride, DDT, chloramphenicol, and sulfonamides. Many types of pesticides other than DDT are thought to contribute to aplastic anemia.

35. **Correct answer: C**
$HgbA_{1c}$ measures the effectiveness of diabetes mellitus therapy. Hemoglobin and glucose have an affinity for each other and join together to form a glycolated hemoglobin. The $HgbA_{1c}$ rises and falls in direct correlation with blood sugars. The American College of Endocrinologists recommends a $HgbA_{1c}$ of less than 6.5%, whereas the American Diabetes Association recommends a $HgbA_{1c}$ less than 7%. Patients with $HgbA_{1c}$s less than 6% are considered nondiabetic.

36. **Correct answer: D**
The traditional treatment of central diabetes insipidus involves the replacement of vasopressin or use of an analogue. The most effective analogue available is desmopressin (DDAVP).

37. **Correct answer: A**
Idiopathic thrombocytopenia purpura (ITP) is the result of a low platelet count. Sometimes platelets are destroyed early and systematically. The cause is thought to be an autoimmune response. Hemorrhages may occur in the brain, which may lead to stroke and an increased intracranial pressure.

38. **Correct answer: B**
The anterior pituitary, or adenohyhypophysis, controls the function of the thyroid gland with TSH (thyroid-stimulating hormone). The anterior pituitary also controls the adrenal cortex with ADH (antidiuretic hormone) and the gonads with LH (luteinizing hormone) or ICSH (interstitial cell-stimulating hormone).

39. **Correct answer: B**
Hyperthermia inhibits the release of thyroxine.

40. **Correct answer: C**
Sickle-cell anemia occurs primarily in the African American population. These people are homozygous for HgS and have more HgS than HgA. This causes some of the cells to form a "sickle" shape—curved with rough edges. A crisis can occur when the low oxygen tension (postulated) causes a proliferation of these cells. The sharp edges of these cells travel through the microcirculation and damage capillaries. A simple thing like cold weather can precipitate massive sickling. Other identified factors include dehydration, vomiting, diarrhea, high altitude, excessive exercise, and stress. When

these cells break apart, they occlude the microcirculation and lower oxygen tension, which initiates more sickling. This is a very painful time for the patient, and oxygen, pain management, and fluids are very important.

41. Correct answer: C
Epogen and Procrit are recombinant erythropoietin, and they are used to correct anemia that can occur with chronic renal failure and an adverse effect would be hypertension. Additional adverse effects include clotting at the site of vascular access, depletion of iron, and increased potassium, creatinine, and BUN.

42. Correct answer: B
Cellular humoral immunity is mediated by B lymphocytes. The B lymphocytes originate in bone marrow and mature there. The B lymphocytes form antibodies (immunoglobulins) that regulate a response to a specific antigen that has bound itself to the B cell's receptor sites. The B cell then forms a specific antibody for that particular antigen. Five different types of immunoglobulins are available: IgG, IgA, IgM, IgE, and IgD. After the antibodies are synthesized, the specific antibody can attach to its antigen and set off the reaction to allow for phagocytosis. The cells retain a "memory" for the specific antigen, and if another exposure occurs, the response will be quicker and stronger.

43. Correct answer: C
ADH (antidiuretic hormone) deals with the functions of thirst and water balance. It is produced by the posterior pituitary gland. When the plasma becomes concentrated, or there is a reduced blood volume, the posterior pituitary gland releases ADH causing water retention and concentration of urine. ADH is regulated by a feedback mechanism in the pituitary gland.

44. Correct answer: B
Signs and symptoms of heat stroke include hot dry skin, flushed face, high body temperature (> 40°C or 104°F), dyspnea, tachycardia, mental status changes, and absence of sweating (unless engaged in activity). This is a medical emergency as the patient's body can no longer maintain thermoregulation.

45. Correct answer: A
All factors except VIII and XII are synthesized in the liver, so that is why liver injuries can bleed so much and are so dangerous.

46. Correct answer: C
Stimulation of the anterior pituitary gland is from the hypothalamus by way of the vascular system.

47. Correct answer: A
Calcitonin is released by the thyroid gland.

48. Correct answer: B
Erythropoietin is a hormone responsible for the synthesis of hemoglobin. Erythropoietin levels increase in response to anemia and low oxygen states and levels decrease in response to hypertransfusion. Levels are also increased in infants with Down syndrome and intrauterine growth restriction. Erythropoietin may also be elevated in infants born to mothers with pregnancy-induced hypertension or diabetes.

49. **Correct answer: D**

    A red blood cell has multiple functions, including carbonic acid dissociation to form bicarbonate ions. The RBC provides oxygen transport via hemoglobin and carbon dioxide transport via carboxyhemoglobin. The RBC buffers protons by binding with hemoglobin to form acid hemoglobin.

50. **Correct answer: B**

    A mean corpuscular hemoglobin (MCH) test measures the average amount (by weight) of hemoglobin in each RBC. A mean corpuscular hemoglobin concentration (MCHC) test measures the average concentration of hemoglobin per single RBC. A mean corpuscular volume (MCV) test measures the average size and volume of a single RBC.

51. **Correct answer: A**

    ABO incompatibility is most often seen in mothers with type O blood, which has an absence of antigens. If the mother is exposed to A and B antigens from the fetus, an ABO incompatibility will exist. The mother can also be exposed to A and B antigens carried in food, bacteria, and pollen. This can make the first pregnancy perilous. ABO incompatibility is less severe than Rh incompatibility and occurs more frequently. ABO incompatibility protects against fetal Rh disease because of rapid destruction of A and B cells. This rapid destruction prevents Rh antigen exposure and resultant maternal antibody production.

52. **Correct answer: B**

    An increase in serum calcium, glucagon, or magnesium stimulates the release of calcitonin. Calcitonin reduces serum calcium levels. Calcitonin targets bone and kidney cells to inhibit bone cell lysis, and it decreases calcium reabsorption by the kidney.

53. **Correct answer: B**

    Seizures are one of the most common presenting symptoms of SIADH. SIADH causes hemodilution and a relative decrease in serum sodium levels. Once the sodium falls below 120, the patient is at great risk for seizures. Excessive urine output and hypotension are symptoms of diabetes insipidus.

54. **Correct answer: D**

    Aminocaproic acid (Amicar) interferes with plasmin and inhibits fibrinolysis. Synthetic antithrombin III inhibits thrombin and can be very useful in DIC.

55. **Correct answer: A**

    Patients who have hemolytic anemia may be fine until they are exposed to a major stressor like infection, trauma, or surgery. A psychological stressor such as divorce may also initiate a crisis. The patient may be overwhelmed, and hemolysis accelerates and may cause tissue hypoxia, ischemia, and progress to necrosis and infarction. Treatment is supportive and targeted to presenting symptoms.

56. **Correct answer: D**

    Immune-mediated HITT usually begins about 5 to 7 days after the initiation of heparin therapy. If a severe reaction develops, the patient will have chest pain due to cardiac ischemia, neurologic impairment and LOC changes, and paresthesias because of cerebral ischemia. The patient may develop pulmonary emboli, dyspnea, extremity pain and pallor due to thrombosis, and possible arterial thrombosis. It usually takes 5–7 days to manifest, but it can take much less.

57. **Correct answer: D**

    Glucagon is released from the alpha cells in the pancreas. Glucagon inhibits glycolysis, increases lipolysis, and increases blood glucose by stimulating glycogenolysis and gluconeogenesis.

58. **Correct answer: D**

    An increase in catecholamines and amino acids with a decrease in serum glucose stimulates the release of glucagon. If one becomes low on serum glucose from exercise, for example, glucagon is released to help produce an increase in blood glucose.

59. **Correct answer: B**

    A high serum magnesium or phosphate level, low serum calcium, with catecholamine release results in secretion of parathyroid hormone. Bone breakdown is accelerated, releasing calcium into the blood. Calcium reabsorption is increased in the intestine, and kidney tubule reabsorption is decreased. Phosphate loss is increased in the urine, which decreases serum phosphate. Parahormone increases reabsorption of magnesium by renal tubules. Renal calculi may develop.

60. **Correct answer: B**

    Some serious side effects of exchange transfusions are air embolism, volume and pressure changes, thromboembolism, bradycardia, and bacterial contamination. Hypothermia, volume overload, transfusion-mediated lung injury, and death are additional serious side effects of exchange transfusions.

61. **Correct answer: A**

    A partial thromboplastin time (PTT) is used to assess intrinsic and common portions of the coagulation cascade. The results may be affected by an absence of clotting factors, anticoagulants, low levels of clotting factors, inhibitors, and an increased use of clotting factors.

62. **Correct answer: A**

    The extrinsic system of the coagulation cascade is initiated by exposure of cell membrane tissue factor from tissue injury. The intrinsic system is initiated by vascular endothelial injury.

63. **Correct answer: B**

    The prothrombin time (PT) is used to assess the extrinsic and common pathways of the coagulation cascade. The test used to assess the intrinsic and common pathways of the coagulation cascade is the partial thromboplastin time (PTT).

64. **Correct answer: C**

    The most important nursing consideration in the infant patient with HHNS is to prevent aspiration. The severe hypokalemia is the result of no intracellular-to-extracellular shift occurring because the patient is not usually acidotic. When the patient is hypokalemic, hypocalcemia and hypomagnesemia also occur. Muscle activity is compromised, and the patient is at high risk for aspiration because of a paralytic ileus.

65. **Correct answer: C**

    Hashimoto's disease, or chronic lymphocytic thyroiditis, is the most common cause of hypothyroidism. Hashimoto's disease is an autoimmune disorder. In Hashimoto's disease the immune system makes antibodies against the thyroid and interferes with production of thyroid hormone.

66. **Correct answer: C**

    A transfusion reaction that usually occurs within 5–30 minutes of the start of the transfusion is known as an acute intravascular hemolytic reaction. The patient may experience chills, fever, tachycardia, hypotension, hematuria, back pain and may exhibit additional signs of shock. The extravascular hemolytic reaction may manifest as fever, low H and H even after transfusion, and elevated bilirubin.

67. **Correct answer: C**

    Pernicious anemia results from a lack of vitamin B_{12}. This disease results from lack of protein intrinsic factor in the stomach that helps the body absorb vitamin B_{12}. This stress on the heart from resultant hypoxia can cause heart murmurs, tachycardias, arrhythmias, hypertrophy, and heart failure. A lack of vitamin B_{12} raises the homocysteine level. High levels of homocysteine add to the buildup of fatty deposits. A lack of vitamin B_{12} can damage nerve cells and cause problems such as parasthesias in hands and feet and problems with ambulation and balance. Memory loss, visual disturbances, and confusion may develop. The condition was named "pernicious" because it was often fatal before the cause was discovered to be a lack of vitamin B_{12}.

68. **Correct answer: D**

    Calcium cannot be utilized by the body without adequate vitamin D levels. Fifteen minutes of daylight on the skin without use of sunblock allows the body to create its own vitamin D. An increased phosphorus level would bind the calcium, making it unavailable.

69. **Correct answer: B**

    The primary effects of aldosterone are to increase reabsorption of water and sodium, which results in an increased extracellular fluid volume. Renal excretion of potassium is increased.

70. **Correct answer: B**

    Aldosterone is secreted by the zona glomerulus of the adrenal cortex.

71. **Correct answer: C**

    Aldosterone secretion is regulated by angiotensin II. When renal blood flow is decreased, angiotensin is released, and it stimulates aldosterone secretion. An increase in potassium ions in extracellular fluid also stimulates the release of aldosterone. Adrenocorticotropic hormone stimulates aldosterone production for short periods of time.

72. **Correct answer: D**

    Pharmacologic antagonists to vitamin K are phenobarbital and hydantoin (anticonvulsants) and heparin and warfarin (anticoagulants). These drugs induce hepatic enzymes and increase vitamin K degradation. Vitamin K transport across the placenta is inhibited, and vitamin K–dependent clotting factors are depressed.

73. **Correct answer: D**

    A factor that suppresses aldosterone production is atrial natriuretic hormone. Hypercalcemia and hypokalemia also suppress aldosterone production.

74. **Correct answer: A**

    Ethan probably has DIC. Disseminated intravascular coagulation is an overstimulation of the clotting cascade. Both the intrinsic and extrinsic pathways are activated at the same time. This causes an acceleration of the clotting process. When the clots lyse, the fibrin split products are anticoagulants. Eventually, all the clotting factors are used up, and no further clots can form. Neonates are at increased risk for DIC secondary to inappropriate levels of anticoagulants and fibrinolytics, along with decreased levels of antithrombin and protein. One of the treatments for DIC is antithrombin III, which sometimes attenuates organ failure and reverse coagulopathy.

75. **Correct answer: B**
Cyclosporine has significant adverse effects which include nephrotoxicity, hypertension, hyperkalemia, leg cramps, headache, seizures, and development of neoplasms.

76. **Correct answer: D**
An antirejection drug classified as antimetabolite is Imuran. Antimetabolites interfere with RNA and DNA synthesis and inhibit T and B lymphocyte proliferation.

77. **Correct answer: D**
Functions of the thyroid gland, adrenal gland, and male and female reproductive glands are regulated by the hypothalamic–pituitary axis. The hypothalamic–pituitary axis releases a number of hormones that inhibit or release several hormones that affect body functions.

78. **Correct answer: B**
The pituitary gland is inferior to the hypothalamus and sits in the sella turcica of the sphenoid bone in the skull.

79. **Correct answer: C**
Cortisol raises the free amino acids in the serum by inhibiting collagen formation and protein synthesis. Cortisol stimulates gastric acid secretion, inhibits loss of sodium from the small intestines, acts as an antidiuretic hormone, and works with epinephrine and norepinephrine to increase blood pressure.

80. **Correct answer: B**
An absolute contraindication for a single-lung, double-lung, or heart-lung transplant is psychiatric illness. Patients with a history of psychiatric illness may be unable to comprehend or follow through a complicated postoperative medication regimen.

81. **Correct answer: C**
Factor VIII deficiency is also known as Von Willebrand's disease. Hemophilia A and B are factor IX deficiencies.

82. **Correct answer: D**
The blood component that contains factor VIII is cryoprecipitate. Cryoprecipitate means it is quick frozen. It contains large amounts of factor VIII. Cryoprecipitate does have disadvantages. It is expensive and there are newer recombinant factor VIII products available. There is the risk of transmission of hepatitis A, hepatitis C, hepatitis G, and HIV.

83. **Correct answer: C**
HHNS develops slowly in type 2 diabetes most often in elderly patients or those with undiagnosed diabetes mellitus. The blood sugars are generally more than 600 mg/dl and can go over 1500 mg/dl with more profound dehydration. The other differentiation between HHNS and DKA is the lack of ketones with HHNS.

84. **Correct answer: B**
Blood sugars over 600 with negative serum ketones and a serum osmolality greater than 310 are typical of hyperglycemic, hyperosmolar, nonketotic syndrome (HHNS). The pH is usually greater than 7.3, and the BUN (blood urea nitrogen) may be elevated. Osmolality is the best predictor of survivability than the blood sugar levels.

85. **Correct answer: C**
Congenital hypothyroidism is manifested by an elevated TSH and a decreased T_4. This disease is usually autosomal recessive, but some cases are autosomal dominant. Congenital hypothyroidism occurs when the thyroid gland fails to develop or function properly. The thyroid gland may be absent, hypoplastic, or displaced. In a few cases the gland is enlarged, but the production of thyroid hormones is deficient or absent.

86. **Correct answer: B**
A fluid that causes decreased platelet aggregation and possible allergic reactions is Dextran. Sometimes Dextran causes acute tubular necrosis because it is made of polymers of high-molecular-weight polysaccharides.

87. **Correct answer: C**
When patients receive multiple transfusions, they are susceptible to increased serum potassium levels. When blood is transfused, sometimes the cells lyse and the intracellular potassium is released. This can also occur as the cells strike the floating ball in the infusion chamber. It is sound practice to monitor electrolytes after every two units of blood given. Remember to monitor the patient for dysrhythmias.

88. **Correct answer: C**
Signs of vitamin D toxicity include azotemia, hypercalcemia, vomiting, and nephrocalcinosis. Vitamin D deficiency also results in hypocalcemia, increased susceptibility to respiratory diseases, lethargy, and seizures.

89. **Correct answer: C**
Kayexalate permanently exchanges 1 gram of medication for 1 mEq of potassium. Other therapies include IV insulin, $D_{50}W$, and sodium bicarbonate. These latter therapies allow quick, effective, short-term correction of the potassium level. Hemodialysis and Kayexalate are the only two methods that permanently remove excess potassium.

90. **Correct answer: C**
Crush injuries can cause a massive release of potassium into the bloodstream. There are approximately 135–145 mEq of potassium in each cell.

91. **Correct answer: C**
A medication that may cause hemolytic anemia is quinidine. In addition, quinidine, procainamide, and acetaminophen may cause hemolytic anemia. Phenobarbital may actually cause aplastic anemia, and furosemide may cause a generalized anemia. Captopril causes pancytopenia.

92. **Correct answer: C**
The fluid of choice to help resuscitate a patient with decompression illness is lactated Ringer's solution. Solutions containing sugar need to be avoided. The patient should be given at least 1 liter over 30 minutes to reduce hemoconcentration and dehydration. Additional boluses of fluid may be necessary. It is likely the patient cannot urinate, so

placement of an indwelling catheter may be necessary. Always place the patient on 100% oxygen.

93. Correct answer: B
Acute hypoglycemia occurs if glucose consumption exceeds glucose production. Lack of food or if the liver is unable to provide glucogenesis, cause a drop in blood glucose can drop to less than 50 mg/dl.

94. Correct answer: B
D_{50}, oral glucose, and treating the cause are the most effective way to treat acute hypoglycemia. The other answers include increased carbohydrate consumption, which would be prohibited. The optimal diet would consist of small frequent meals and reduced carbohydrates.

95. Correct answer: B
The anion gap measures anions not generally measured in routine labs. It is an estimate of the degree of lactic acidosis. The formula for figuring the anion gap is $Na - (HCO_3 + Cl)$. The normal level is 10–20 mEq/L. With diabetic ketoacidosis the anion gap is greater than 30 mEq/L.

96. Correct answer: D
Cryoprecipitate, as mentioned previously, does carry factors VIII, XIII, and fibrinogen. There is a risk of disease transmission and transfusion reactions.

97. Correct answer: B
Possible causes of thrombocytopenia could include portal hypertension. Other potential causes include sepsis, viral infection, burns, and radiation therapy. Medications such as thiazides, furosemide, penicillins, sulfonomides, ranitidine, and heparin may cause thrombocytopenia. Chemotherapy is another cause.

98. Correct answer: C
A sodium bicarbonate drip should be anticipated to replace the HCO_3. This helps to resolve the metabolic acidosis. Boluses would be given only if the pH was very low. The insulin drip will not directly correct the HCO_3.

99. Correct answer: D
Your patient is having an Addisonian crisis. Subclinical adrenal insufficiency may coexist with myxedema. The treatment of choice is intravenous hydrocortisone therapy.

100. Correct answer: B
Connie has secondary hyperparathyroidism. In ESRD, vitamin D synthesis is decreased, thus causing hypocalcemia. The calcium is also bound to phosphorus, further reducing the calcium levels. This decrease stimulates the parathyroid glands to secrete parathyroid hormone in an attempt to correct the calcium levels.

101. Correct answer: A
HIT is heparin-induced thrombocytopenia, so it is best to eliminate the use of heparin.

102. Correct answer: B
Type II HIT patients are at great risk for developing pericarditis. Type II HIT is sometimes called "white clot syndrome." Thrombi are primarily venous in origin and can lead to DVT, pulmonary emboli, thrombotic stroke, limb ischemia, and myocardial infarction.

103. **Correct answer: C**

    Anterior pituitary and hypothalamus regulate thyroid function. The anterior pituitary gland secretes TSH (thyroid-stimulating hormone) and the hypothalamus regulates the anterior pituitary gland with thyrotropin-releasing hormone (TRH).

104. **Correct answer: B**

    Pheochromocytoma is a tumor of the adrenal medulla. These tumors are rarely malignant. They cause release of large amounts of catecholamines such as dopamine, epinephrine, and norepinephrine.

105. **Correct answer: C**

    The best option for pheochromocytoma is surgical removal of the tumor. Alpha-adrenergic blockers or beta-adrenergic blockers may be used to treat hypertension until surgery can be done.

106. **Correct answer: D**

    Hypertension with pheochromocytoma can be triggered by foods such as cheese, alcohol, yogurt, and caffeine. It is important to give the patient a list of foods to avoid. Crises often occur after life events where these foods might be consumed.

107. **Correct answer: A**

    Treatment should include clotting factors and antivenin. Rattlesnakes evenomate with an enzyme called hyaluronidase that breaks down the hyaluronic acid barriers on cells. The cells lyse and exudative products enter the bloodstream. Treatment is very similar to a patient with DIC because fibrin split products (anticoagulants) are released. The patient may have to receive multiple vials of antivenin.

108. **Correct answer: D**

    Damage to the tissues and vessels as a result of a snake bite initiates the extrinsic cascade. Thromboplastin and factor VII are released and are activated in the presence of calcium.

109. **Correct answer: D**

    Hypoparathyroidism is usually caused by damage (i.e., surgery) to the parathyroid gland. This damage leads to increased phosphotemia and lowered calcium.

110. **Correct answer: B**

    A calcium level of 11.9 mg/dl indicates hyperparathyroidism. Hyperparathyroidism can be either primary or secondary in nature. Primary hyperparathyroidism is the excess secretion of PTH (parathyroid hormone) and may be related to a breakdown of the feedback system to the glands or overgrowth of the gland. Secondary hyperparathyroidism is generally related to a chronic disorder such as chronic renal failure or a malabsorption state.

111. **Correct answer: D**

    Treatment of thyrotoxic crisis includes PTH to decrease thyroid-stimulating hormone and thyroid hormones, plus treatment based on presenting symptoms.

112. **Correct answer: B**

    Thyroid medications should be taken on an empty stomach 30 minutes before breakfast, at the same time every day. Other teaching points include regular follow-up labs of TSH and T_4, symptoms of myxedema and hyperthyroidism. Taking thyroid medication in the evening can lead to insomnia.

113. **Correct answer: D**

A TSH (thyroid-stimulating hormone) level of 0.001 indicates hyperthyroidism or thyrotoxicosis. Causes can include goiter, Graves' disease, thyroid carcinoma, and TSH secreting pituitary adenoma. Hyperthyroidism without toxicosis is most often related to excessive intake of thyroid hormones.

114. **Correct answer: B**

This patient should also receive platelet infusions. PRBCs contain no platelets and platelets must be given to aid in hemostasis.

115. **Correct answer: C**

The Somoygi effect is nocturnal hypoglycemia with rebound hyperglycemia. It is more common in type 1 diabetics, especially children. The Dawn phenomenon is morning hyperglycemia without nocturnal hypoglycemia caused by growth hormone secretion in the early morning hours.

116. **Correct answer: C**

Drake has HHNS. Normal saline should be given in large volumes until depletion is corrected and then D_5NS once blood glucose is in the 250–300 mg/dl range. An insulin drip with a sliding scale and hourly glucose monitoring would probably be ordered. Frequent electrolyte monitoring would also be performed. If the patient was given D_5 ½NS too early in the treatment, it could lead to cerebral edema.

117. **Correct answer: A**

A widening QRS, peaked T waves would be seen on an EKG if the patient was hyperkalemic. If the condition becomes severe, the patient can develop asystole.

118. **Correct answer: A**

Hepatitis D is detectable only with a concurrent HBV infection. Hepatitis D (HDV) can only replicate when hepatitis B (HBV) is present. When HDV is present, either as a coinfection or a superinfection, liver disease and progression are more rapid and severe. IGM rises early in infection and may remain chronically high. IgG rises slowing during infection but continues for life. HDV replication is only when HBV is present.

119. **Correct answer: C**

The correct order of response of the renin-angiotensin mechanism when there is a decrease in blood flow to the kidneys is renin, angiotensinogen, angiotensin I, angiotensin I converting enzyme, angiotensin II, and aldosterone. The kidneys perceive a drop in blood flow leading to the release of renin from the juxtoglomerular cells of the nephron. This stimulates the release of angiotensinogen, which stimulates the release of angiotensin I. If the blood pressure is not corrected, the lungs release angiotensin I converting enzyme that in turn causes the secretion of angiotensin II. Angiotensin II causes the release of aldosterone from the adrenal glands causing the retention of sodium and water retention and increased blood pressure.

120. **Correct answer: B**

Anything that causes a perceived drop in renal blood flow triggers the renin angiotensin mechanism. Renin release can also be triggered by sodium and volume depletion such as seen with diuretic use.

121. **Correct answer: C**

    Renin is stored in a crystalline form in the juxtoglomerular cells of the kidneys. When the kidneys perceive a decreased blood flow the sympathetic response triggers the release of renin, which converts angiotensinogen to angiotensin I, a mild vasoconstrictor. If the problem is not resolved the lungs release angiotensin I converting enzyme to create angiotensin II, a powerful vasoconstrictor. Angiotensin II triggers the release of aldosterone from the adrenal glands, which causes sodium and water retention thereby increasing the blood pressure.

122. **Correct answer: A**

    Winona's presentation of confusion, hyptonia, and seizures is indicative of spinal cord involvement. A spinal tap would provide proof of the presence of blast cells in the spinal fluid. Rapid, aggressive chemotherapy treatment is indicated.

123. **Correct answer: C**

    An $HgbA_{1c}$ of 6–7% will mean Laurie's glucose was 100–150 mg/dl over a 3-month period. Four to 5% is normal, and 7–8% and 8–9% or more are indicative of poorly controlled diabetes mellitus.

124. **Correct answer: B**

    Norepinephrine is released by the hypothalamus in response to chemical and temperature receptors in the skin, face, and along the spinal column. Norepinephrine triggers a cascade of actions within the body to retain or create heat in the core. The efficiency of this cascade is impaired by weight, disease process, and respiratory function. Peripheral vasoconstriction shunts blood flow to internal organs to control heat loss through the abdomen. Norepinephrine also causes pulmonary vasoconstriction that inhibits normal blood flow through the lungs, inhibiting blood oxygenation. The best treatment for hypothermia or cold stress is appropriate and timely prevention.

125. **Correct answer: B**

    The patient most likely to develop DKA is the one who is noncompliant with cellulitis. DKA is more common in insulin-dependent diabetics, especially those with an illness or infection such as cellulitis. However, 20–30% of DKA patients have no identified precipitating factors. A well-controlled diabetic is at low risk for DKA. Type 2 diabetics are more likely to develop HHNS.

126. **Correct answer: C**

    An irregularly shaped lump near the infraclavicular border and respiratory distress with dry cough is suspicious for lymphoma. The ED nurse should ask if there has been any abdominal pain or distension, which might be indicative of hepatosplenomegaly. Rapid tumor growth is associated with Burkitt's non-Hodgkin lymphoma. Additional questions will assist in determining which type of lymphoma may be present. A sudden weight loss, fever, and nausea/vomiting with decreased appetite have been associated with lymphomas. The nurse's findings and history assessment should be reported to the physician immediately. As this patient is also suffering respiratory distress, the physician may perform a biopsy to determine type of lymphoma and additional tests to determine spread of disease.

127. **Correct answer: C**

    Injury or infection as well as manipulation of the thyroid gland can trigger a thyroid storm and thyrotoxicosis.

128. **Correct answer: A**

    Propranolol (Inderal) is used for a patient having a thyrotoxic crisis. Propranolol is a beta-blocker and decreases the effects of the sympathetic stimulation of thyrotoxic crisis. It controls heart rate, hypertension, and oxygen consumption.

129. **Correct answer: D**

    Thyrotoxic crisis symptoms include hypertension, hyperthermia, flushing, tachycardia (especially atrial tachyarrhythmias), high output heart failure, nausea and vomiting, psychosis, and delirium. Treatment includes supportive care and medications to block catecholamine effects.

130. **Correct answer: C**

    Blood component (factor) replacement therapy for DIC does not include amicar. Amicar is used to inhibit fibrinolysis, not replace clotting factors. It is used in the treatment of DIC, but it may change a simple bleeding issue into DIC. It must be used in combination with heparin. DIC is usually treated with FFP, cryoprecipitate, and platelets. Cryoprecipitate contains more than 5–10 times more fibrinogen than FFP. A good rule of thumb is to give 10 units of cryoprecipitate for each 3 units of FFP. If the patient is actively bleeding, platelets are commonly used.

131. **Correct answer: B**

    Trousseau's sign is known as carpal-pedal spasm and is seen with decreased calcium levels. Hypocalcemia can occur with end-stage renal disease (increased phosphorus) and decreased vitamin D levels. It is also seen in patients who receive 3 or more units of red blood cells that are treated with calcium citrate.

132. **Correct answer: C**

    Chvostek's sign is seen with hypocalcemia. It is elicited by tapping the cheek over the zygomatic arch and causes facial twitching. The QT interval would be prolonged with hypocalcemia. Cullen's sign is ecchymosis around the umbilicus and is often seen with pancreatitis.

133. **Correct answer: A**

    Thyroxine is responsible for the symptoms of hypothyroidism. The decreased T_4 leads to hypothyroid symptoms of cold, dry skin, hair loss, periorbital edema, and possible thyroid enlargement.

134. **Correct answer: D**

    The adrenal medulla produces 75–85% of the catecholamine epinephrine and 25% of norepinephrine from phenylalanine.

135. **Correct answer: B**

    The origins of microvascular disease associated with diabetes mellitus are due to changes in the capillary basement membrane causing hypoxia on the cellular level. Prolonged hyperglycemia thickens the capillary basement membrane. This thickening leads to decreased blood flow, hypoxia, and a lack of nutrients at the cellular level. The eye and kidney are the organs most susceptible to this process.

136. **Correct answer: B**

    Peanut butter contains high amounts of folic acid. Additional foods high in folic acid include red beans, broccoli, asparagus, liver, and beef.

137. **Correct answer: C**
Coronary artery disease, cerebral vascular accident, and peripheral vascular disease are the three major problems associated with macrovascular disease seen in type 2 diabetes mellitus. Mortality or morbidity in these patients is due to macrovascular changes. Diabetes leads to early atherosclerosis and atherosclerotic heart disease. The other problems listed (retinopathy and peripheral neuropathy and diabetic nephropathy) are microvascular diseases.

138. **Correct answer: C**
NASH (nonalcohol steatohepatitis) shows fatty liver infiltrates and is often seen with insulin resistance, obesity, and increased triglycerides. NASH may progress to cirrhosis if no lifestyle changes are made.

139. **Correct answer: A**
The role of glucophage in the body is as an antihyperglycemic agent, which improves glucose tolerance in patients with type 2 diabetes. Glucophage (Metformin) decreases liver glucose production and also acts to decrease intestinal absorption of glucose.

140. **Correct answer: A**
Epogen and Procrit are recombinant erythropoietin and are used to correct anemia. Adverse effects include clotting at the site of vascular access, depletion of iron, and may cause increases of potassium, creatinine, and BUN.

141. **Correct answer: B**
Clopidogrel (Plavix) interferes with phenytoin, tamoxifen and tolbutamide, fluvastin, toresemide, and warfarin. It also may affect nonsteroidal anti-inflammatories. Plavix does not seem to affect estrogen, cimetidine, or phenobarbital.

142. **Correct answer: D**
Insulin secretion is controlled by chemicals such as glucose and amino acids. Hormones (such as GI hormones) and neuronal controlled prostaglandin also control insulin secretion.

143. **Correct answer: A**
Risk factors for the development of diabetes mellitus include blood pressure greater than 140/90 or higher than accepted for age, first-degree relative with diabetes mellitus, non–White ancestry, obesity (BMI greater than 30), and HDL (high-density lipoproteins) less than 35.

144. **Correct answer: B**
Insulin resistance predisposes the patient to elevated blood glucose and increased insulin production. VLDL (very-low-density lipoproteins) production increases with hyperinsulinemia.

145. **Correct answer: C**
Low-molecular-weight heparin is more stable than unfractionated heparin. LMWH (i.e., Lovenox) is so stable and predictable that PTTs are not required. It is also easy to administer at home.

146. **Correct answer: A**
Hemoglobin is phagocytized primarily in the liver. Hemoglobin is composed of two parts. The first part is "heme" that causes the reddish color and contains iron and

porphyrin. The second part is a protein called "globin." Hemoglobin combines with oxygen to form oxyhemoglobin. Hemoglobin also binds with CO_2 and carries it to alveoli to be expired. When the hemoglobin is phagocytized in the liver, it breaks down into the heme and globin.

147. **Correct answer: B**

    The pancreas is located in the left upper quadrant of the abdomen and sits behind the stomach near the spleen and duodenum. This is a basic question, but one that has caught many an unwary nurse.

148. **Correct answer: B**

    The parathyroid glands are located posterior to the thyroid gland and may consist of four to six small glands. The parathyroid glands produce PTH (parathyroid hormone) that regulates serum calcium, magnesium, and phosphorus levels. PTH also stimulates the kidney to produce bioavailable vitamin D.

149. **Correct answer: B**

    The thyroid gland is located below the larynx on either side of the trachea.

150. **Correct answer: C**

    Numerous physical changes occur with Cushing syndrome or Cushing disease: thinning hair, acne, moon facies, increased body hair, buffalo hump on the upper back, purple striae on the trunk, truncal obesity with thin extremities, and easy bruising.

151. **Correct answer: B**

    The anterior pituitary gland produces numerous hormones that include TSH, LH, FSH, ACTH, and melanocyte-stimulating hormone. Substance P is a hormone released by the hypothalamus. Vasopressin and oxytocin are released by the posterior pituitary gland.

152. **Correct answer: C**

    Oat cell carcinomas are primarily found in the bronchial wall. Oat cell carcinoma is a small cell carcinoma. On CXR, a central mass will be seen. This type of carcinoma easily spreads to the brain, bone, liver, and adrenal glands. Prognosis is very poor.

153. **Correct answer: A**

    DIC is usually fatal if untreated because the patient exsanguinates.

154. **Correct answer: A**

    Cushing syndrome is usually seen with Cushing disease. Anticipated diagnostic tests include computerized tomography of the brain, chest, and abdomen, 24-hour urine cortisol levels, ACTH serum concentrations. It is important to rule out tumors of the pituitary gland, chest (small cell cancer of the lung), adrenal tumors, and pheochromocytomas. These tumors cause excessive ACTH production leading to physical changes seen with Cushing syndrome such as moon facies, buffalo hump, truncal obesity, and purple striae on the abdomen.

155. **Correct answer: A**

    An insulin drip moves potassium back into the intracellular space. Potassium is pulled from the intracellular space due to metabolic acidosis. The insulin drip helps correct the metabolic acidosis, allowing the potassium to return to normal levels.

156. **Correct answer: C**
    Back pain or abdominal pain with itching can be indicators of acute rejection of the liver. Additional indicators include elevated liver enzymes, elevated bilirubin, jaundice, and elevated ammonia levels (a late sign). The itching is a result of bilirubin deposits in the skin.

157. **Correct answer: B**
    Signs and symptoms of DKA include polyuria, polydipsia, and polyphagia, known as the "3Ps." The fruity breath is from ketone production when fatty acids are broken down. Dehydration is due to the osmotic diuresis. Fatigue is due to potassium shifting from inside the cell to the intravascular space.

158. **Correct answer: B**
    The ACT (activated coagulation time) is more sensitive to factor VIII and heparin than whole blood clotting time. The test is easy to do and is reliable. The ACT measures the ability of the blood to clot. Fresh, whole blood is added to a test tube that contains an activator. The activator can be glass particles, kayolin, or diatomaceous earth. The result is the time it takes for a clot to form.

159. **Correct answer: C**
    The most common cause of a fatal transfusion reaction is mismatched blood. Mismatched blood causes a hemolytic reaction resulting in systemic cellular lysis. The overwhelming destruction of cells cannot be corrected rapidly enough by the bone marrow.

160. **Correct answer: A**
    Rejection of a transplanted organ usually occurs as a result of cellular immunity. The function of T cells is cellular immunity. These cells recognize the transplanted organ cells as foreign resulting in a mounted attack leading to rejection. Immunosuppressive drugs suppress this normal response.

161. **Correct answer: C**
    Organ rejection that occurs 3–5 days after transplant that is antibody mediated with fever and oliguria is known as an accelerated acute rejection. This is the standardized definition of this type of rejection.

162. **Correct answer: C**
    The most common precipitating factor in the development of diabetic ketoacidosis is hyperglycemia with concurrent illness or injury. DKA is seen with illness or injury such as infection, surgery, trauma, or UTI. DKA is defined as a fasting blood sugar greater than 250 mg/dl to approximately 1000 mg/dl.

163. **Correct answer: B**
    The transplanted kidney is placed in the pelvic area. Pelvic pain is an ominous sign. Patients that have undergone kidney transplants should be educated to notify their physicians immediately if suffering from pelvic pain as it is a symptom of rejection.

164. **Correct answer: B**
    A mnemonic often used to help assess a patient's pain level is PQRST:
    P: provoke (or palliate)
    Q: quality

R: radiation (or region)
S: severity (use a 1 to 10 scale)
T: time (onset, duration, constant)

165. **Correct answer: C**
Graves' disease is a condition of increased thyroid function, not hypothyroidism, that leads to hyperthyroidism, goiter, and exophthalmos. It is generally an autoimmune disease that can be seen at any age but is most common in the 30–40 year old woman. It may be brought on by stress, medications, and smoking.

166. **Correct answer: D**
Radioactive iodine is the first-line therapy for Graves' disease in the United States. The radioactive iodine effectively destroys the thyroid gland. The patient must then be monitored for signs of hypothyroidism. Methimazole is the generic for Tapazole. Levothyroxine is for hypothyroidism.

167. **Correct answer: B**
A 69 year old woman with hypothyroidism and pneumonia is likely to develop myxedema coma. Myxedema coma is a rare but life-threatening illness seen in older, long-term hypothyroid patients. The cause of myxedema is often infection such as urosepsis or pneumonia. Some medications such as amiodarone, barbiturates, lithium, and beta-blockers can also lead to myxedema.

168. **Correct answer: D**
An arterial gas embolism is the likely cause of this patient's death. An AGE causes tearing of alveoli, which in turn releases gas into the pulmonary capillaries. The bubbles travel through the circulation and may cause symptoms similar to those of a stroke. Symptoms of AGE usually occur within minutes of surfacing, whereas symptoms of decompression sickness may appear hours after the dive.

169. **Correct answer: D**
A welder is the least likely individual to suffer injury related to decompression illness, otherwise known as the bends. SCUBA divers, pilots, astronauts, and anyone who is a compressed-air worker is at risk. The primary risk for DCI is a reduction in ambient pressure.

170. **Correct answer: B**
A risk factor for the development of decompression illness (DCI) includes obesity. Gas bubbles may be trapped in the tissues for longer periods of time. Not all risk factors for DCI have been identified. However, the known risk factors include rapid ascents, cold water, alcohol use, dehydration, heavy exercise at depth, exercise immediately after surfacing, and existing pulmonary disease.

171. **Correct answer: A**
Caisson disease is another name for the bends. Although this illness may be caused by excess nitrogen bubbles in tissues, other gases may cause this condition. Symptoms of Caisson disease include fatigue, a rash over the torso, pruritis, pain in the joints, muscle weakness, dyspnea, inability to urinate, numbness and tingling, mental status changes, and death.

SECTION 13: MEDICAL EMERGENCIES REFERENCES

Andresen, C., Moalli, M., Turner, C., Berryman, E., Pero, R., & Bagi, C. M. (2008). Bone parameters are improved with intermittent dosing of vitamin D_3 and calcitonin. *Calcified Tissue International, 83*(6), 393–403.

Aster, R. H., & Bougie, D. W. (2007). Drug-induced immune thrombocytopenia: Current concepts. *New England Journal of Medicine, 357*(6), 580–587.

Bacigalupo, A., & Passweg, J. (2009). Diagnosis and treatment of acquired aplastic anemia. *Hematology/Oncology Clinics of North America, 23*(2), 159–170.

Balasubramanian, S., & Ganesh, R. (2008). Vitamin D deficiency in exclusively breast-fed infants. *Indian Journal of Medical Research, 127*(3), 250–255.

Berg, R., Talving, P., & Inaba, K. (2011). Cardiac rupture following blunt trauma. *Trauma, 13*(1), 35–45.

Bhullar, I. S., Braman, R., & Block, E. F. J. (2007). Recombinant factor VII as an adjunct to control of hemorrhage from chest trauma in a Jehovah's Witness. *American Surgeon, 73*(8), 818–819.

Biagini, E., Spirito, P., Leone, O., Picchio, F. M., Coccolo, F., Ragni, L., . . . Rapezzi, C. (2008). Heart transplantation in hypertrophic cardiomyopathy. *American Journal of Cardiology, 101*(3), 387.

Bjerkeset, O., Romild, U., Smith, G., Davey, & Hveem, K. (2011). The associations of high levels of C-reactive protein with depression and myocardial infarction in 9258 women and men from the HUNT population study. *Psychological Medicine, 41*(2), 345–352.

Bolton-Maggs, P. H. (2009). Factor XI deficiency: Resolving the enigma? *Hematology, 1*, 97–105.

Brimioulle, S., Orellana-Jimenez, C., Aminian, A., & Vincent, J. L. (2008). Hyponatremia in neurological patients: Cerebral salt wasting versus inappropriate antidiuretic hormone secretion. *Intensive Care Medicine, 34*(1), 125–131.

Burchett, M. L. R., Hanna, C. E., & Steiner, R. D. (2009). Endocrine and metabolic diseases. In C. E. Burns, A. M. Dunn, M. A. Brady, N. B. Starr, & C. G. Blosser (Eds.), *Pediatric primary care* (4th ed., pp. 584–611). St. Louis, MO: Saunders Elsevier.

Burns, S. M. (Ed.). (2007). *American Association of Critical-Care Nurses (AACN): AACN protocols for practice: Healing environments* (2nd ed.). Sudbury, MA: Jones and Bartlett.

Cadogan, M. P. (2010). CPR decision making and older adults: Clinical implications. *Journal of Gerontological Nursing, 36*(12), 10–15.

Cassandra, H. (2009). Enterovirus triggers type 1 diabetes mellitus. *Nurse Educator, 34*(4), 147.

Chernecky, C., & Berger, B. (2004). *Laboratory tests and diagnostic procedures* (4th ed.). Philadelphia, PA: Saunders.

Clark, N., Witt, D., & Delate, T. (2008). The clinical consequence of subtherapeutic anticoagulation: The low INR study (LINeRS). *Journal of Thrombosis and Thrombolysis, 25*(1), 127–128.

Crenner, C. (2008). The troubled dream of genetic medicine: Ethnicity and innovation in Tay-Sachs, cystic fibrosis, and sickle cell disease. *Journal of the History of Medicine and Allied Sciences, 63*(1), 124–126.

Cullen, K. W., & Buzek, B. B. (2009). Knowledge about type 2 diabetes risk and prevention of African-American and Hispanic adults and adolescents with family history of type 2 diabetes. *Diabetes Educator, 35*(5), 836–839.

Danes, A. F., Cuenca, L. G., Rodriguez Bueno, S., Mendarte Barrenechea, L., & Ronsano, J. B. (2008). Efficacy and tolerability of human fibrinogen concentrate administration to patients with acquired fibrinogen deficiency and active or in high-risk severe bleeding. *Vox Sanguinis, 94*(3), 221–226.

Dewar, D. C., Butcher, N. E., King, K. L., & Balogh, Z. J. (2011). Post injury multiple organ failure. *Trauma, 13*(1), 81–91.

Dhaliwal, G., Cornett, P. A., & Tierney, L. M. (2004). Hemolytic anemia. *American Family Physician, 69*(11), 2599–2606.

Domen, R. E., & Hoeltge, G. A. (2003). Allergic transfusion reactions: An evaluation of 273 consecutive reactions. *Archives of Pathology & Laboratory Medicine, 127*(3), 316–320.

Doyle, P., Sajid, M., O'Brien, T., Dubois, K., Engel, J. C., Mackey, Z. B., & Reed, S. (2008). Drugs targeting parasite lysosomes. *Current Pharmaceutical Design, 14*(9), 889–900.

Dunn, J. P., & Jagasia, S. M. (2007). Case study: Management of type 2 diabetes after bariatric surgery. *Clinical Diabetes, 25*(3), 112–114.

Dvorak, C. C., & Cowan, M. J. (2008). Hematopoietic stem cell transplantation for primary immunodeficiency disease. *Bone Marrow Transplantation, 41*(2), 119–126.

Eldin, W. S., Ragheb, A., Klassen, J., & Shoker, A. (2008). Evidence for increased risk of prediabetes in the uremic patient. *Nephron, 108*(1), c47–c55.

Emergency Nurses Association, & Newberry, L. (2003). *Sheehy's emergency nursing: Principles and practice* (5th ed.). St. Louis, MO: Mosby/Elsevier.

Ensenauer, R. E., Michels, V. V., & Reinke, S. S. (2005). Genetic testing: Practical, ethical, and counseling considerations. *Mayo Clinic Proceedings, 80*(1), 63–73.

Evangelopoulos, D. S., Deyle, S., Zimmermann, H., & Exadaktylos, A. K. (2011). Full-body radiography (LODOX Statscan) in trauma and emergency medicine: a report from the first European installation site. *Trauma, 13*(1), 5–15.

Finch, R. (2009). Antimicrobials: Past, present and uncertain future. *Clinical Medicine, 9*(3), 257–258.

Gambol, P. (2007). Maternal phenylketonuria syndrome and case-management implications. *Journal of Pediatric Nursing, 22*(2), 129–138.

Grabowski, G. (2008). Lysosomal storage disease 1: Phenotype, diagnosis, and treatment of Gaucher's disease. *Lancet, 372*(9645), 1263–1271.

Gurm, H. S., & Eagle, K. A. (2008). Use of anticoagulants in ST-segment elevation myocardial infarction patients: A focus on low-molecular-weight heparin. *Cardiovascular Drugs and Therapy, 22*(1), 59–69.

Hedner, U., & Brun, N. C. (2007). Recombinant factor VIIa (rFVIIa): Its potential role as a hemostatic agent. *Neuroradiology, 49*(10), 789–793.

Hernan, A., Lopez, M., Debes, J. D., & Dickstein, G. (2007). Wilson's disease: What lies beneath. *Digestive Diseases and Sciences, 52*(4), 941–942.

James, A. H. (2007). Heparin-induced thrombocytopenia: A quick review of recent studies. *Journal of Respiratory Diseases, 28*(9), 396.

Johnsen, P., Townsend, J., Bøhn, T., Simonsen, G. S., Sundsfjord, A., & Nielsen, K. M. (2009). Factors affecting the reversal of antimicrobial-drug resistance. *Lancet Infectious Diseases, 9*(6), 357–364.

Jones & Bartlett Learning. (2011). *2011 nurse's drug handbook* (10th ed.). Sudbury, MA: Jones & Bartlett Learning.

Jones, K. L. (2006). *Smith's recognizable patterns of human malformation* (6th ed.). Philadelphia, PA: Elsevier.

Kamoun, M., & Grossman, R. A. (2008). Kidney-transplant rejection and anti-MICA antibodies. *New England Journal of Medicine, 358*(2), 196.

Kiernan, P. D., Khandhar, S. J., Fortes, D. L., Sheridan, M. J., & Hetrick, V. (2010). Thoracic esophageal perforations. *American Surgeon, 76*(12), 1355–1362.

Krajcik, S., Haniskova, T., & Mikus, P. (2011). Pneumonia in older people. *Reviews in Clinical Gerontology, 21*(1), 16–27.

Krishnamoorthy, P., Alyaarubi, S., Abish, S., Gale, M., Albuquerque, P., & Jabado, N. (2006). Primary hyperparathyroidism mimicking vaso-occlusive crises in sickle cell disease. *Pediatrics, 118*(2), 786–787.

Labbé, E., Herbert, D., & Haynes, J. (2005). Physicians' attitude and practices in sickle cell disease pain management. *Journal of Palliative Care, 21*(4), 246–251.

Levi, M., & Cate, H. T. (1999). Disseminated intravascular coagulation. *New England Journal of Medicine, 341*(8), 586–592.

Lewis, A., Courtney, C., & Atkinson, A. (2009). All patients with "idiopathic" hypopituitarism should be screened for hemochromatosis. *Pituitary, 12*(3), 273–275.

Lisman, T., & Leebeek, F. W. G. (2007). Hemostatic alterations in liver disease: A review on pathophysiology, clinical consequences, and treatment. *Digestive Surgery, 24*(4), 250–258.

Mäntyselkä, P., Korniloff, K., Saaristo, T., Koponen, H., Eriksson, J., Puolijoki, H., . . . Vanhala, M. (2011). Association of depressive symptoms with impaired glucose regulation, screen-detected, and previously known type 2 diabetes: Findings from the Finnish. *Diabetes Care, 34*(1), 71–76.

McNally, P. (2001). *GI/liver secrets* (2nd ed.). Philadelphia, PA: Hanley & Belfus/Elsevier.

Mitka, M. (2007). Dual antithrombotic therapy's increased risks not always offset by benefit. *Journal of the American Medical Association, 298*(13), 1504.

Mongardon, N., Bruneel, F., Henry-Lagarrigue, Legriel, S., Revault d'Allonnes, L., Guezennec, P., . . . Bedos, J. P. (2007). Shock during heparin-induced thrombocytopenia: Look for adrenal insufficiency! *Intensive Care Medicine, 33*(3), 547–548.

Norris, W. E. (2004). Acute hepatic sequestration in sickle cell disease. *Journal of the National Medical Association, 96*(9), 1235–1239.

Olson, J. D., Brandt, J. T., Chandler, W. L., Van Cott, E. M., Cunningham, M. T., Hayes, T. E., . . . Wang, E. C. (2007). Laboratory reporting of the International Normalized Ratio: Progress and problems. *Archives of Pathology & Laboratory Medicine, 131*(11), 1641–1617.

Pagana, K. D., & Pagana, J. (2005). *Mosby's Manual of diagnostic and laboratory tests* (3rd ed.). St. Louis, MO: Mosby/Elsevier.

Prasad, V. K., & Kurtzberg, J. (2008). Emerging trends in transplantation of inherited metabolic diseases. *Bone Marrow Transplantation, 41*(2), 99–108.

Prescribing reference. (2009). *NPPR: Nurse Practitioner's Prescribing Reference, 16*(2).

Sarkissian, C., Gámez, A., & Scriver, C. (2009). What we know that could influence future treatment of phenylketonuria. *Journal of Inherited Metabolic Disease, 32*(1), 3–9.

Shimshi, M., & Davies, T. F. (2010). Hypothyroidism. In R. E. Rakel & E. T. Bope (Eds.), *Conn's current therapy 2010* (pp. 672–676). Philadelphia, PA: Saunders Elsevier.

Shorr, A. K., Helman, D. L., Davies, D. B., & Nathan, S. D. (2004). Sarcoidosis, race, and short-term outcomes following lung transplantation. *Chest, 125*(3), 990–996.

Sievert, A., Uber, W., Laws, S., & Cochran, J. (2011). Improvement in long-term ECMO by detailed monitoring of anticoagulation: A case report. *Perfusion, 26*(1), 59–64.

Smeltzer, S., & Bare, B. G. (2003). *Brunner and Suddarth's textbook of medical–surgical nursing* (10th ed.). Philadelphia, PA: Lippincott Williams & Wilkins.

Stewart, L. J., Johnston, R. B. Jr., & Liu, A. H. (2009). Immunodeficiency. In W. W. Hay, Jr., M. J. Levin, J. M. Sondheimer, & R. R. Deterding (Eds.), *Lange current diagnosis and treatment in pediatrics* (19th ed., pp. 891–910). New York, NY: McGraw–Hill Medical.

Steyn, N. P., Lambert, E. V., & Tabana, H. (2009). Conference on "Multidisciplinary approaches to nutritional problems." Symposium on "Diabetes and health." Nutrition interventions for the prevention of type 2 diabetes. *Proceedings of the Nutrition Society, 68*(1), 55–70.

Swanson, K., Dwyre, D. M., Krochmal, J., & Raife, T. J. (2006). Transfusion-related acute lung injury (TRALI): Current clinical and pathophysiologic considerations. *Lung, 184*(3), 177–185.

Takaro, T. K., Krieger, J., Song, L., Sharify, D., & Beaudet, N. (2011). The breathe-easy home: The impact of asthma-friendly home construction on clinical outcomes and trigger exposure. *American Journal of Public Health, 101*(1), 55–62.

Tweet, M. S., & Polga, K. M. (2010). 44-year-old man with shortness of breath, fatigue, and paresthesia. *Mayo Clinic Proceedings, 85*(12), 1148–1151.

Unkle, D. W. (2007). Heparin-induced thrombocytopenia. *Orthopaedic Nursing, 26*(6), 383–387.

Vandergheynst, F., & Decaux, G. (2008). Lack of elevation of urinary albumin excretion among patients with chronic syndromes of inappropriate antidiuresis. *Nephrology, Dialysis, Transplantation, 23*(7), 2399–2401.

von Köckritz-Blickwede, M., & Nizet, V. (2009). Innate immunity turned inside-out: Antimicrobial defense by phagocyte extracellular traps. *Journal of Molecular Medicine, 87*(8), 775–783.

Whiteman, M. (2011). Hydrogen sulfide and inflammation: The good, the bad, the ugly and the promising. *Expert Review of Clinical Pharmacology, 4*(1), 13–32.

Young, N. S., Scheinberg, P., & Calado, R. T. (2008). Aplastic anemia. *Current Opinion in Hematology, 15*(3), 162–168.

SECTION 14:

Psychosocial

1. A false perception that is not grounded in reality and not accounted for by external stimuli is called
   A. A fugue
   B. A hallucination
   C. An idea of reference
   D. Disorientation

2. The false belief that something is wrong with one's body or body part is called
   A. Malingering
   B. Hypochondriasis
   C. Transference
   D. Somatic delusion

3. When you came on shift you learned that a fellow nurse, who is only 48 years old, was diagnosed with Korsakoff's syndrome. You are shocked at the diagnosis because Korsakoff's syndrome is a
   A. Fatal form of brain tumor that usually causes death within months
   B. Type of acute pancreatitis caused by long-term alcohol abuse
   C. Type of organic brain syndrome
   D. Severe form of intestinal cancer

4. You are discussing postdischarge psychiatric resources with the patient's family. You note they are using the terms "psychological emergency" and "crisis" interchangeably. To clarify this issue you tell the family that
   A. A crisis is an immediate danger to someone else, and an emergency is a suicide attempt
   B. A crisis develops over time as a result of a psychological stressor, and an emergency is an immediate situation that if not corrected will result in harm to self or others
   C. A crisis occurs when no intervention will be effective, and an emergency is when interventions have the greatest impact
   D. A crisis is sudden and precedes a psychological emergency when lives may be threatened

5. Marlene was transported to the ED after a suicide attempt. She took more than sixty 500-mg acetaminophen tablets with alcohol. While caring for her you notice multiple 3- to 4-inch thin scars on her thighs and abdomen. What is your best response to this discovery?
   A. Tell her husband so he can deal with it
   B. Ask her what happened in a nonjudgmental way
   C. Tell her how lucky she is to be alive
   D. Tell her this behavior is not acceptable

6. Your patient is a college student and was admitted to the ED after ingesting about 50 extra-strength acetaminophen tablets. Until now he has refused to say why he ingested the drug. About an hour after arrival you find him crying. When you ask him why he is crying, he tells you he was sexually assaulted by an unknown male 3 weeks ago and he is afraid this will brand him a homosexual. Which of the following responses is the most therapeutic?
   A. "Don't worry, you'll get over this and be okay"
   B. "Let me get the psychologist to come talk with you tomorrow"
   C. "Why do you believe this will make you a homosexual?"
   D. "What is wrong with being a homosexual?"

7. Alcohol abuse may lead to a deficiency in micronutrients that in turn may cause depression and suicidal behavior. One of these micronutrients is
   A. Potassium
   B. Copper
   C. Sodium
   D. Selenium

8. Morgan is a 20 year old admitted for observation after fighting at a friend's house. She has a right fractured humerus, a right Colle's fracture, mild concussion, and right orbital fracture. When paramedics arrived she was found talking to herself, resisted medical care, and stated she could heal herself. During your assessment you find Morgan is withdrawn, irritable, fatigued, and indecisive about what to do with her clothing. You should
   A. Request a drug screen
   B. Request a psychological evaluation for schizophrenia
   C. Request social worker to assess Morgan's home life
   D. Evaluate Morgan for feelings of suicide

9. Binge eating, mutilation, obesity, drug abuse, and alcoholism are all examples of
   A. Self-destructive behavior
   B. Psychotic behavior
   C. Neurosis
   D. Immaturity

10. As the educator for a busy emergency department, you note an increased frequency of patients with underlying mental disorders being admitted. You overhear some negative comments regarding nursing assignments for these patients. You ask the nurses to complete a self-awareness survey regarding their beliefs and understanding of mental health issues. You will use this information to
    A. Determine which nurses should never care for patients with mental health issues
    B. Change nursing assignments immediately
    C. Determine which nurses should be written up and counseled
    D. Create an education program for the nurses to increase understanding of mental health issues and how to access resources

11. Your staff in the ED has just completed a code lasting 2 hours for a 21 year old rape and trauma victim. Due to overwhelming injuries the patient did not survive. Chaplain services are called in to assist with a nursing staff debriefing. Staff members experiencing which of the following emotions are at highest risk for psychological stress?
    A. Anger
    B. Fear
    C. Anxiety
    D. Denial

12. "Sugar" is a gang member and heavy alcohol abuser. During a fight almost 24 hours ago Sugar was shot in the leg and hand. His gang members left him at the entrance to the ED with a note explaining about the injuries sustained the previous night. You observe Sugar thrashing around in the bed, and he is suddenly awake when you enter the room. He is shaking, has vomited, and is tachycardic, hypertensive, and talking to people not in the room. You suspect he is
    A. Exhibiting signs of paranoid schizophrenia
    B. Experiencing delirium tremens
    C. Experiencing sepsis
    D. Experiencing drug withdrawal

13. Within a Chinese family cultural values and practices may include which of the following beliefs?
    A. Chi is an external energy
    B. Disease is caused by disharmony with society
    C. Medicinal herbs are important
    D. Family involvement in limited

14. Signs and symptoms of anorexia nervosa may include
    A. Tachycardia
    B. Absent menses
    C. Hyperthermia
    D. Hyperactivity

15. Your patient is being evaluated for adult ADHD. Which of the following conditions or abnormalities is expected to be present if he has ADHD?
    A. A cousin with hyperthyroidism
    B. Eye problems
    C. A heart murmur
    D. None

16. Karl is waiting for emergency surgery for a fractured tibia. Despite being heavily medicated for pain, he continually demands to have his cell phone and a computer pad in his room. His wife says Karl spends too much time on the computer at home. Karl insists he only spends about an hour after work on the computer and texting his friends. Karl probably suffers from
    A. Internet addiction
    B. Bipolar disorder
    C. Depression anxiety
    D. Separation anxiety

17. Which of the following statements is untrue regarding responses to posttraumatic stress disorder?
    A. Patients are less likely to socialize
    B. Patients may have increased ability to complete home or work tasks
    C. Patients may become irritable and hostile
    D. Patients may exhibit regressive behaviors

18. Which of the following statements is true about posttraumatic stress disorder?
    A. Only war veterans experience PTSD
    B. PTSD is easy to diagnose
    C. Multiple traumatic events heighten the risk of PTSD
    D. Patients become less aggressive

19. Joanne is the sole survivor of a car versus train crash that killed her immediate family. While being treated for her injuries her behavior and moods rapidly change. Which of the following behaviors is of most concern to the staff and indicates possible suicidal behavior?
    A. Yelling at the staff
    B. Withdrawal from conversation and interactions with others
    C. Drug seeking with multiple requests for pain medications and sedatives
    D. Crying and statements about feeling helpless

20. Marge and Harold are the parents of a 19 year old with leukemia. Their daughter just died in the ED. Initially, the parents say little while in the waiting room and have a glazed expression while at their daughter's bedside. As an ED nurse you recognize their response as
    A. Adaptation to the ED environment
    B. The initial steps to coping
    C. The initial response to a crisis
    D. Normal and does not need to be addressed

21. During discharge teaching you notice multiple bruises on the arms and reddened areas on the neck of the patient's older sister. You suspect she is being physically abused. What other indicator would support your assessment?
    A. Extroverted behavior
    B. Denial of abuse when asked directly
    C. She volunteers information
    D. Hesitance to discuss home situation

22. You are caring for a patient who was the driver in a motor vehicle accident in which a child was killed. She is combative and restless, hyperventilating, tachycardic, and has an elevated blood pressure. She states, "I've got to leave here... they'll arrest me...they'll lock me up...I can't believe this... there is no way out." You should tell her
    A. "They should arrest you, you killed a child"
    B. "Calm down. It wasn't your fault"
    C. "Stop it. You are working yourself up. Look at me and focus on what I am telling you to do"
    D. "Just relax. They can't arrest you because you are a patient here"

23. Your patient, a drug abuser with cirrhosis, has returned again to the ED after failing rehabilitation. Although you previously had a friendly and open relationship, he will not look at you and only answers minimally to questions. You tell him
    A. "I can't believe you wasted the opportunity at the rehabilitation center"
    B. "I know you want to stay drug free but now you will have a permanent criminal record"
    C. "Why don't we work together to find new resources for you to use when you are tempted to take one of these drugs"
    D. "I am proud of how long you stayed sober. Let's try again"

24. Carla was admitted to the ED after fainting at work secondary to bradycardia and malnutrition. She is 67 inches tall but weighs only 93 pounds. You find her crying, sitting on the edge of her gurney. She tells you that she is worried the intravenous fluid will make her gain weight. What is the most effective way to manage this problem?
    A. Have her boyfriend talk to her
    B. Ask if she wants to speak to her minister
    C. Ask the physician for a dietary consult
    D. Ask for a patient conference with the healthcare team and family

25. You are obtaining a patient's history when you notice multiple rotted teeth. You suspect bulimia nervosa. The patient tells you she regularly purges after meals so she can meet the weight standards for her job. What family dynamics would you expect to find associated with bulimia nervosa?
    A. No significant family dynamics are noted with bulimia nervosa
    B. A family history of drug abuse or psychiatric disorders
    C. A strong sense of ego
    D. Poor scholastic performance

26. Joan was at a party with some friends where she consumed alcohol and a mix of over-the-counter and prescription medications. She is now comatose and on life support. She is not expected to survive. Her husband is devastated and angry. He challenges everything you say and keeps copious notes about her care. You are concerned he may plan to sue you or the hospital. Which of the following actions should be your priority?
    A. Try to get a hold of his notebook and make copies
    B. Contact the nursing supervisor or your nurse manager with your concerns
    C. Contact your malpractice carrier for advice
    D. Ask to change assignments

27. Depression often devastates families and often goes undiagnosed and misunderstood by families, the public, and the medical community. Which of the following is also true regarding depression?
    A. Depression is seen only in maltreated individuals
    B. Depression is easy to diagnose
    C. The elderly do not respond to antidepressant therapy
    D. Depression is recurrent and may increase in severity

28. In the United States Asperger's syndrome is considered to be which of the following types of disorders?
    A. Developmental delay disorder
    B. Autistic spectrum disorder
    C. Pervasive developmental disorder
    D. Attention deficit disorder

29. Wanda has sickle-cell anemia and is a frequent patient in your ED. You were told in report that Wanda's siblings were escorted out of the unit for arguing in the hallway about financial difficulties and responsibilities. During your assessment Wanda appears to have difficulty concentrating on your questions and is withdrawn and restless. When attempting to engage her in activities, she refuses and states that she "wants to be alone." You should
    A. Respect her wishes and go care for your other patient
    B. Leave the room to contact her husband
    C. Straighten her room while looking for sharp objects or potential dangers
    D. Leave the room to contact the hematologist and the doctor

30. Dorothy was admitted to the ED for appendicitis. She is grimacing and will not allow you to assess her abdomen. The physician ordered IM Demerol for pain. Approximately 10 minutes after administration of the Demerol, Dorothy is combative, has pulled her IV out, has torn off her IV dressing, and is screaming at the staff. Your next action should be to
    A. Apply restraints by yourself as additional staff may scare her
    B. Wear personal protective equipment to enter her room to apply restraints
    C. Call security to help subdue Dorothy
    D. Use a Posey restraint system to subdue Dorothy

31. Linda is the lone survivor of a car crash that killed her parents and two siblings. She has sustained a hemothorax and bilateral broken legs. She had a chest tube placed and vital signs are stable. She has been alert and oriented ×4 throughout her treatment and is extremely depressed and withdrawn. You are discussing medications, impending surgical procedures, psychiatric therapy, and the increased risk of suicide and suicidal behavior with Linda's distant relatives. The family makes each of the following statements regarding Linda's possibility of suicide. Which of the statements is inaccurate and needs to be corrected?
    A. "If Linda is considering suicide, she will make statements or give warnings of suicide"
    B. "We should trust our instincts if we feel Linda is in danger"
    C. "As she recovers from her depression, she is at greater risk of suicide"
    D. "If she talks about suicide or asks about pills, then she is just voicing the thought and will not attempt suicide"

32. The fear of crowds is known as
    A. Acrophobia
    B. Agoraphobia
    C. Arachnophobia
    D. Aschizophobia

33. Your patient is explaining his history to you when he simply stops speaking and looks around the room. His behavior is known as
    A. Rude
    B. Affect
    C. Blocking
    D. Amnesia

34. Simultaneous existence of contradictory or contrasting emotions toward a person or object is known as
    A. Apathy
    B. Double bind
    C. Depersonalization
    D. Ambivalence

35. Which of the following medications is not considered an antimanic drug?
    A. Klonopin
    B. Tegretol
    C. Lithium
    D. Tofranil

36. Which of the following is classified as an antianxiety drug?
    A. Restoril
    B. Elivil
    C. Sinequan
    D. Tofranil

37. Your patient cut his forearm and requires several stitches. He begins to hallucinate midway through the procedure. He is demanding, loud, and very insistent. His behavior worsens and disrupts the staff. You could categorize his behavior as
    A. Paranoid
    B. Self-absorbed
    C. Deteriorating
    D. Overanxious

38. Your patient's family is frustrated that their family member has not improved during the week since being placed on Elavil. The patient has remained depressed, so the family brought the patient to the ED to determine the cause of the continuing depression. As an ED nurse you know
    A. The Elavil dose is not high enough to be therapeutic
    B. Elavil is causing an idiosyncratic reaction in this patient
    C. The patient must not be taking the medication
    D. Elavil may take up to 3 weeks to become effective

39. A patient undergoing an assessment for an ear injury becomes agitated because his friend was not allowed to accompany him to the treatment area. Despite reassurances that the exam will not take long, the patient throws the exam chair into the wall and begins disconnecting the suction and oxygen apparatus from the wall. Your first priority is to
    A. Call a code
    B. Be firm and establish clear limits on behavior
    C. Leave the room
    D. Sedate the patient

40. Which of the following drugs is classified as an MAO inhibitor?
    A. Nardil
    B. Cogentin
    C. Artane
    D. Akineton

41. A side effect after administration of an antipsychotic drug that causes muscle spasms is known as
    A. Dystonia
    B. Expression
    C. Latency
    D. Delusion

42. Your patient has been taking an antipsychotic medication. She is now suffering from drooling, muscle tremors, and has difficulty walking. This patient is exhibiting
    A. Boundry effects
    B. Extrapyramidal effects
    C. Dystonic effects
    D. Latent effects

43. If a patient shows a lack of concern about his or her condition or physical symptoms, this condition is known as
    A. Introspection
    B. Labelle indifference
    C. Negativism
    D. Validation negativity

44. Your 22 year old patient inhaled a large amount of cocaine. He is now complaining of paresthesias and "something small like little pieces of rock crawling under my skin." This condition is a type of psychosis and is known as
    A. Magnan's sign
    B. Drummond's sign
    C. Cullen's sign
    D. Wilder's sign

SECTION 14: PSYCHOSOCIAL ANSWERS

1. **Correct answer: B**
   A false perception that is not grounded in reality and not accounted for by external stimuli is called a hallucination.

2. **Correct answer: D**
   The false belief that something is wrong with one's body or body part is called somatic delusion. Malingering is the deliberate manufacturing of an illness to prolong treatment. Hypochondriasis is morbid concern with one's body or health in the absence of a physical cause.

3. **Correct answer: C**
   Korsakoff's syndrome is a type of organic brain syndrome caused by long-term alcohol abuse and thiamine and B complex vitamin deficiencies.

4. **Correct answer: B**
   A crisis develops over time as a result of a psychological stressor, and an emergency is an immediate situation that if not corrected will result in harm to self or others. A psychological crisis may precede an emergency, but not always. Although there is no specific definition for either term, an accepted criterion is that a crisis is a less immediate situation that has developed over time in the presence of a psychological situation. Coping mechanisms may be partially effective but do not address the situation directly and lead to a conclusion of the problem. A crisis may develop into an emergency if coping mechanisms fail or additional stressors appear. A psychological emergency is a sense of urgency that if the situation is not resolved, anxiety may be intolerable and may lead to feelings of being overwhelmed. Coping skills have completely failed and patient recognizes the need for help to alleviate the stressors. Suicide calls, notes, and messages meet these criteria.

5. **Correct answer: B**
   When suspect scars are noted on patients who have attempted suicide, it is important to ask what happened in a nonjudgmental way. This approach allows the patient the option of discussing her feelings or the cause of her self-abuse. She should also be receiving psychiatric help, and both the physician and the psychologist/psychiatrist need to know about the cutting. Many individuals cut themselves to relieve perceived pain and stress in their lives. Telling her husband so he can deal with the situation, telling her how lucky she is to be alive, and telling her this behavior is not acceptable negate her feelings and may lead to further cutting and suicide attempts.

6. **Correct answer: C**
   This patient has opened up to you, and it is important to maintain the communication. Finding out why he feels homosexuality is bad gives insight to the suicide attempt. There are many other legal and ethical issues that have to be handled with this case. It is obvious he will need psychological counseling. After your conversation you must follow your hospital's policy/procedure manual's about reporting such incidents. "Don't worry, you'll get over this and be okay" and "Let me get the psychologist to come talk with you tomorrow" are not therapeutic, and they negate his feelings. Asking, "What is wrong with being a homosexual?" could be perceived as threatening.

7. **Correct answer: D**

   Alcohol abuse may cause a loss of selenium. Selenium is a trace element necessary for brain function. Research has shown that selenium deficiency in individuals who abuse alcohol may contribute to the development of depression and suicidal behavior.

8. **Correct answer: D**

   You should first evaluate Morgan's feelings, paying close attention to any statements indicating a risk for suicide or injury to staff. Morgan is now exhibiting signs of depression after a manic episode. Patients with psychotic elements exhibited with mania, depression, or both may be misdiagnosed with schizophrenia, anxiety disorder, and/ or drug abuse. Patients with bipolar disorder may swing between moods over minutes, hours, or days. Symptoms include hallucinations, delusions, and aggressive or violent behavior. Careful history may reveal a trend of manic and depressive episodes that would clarify Morgan's true condition and lead to faster and correct treatment. A social worker should be involved, but ensuring immediate patient and staff safety is the primary concern.

9. **Correct answer: A**

   Binge eating, mutilation, obesity, drug abuse, and alcoholism are all examples of self-destructive behavior. Self-destructive behaviors are those that over time will shorten or threaten length and quality of life.

10. **Correct answer: D**

    Surveys can be used to anonymously identify staff perceptions and determine educational opportunities. Mental health issues impact every person at some point in their lives. Whether due to a catastrophic event or ongoing psychological issues, it is important that nurses understand their own biases regarding mental health and be able to identify resources when caring for this population. If the nurses believe the survey will be used punitively, then data may be skewed to what the staff believe the surveyor is looking for, not the truth. Instead of changing assignments immediately, it is best to use the opportunity for education and professional growth.

11. **Correct answer: C**

    Anger, fear, and denial are normal emotions in this situation, but staff members who feel anxiety are at the greatest risk. Anxiety is a common emotion found in psychological emergencies. Anxiety involves uncertainty of the unknown and may limit the person's ability to identify resources or initiate appropriate coping mechanisms. Debriefings after codes, both successful and unsuccessful, are therapeutic and allow staff to verbalize emotions in a safe and stabile environment. As a team, the staff may identify ways to support families and each other during crisis and emergency situations.

12. **Correct answer: B**

    The timing of Sugar's symptoms is consistent with alcohol withdrawal or delirium tremens (DTs). DTs usually are seen 12 to 24 hours after last ingestion of alcohol as blood alcohol levels drop. Effects may peak up to 15 days after DTs begin. Fluids, vitamins, nutrition, and short-term pharmacologic treatments are appropriate. The severity of symptoms is affected by the amount and duration of alcohol ingestion as well as underlying physical health, other drugs, and existing psychological status. There are no indications at this time that the patient is septic or has schizophrenia. There may be underlying drug withdrawal symptoms.

13. **Correct answer: C**

    Many cultures may have beliefs and practices that may influence medical management of the patient in the hospital setting. The Chinese often use medicinal herbs and religious beliefs regarding internal energy known as a person's chi to manage health. Cultural beliefs must be acknowledged as influential in patient care regardless of staff beliefs.

14. **Correct answer: B**

    Patients with anorexia nervosa may have a diminished or absent menses. Other signs and symptoms may include bradycardia, hypothermia, fatigue, GERD, electrolyte abnormalities, hair loss, and loss of tooth enamel.

15. **Correct answer: D**

    In most cases no additional abnormalities are found in patients with ADHD. However, if there is a family history of ADHD, there is a higher probability of an individual having ADHD.

16. **Correct answer: A**

    There is actually a diagnosis of Internet addiction. The American Psychiatric Association is currently developing criteria for this diagnosis. Criteria currently recognized are lying about time spent on the Internet, avoiding friends or family to be on the Internet, anxiety when the Internet is not available, and increasing hours spent on the Internet. Academic and work performance often suffers. Internet addiction rehabilitation centers are becoming more prevalent. Karl needs a referral to a mental health practitioner. At present, it is believed that approximately 9 million Americans fulfill the criteria for IA and 30% of those with IA have one or more comorbid psychiatric disorders.

17. **Correct answer: B**

    Patients with PTSD may have diminished concentration and are unable to concentrate on home or work tasks. Patients often regress, have increased anxiety, become aggressive, suffer panic attacks, avoid family, and reenact the event frequently. Patients with PTSD are more likely to attempt suicide than their peers without PTSD.

18. **Correct answer: C**

    Posttraumatic stress disorder may result in many different symptoms. If the patient experiences multiple traumatic events, the risk for developing PTSD increases. Additional causes of PTSD can include physical or sexual abuse, neglect, harrassment, death of a significant other, accidents, war, terrorist attacks, disasters, or life-threatening illnesses/injuries. PTSD may also be caused by witnessed domestic violence, suicide, or murder.

19. **Correct answer: D**

    Feelings of helplessness or hopelessness indicate psychotic emergencies. Extreme anxiety or ability to recognize options should alert staff and family to a greater risk of suicide because suicide may be seen by the patient or individual as the only option and are a warning of suicide. The other statements indicate depression and/or levels of grief and emotional expression.

20. **Correct answer: C**

    The death of their daughter is causing the parents to experiencing the initial response to a crisis. The death may have been expected eventually but now involves an environment and circumstances beyond the parent's experience or ability to cope. The crisis may last for weeks depending on available support systems, the healthcare team, parent education, culture, and spiritual intervention.

21. **Correct answer: B**
Abuse may be suspected if the sister denies abuse in the presence of bruising, injury to bones, and around the throat. Many abused women and children have stories of a positive home life and excuses to explain injuries due to clumsiness. Due to the likely introverted personalities of abused individuals, it is important to establish a safe zone and trust to encourage honest communication and to begin assistance to escape the abuse.

22. **Correct answer: C**
The goal at this point is to regulate the patient's breathing and stabilize vital signs. Using a firm and quiet voice with simple sentences can help the severely anxious patient focus and diffuse the anxiety. Severely anxious individuals are less able to see options and cope at this stage. Goals should include decreasing an unnecessary stress and remaining available to the patient for communication. The other answers speak to facts not known or are judgmental and may increase fear or lead to false hope.

23. **Correct answer: C**
"Why don't we work together to find new resources for you to use when you are tempted to take one of these drugs" is the appropriate statement. Sometimes patients are "frequent flyers" and relationships are developed with certain ED staff. The patient may feel as if he has failed the nurse by not remaining sober and that assistance may be withdrawn. This statement does not judge the patient and shows the patient that help is still available by initiating communication and encouraging the patient to talk about his struggles with staying away from drugs.

24. **Correct answer: D**
Carla has anorexia. It is very difficult to treat anorexia nervosa and often requires a team approach. This patient and her significant others may need psychological counseling as well as medical and nutritional assistance. The important concern for the ED nurse is the impact anorexia has on the body and the patient's recovery. The typical anorexic may have multiple complications of one or more body systems. She may have symptoms such as cardiac arrhythmias, EKG abnormalities, amenorrhea, esophagitis, anemia, dehydration, electrolyte imbalances, peripheral neuropathy, hematuria, and osteopenia.

25. **Correct answer: B**
Family dynamics you would expect to find associated with bulimia nervosa include a strong family history of similar disorders, drug abuse, and psychiatric disorders. Bulimia nervosa is often seen in patients who are overachievers, trying to please those around them. These patients often do very well in school and have above average intelligence. They also have poor self-esteem or self-image problems.

26. **Correct answer: B**
Any time you have concerns about a patient's or family's behavior, it is best to notify administration as soon as possible. Note taking does not necessarily mean a law suit. Taking the notebook is illegal. Contacting your malpractice carrier is possibly overreacting to a situation where a lawsuit has not been considered. Changing assignments

may give the husband more anxiety and suspicion that something is wrong with the care you have already provided. The best defense is to keep the husband informed of his wife's condition. Another valid response to this situation is to have a patient conference and involve the husband with the entire ED healthcare team.

27. **Correct answer: D**
Depression is recurrent and may increase in severity. Many cases are reported that after the first depressive episode, as many as 40% of individuals will experience another episode within 2 years. Often, these patients are diagnosed with multiple psychiatric disorders such as anxiety disorder, dysthymic disorders, disruptive behavior, or substance abuse. Depression may be seen in any patient, although environmental factors such as maltreatment can contribute to risk of depression. A patient with chronic illness, infection, or biochemical factors is also at risk for depression. Depression is difficult to diagnose unless there is an understanding of depression and risk factors. Unfortunately, depression can be just as severe in children and teens as in adults and is associated with approximately 80% of childhood and teen suicides. Undiagnosed and untreated depression can continue into adulthood impacting personal and professional relationships and the ability to function successfully in society.

28. **Correct answer: C**
Asperger's syndrome is a pervasive developmental disorder. Patients affected by this disorder are eccentric in their behavior and social interactions. Men are most affected by this disorder by a 4:1 ratio over women. There is no known cause of Asperger's syndrome, but it often occurs with fragile X syndrome, hypothyroidism, and neurofibromatosis. The condition is generally diagnosed between 3 and 11 years of age. About one-fourth of those affected grow out of their condition by adulthood.

29. **Correct answer: C**
Wanda is exhibiting signs of depression and should not be left alone until you have determined she is not a danger to herself or others. While straightening her room you should note any potential items that could be used by Wanda to harm herself or others. If the items can be removed, do so. If not, attempt to lessen the danger. Wanda's depression may have been brought on by many factors such as her prolonged and recurrent illness, family financial and emotional stress, and feelings of guilt or anger regarding her frequent hospital visits. Only after ensuring Wanda's safety should the nurse leave the room to contact the physician, social worker, case manager, charge nurse, and manager. Should Wanda's mental health continue to deteriorate, she may need constant observation for suicide or restraints applied. Wanda's husband will need to be contacted and updated, but it is important that the staff have a clear plan of action with him This includes family support, financial guidance, specialist support, and, most important, a plan for Wanda's mental and physical health.

30. **Correct answer: B**
When entering Dorothy's room or any patient's room to apply restraints, wear appropriate personal protective equipment to protect yourself against exposure to bodily fluids. Dorothy most likely has had a psychotic reaction to the Demerol and has exposed her IV site and removed her IV—a potential for exposure to bodily fluids. When attempting to place restraints on a combative patient, regardless of the age, at least four staff members should be present—one for each limb. The family should not be asked to participate in placement of the restraints as they are untrained and it may

be seen as a betrayal by the patient. Instead, family members should remain at a safe distance to avoid injury or interference with healthcare providers. A Posey is not the best choice because it leaves the patient's hands free to continue pulling on IV lines. Whenever restraints are in use, be vigilant to document continued need of restraints, type used, time placed, vital signs including airway, breathing and circulation before and after restraints are placed, time of removal, and reassessments. Be sure to follow your facility's restraint protocols and policies. Patient and staff safety is paramount.

31. **Correct answer: D**
The statement, "If she talks about suicide or asks about pills, then she is just voicing the thought and will not attempt suicide," needs to be corrected. Careful consideration and observation should be given to any person voicing any thought or plan regarding suicide. Many individuals provide warning to suicidal thoughts to providing those in the family or in proximity the opportunity to intervene. Warnings are often cries for help and intervention. Family members should pay close attention to any impression or instinct that the person is considering suicide. As individuals enter and exit depression, they are at greatest risk for suicide because they have sufficient mental focus to form a plan and energy or motivation to carry it out.

32. **Correct answer: B**
The fear of crowds is known as agoraphobia. A phobia is a fear or dread of an act, an object, or a situation that is usually not realistically dangerous. However, the patient perceives that danger exists.

33. **Correct answer: C**
When a patient simply stops talking and there is a gap or interruption in speech that is related to absent thoughts or distractions, it is known as blocking.

34. **Correct answer: D**
Simultaneous existence of contradictory or contrasting emotions toward a person or object is known as ambivalence.

35. **Correct answer: D**
Tofranil is an antidepressant. Tegretol, klonopin, and lithium are all antimanic drugs.

36. **Correct answer: A**
Restoril is classified as an antianxiety drug. Elivil, sinequan, and tofranil are all classified as tricyclic medications.

37. **Correct answer: C**
Because this patient's behavior is escalating, the correct assessment is deteriorating. The patient may be exhibiting some paranoid tendencies, but the cause of the hallucinations is unknown at this time.

38. **Correct answer: D**
Elavil and tricyclics in general may take up to 3 weeks to become effective. It is appropriate to reassure the patient and the family and make certain all parties verbalize understanding.

39. **Correct answer: B**
This patient is acting out his frustration. It is important to act immediately to set firm clear goals and limits to behavior. It is crucial you remain with the patient until he

calms down, then attempt to discuss his feelings. Obviously, if you believe you or the patient is in imminent danger, call for help.

40. **Correct answer: A**
    Nardil is classified as an MAO inhibitor. Parnate and marplan are also MAO inhibitors. Cogentin, artane, and akineton are antiparkinson drugs.

41. **Correct answer: A**
    A side effect after administration of an antipsychotic drug that causes muscle spasms is known as dystonia.

42. **Correct answer: B**
    The patient's drooling, muscle tremors, and difficulty walking are similar to those of patients who suffer from Parkinson's disease and are known as extrapyramidal effects.

43. **Correct answer: B**
    If a patient shows a lack of concern about his or her condition or physical symptoms, this condition is known as labelle indifference. This is very important to the ED nurse because it is likely the symptom(s) arise from hysteria rather than an organic cause.

44. **Correct answer: B**
    This condition is a type of psychosis and is known as Drummond's sign. Cocaine users have paresthesias, psychoses, and imagine they have a foreign body, in the shape of a powder or fine sand, under the skin that is constantly changing its position.

SECTION 14: PSYCHOSOCIAL REFERENCES

Baker, A. L., Kavanagh, D. J., Kay-Lambkin, F. J., Hunt, S. A., Lewin, T. J., Carr, V. J., & Connolly, J. (2010). Randomized controlled trial of cognitive-behavioural therapy for coexisting depression and alcohol problems: Short-term outcome. *Addiction, 105*(1), 87–99.

Buxton, J. A., & Dove, N. A. (2008). The burden and management of crystal meth use. *CMAJ: Canadian Medical Association Journal, 178*(12), 1537–1539.

Cruickshank, C. C., & Dyer, K. R. (2009). A review of the clinical pharmacology of methamphetamine. *Addiction, 104*(7), 1085–1099.

Czincz, J., & Hechanova, R. (2009). Internet addiction: Debating the diagnosis. *Journal of Technology in Human Services, 27*(4), 257–272.

Emergency Nurses Association, Newberry, L., & Criddle, L. M. (2007). *Sheehy's manual of emergency care* (6th ed.). St. Louis, MO: Mosby.

Fortson, B. L., Scotti, J. R., Chen, Y.-C., Malone, J., & Del Ben, K. S. (2007). Internet use, abuse, and dependence among students at a Southeastern regional university. *Journal of American College Health, 56*(2), 137–144.

Gasparis Vonfrolio, L., & Noone, J. (1997). *Emergency nursing examination review* (3rd ed.). Staten Island, NY: Power Publications.

Hardin, S. R., & Kaplow, R. (2010). *Cardiac surgery essentials for critical care nursing*. Sudbury, MA: Jones & Bartlett Learning.

Hernandez, L., Eaton, C. A., Fairlie, A. M., Chun, T. H., & Spirito, A. (2010). Ethnic group differences in substance use, depression, peer relationships, and parenting among adolescents receiving brief alcohol counseling. *Journal of Ethnicity in Substance Abuse, 9*(1), 14–27.

Holleran, R. S. (2005). *Emergency transport nursing* (4th ed.). St. Louis, MO: Mosby.

Jacobs, B. B., & Hoyt, K. S. (2007). *Trauma nursing core course provider manual* (6th ed.). Bedford, IL: Emergency Nurses Association.

Jones & Bartlett Learning. (2011). *2011 nurse's drug handbook* (10th ed.). Sudbury, MA: Jones & Bartlett Learning.

Lippincott. (2010). *Professional guide to signs and symptoms* (6th ed.). New York, NY: Lippincott.

National Institute of Mental Health. (2009). How is bipolar disorder treated? *National Institute of Mental Health Online*. Retrieved August 18, 2010, from http://www.nimh.nih.gov/health/publications/bipolar-disorder/how-is-bipolar-disorder-treated.shtml.

National Institute on Drug Abuse. (2010). *NIDA InfoFacts: Methamphetamine*. Retrieved July 7, 2010, from http://www.nida.nih.gov/infofacts/methamphetamine.html.

Proehl, J. A. (2008). *Emergency nursing procedures* (4th ed.). St. Louis, MO: Saunders.

Rouget, B. W., & Aubry, J. M. (2007). Efficacy of psychoeducational approaches on bipolar disorders: A review of the literature. *Journal of Affective Disorders, 98*(1–2), 11–27.

Sher, L. (2008). Depression and suicidal behavior in alcohol abusing adolescents: Possible role of selenium deficiency. *Minerva Pediatrica, 60*(2), 201–209.

Tao, R., Huang, X., Wang, J., Zhang, H., Zhang, Y., & Li, M. (2010). Proposed diagnostic criteria for Internet addiction. *Addiction, 105*(3), 556–564.

Treasure, J., Claudino, A. M., & Zucker, N. (2010). Eating disorders. *Lancet, 375*(9714), 583–593.

U.S. Drug Enforcement Administration. (2010). Drug abuse prevention and control. *United States Drug Enforcement Administration Online*. Retrieved July 7, 2010, from http://www.usdoj.gov/dea/pubs/csa.html.

Urdern, L. D., Stacy, K. M., & Lough, M. E. (2005). *Thelan's critical care nursing* (5th ed.). St. Louis, MO: Mosby.

Watson, S., & Gorski, K. A. (2011). *Invasive cardiology* (3rd ed.). Sudbury, MA: Jones & Bartlett Learning.

Yacoubian, G. S. Jr., & Peters, R. J. (2007). An exploration of recent club drug use among rave attendees. *Journal of Drug Education, 37*(2), 145–161.